Public Health
in
America

This is a volume in the Arno Press series

PUBLIC HEALTH
IN
AMERICA

Advisory Editor

Barbara Gutmann Rosenkrantz

Editorial Board

Leona Baumgartner
James H. Cassedy
Arthur Jack Viseltear

See last pages of this volume
for a complete list of titles.

SELECTIONS FROM THE JOURNAL
OF THE MASSACHUSETTS ASSOCIATION
OF BOARDS OF HEALTH
(1891-1904)

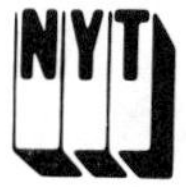

ARNO PRESS

A New York Times Company

New York / 1977

Editorial Supervision: JOSEPH CELLINI

Reprint Edition 1977 by Arno Press Inc.

PUBLIC HEALTH IN AMERICA
ISBN for complete set: 0-405-09804-9
See last pages of this volume for titles.

Manufactured in the United States of America

Library of Congress Cataloging in Publication Data
Main entry under title:

Selections from the journal of the Massachusetts
    Association of Boards of Health (1891-1904).

    (Public health in America)
    1. Public health--Massachusetts--Addresses,
essays, lectures. 2. Massachusetts Association of
Boards of Health. 3. Public health--Massachusetts
--History--Sources. I. American journal of public
hygiene. II. Series.
RA447.M4S44   614'.09744   76-40669
ISBN 0-405-09878-2

CONTENTS

MASSACHUSETTS ASSOCIATION OF BOARDS OF HEALTH.

ORGANIZED 1890.

| Vol. I. | January, 1891 | No. 1. |

This Association, as a Body, is not responsible for statements or opinions of any of its members.

PRELIMINARY MEETING.

IN response to the following circular

OFFICE OF THE BOARD OF HEALTH,
Worcester, Mass., Nov. 8, 1889.

TO THE BOARD OF HEALTH IN ————.

Gentlemen : — It has been suggested that a Society could be formed to advantage, comprising the various Boards of Health throughout the state of Massachusetts.

This Society should hold meetings annually, or oftener, in different places, at which a dinner could be served. The objects should be :

1st. To discuss topics, and hear papers of sanitary interest.

2d. To aid legislation and secure uniform interpretation and enforcement of existing statutes.

3d. To compare the rules of local boards and city ordinances, for the purpose of advance in sanitary matters.

4th. To secure co-operation between local boards, for the suppression of disease, especially epidemics, and for the abatement of nuisances.

5th. To establish pleasant and helpful social relations among the Boards of Health through the state.

Will you please send your opinion of this matter as early as convenient, and any suggestions that you may like to offer?

Very truly yours,

L. F. WOODWARD, M.D.,
Chairman of Worcester Board of Health.

thirty-five gentlemen connected with twenty-four Boards of Health in the state, met at Huntington Hall, Institute of Technology Building, Boston, on Saturday, Jan. 11, 1890, at two P.M. Dr. S. H. Durgin, of Boston, was chosen Chairman, and Dr. J. B. Field, of Lowell, Secretary, for the purposes of temporary organization. Dr. L. F.

Woodward, of Worcester, then explained the origin of the proposed organization. The Worcester Board of Health had sent to every city and town in the state of over two thousand population, a circular relative to the formation of an association of Boards of Health. The replies to this circular were so favorable that the Boston Board of Health issued a call for the present meeting.

After a general and informal discussion of the needs, work and benefits of such an organization, the following gentlemen were chosen a committee to draft a Constitution and By-Laws and to nominate a list of officers, with instructions to report within sixty days: L. F. Woodward, M.D., H. P. Walcott, M.D., S. H. Durgin, M.D., J. A. Gage, M.D., W. K. Knowles, M.D., J. B. Field, M.D.

Mr. BABBITT, *of Boston :* — I move that the next meeting be held in Boston as soon as the above committee is ready to report, and that the Boston Board of Health shall have charge of the arrangements for the same, at which a subscription dinner, costing not more than $1.50 per plate, shall be given.

The motion was adopted with applause.

Adjourned, subject to call of Boston Board of Health.

FIRST REGULAR MEETING.

The first regular meeting of the organization was held at the Revere House, Boston, March 19, 1890, and was called to order by the temporary Chairman, Dr. Durgin.

The records of the preliminary meeting were read and approved.

The Committee on Constitution made its report, and submitted a draft of a Constitution, which, after a few amendments suggested by the members present, was adopted.

The Committee on Nominations of Officers for the ensuing year submitted its report, which was accepted, and the following nominees were unanimously elected :

President, HENRY P. WALCOTT, M.D.   (Chairman of State Board of Health and member of Cambridge Board of Health.)

First Vice-President, SAMUEL H. DURGIN, M.D.   (Chairman of Boston Board of Health.)

Second Vice-President, SAMUEL W. ABBOTT, M.D.   (Secretary of State Board of Health and member of Wakefield Board of Health.)

Secretary, LEMUEL F. WOODWARD, M.D. (Chairman of Worcester Board of Health.)

Treasurer, JAMES B. FIELD, M.D. (Chairman.)

Executive Committee, the preceding officers *ex-officio:* For two years — J. E. CLARK, M.D., Medford; W. H. CHAPIN, M.D., Springfield; W. K. KNOWLES, M.D., Everett; E. A. SAWYER, M.D., Gardner; W. S. FRENCH, West Newton. For one year — C. H. MORROW, M.D., Gloucester; A. G. GRIFFIN, M.D., Malden; M. R. DONOVAN, M.D., Lynn; G. L. TOBEY, M.D., Lancaster; H. HARLOW, Plymouth.,

Dr. Walcott on taking the chair, after thanking the Association for the honor conferred upon him by making him its first President, made a few remarks upon the objects and work of the Association, and the necessity for united, energetic and intelligent action by its members.

THE PRESIDENT stated that he would appoint the Committee on Papers and Publications at the next meeting.

Mr. BABBITT — I move that the Secretary be instructed, in behalf of the Association, to extend its sincere thanks to Gen. Francis A. Walker for the use of Huntington Hall at the preliminary meeting of the Association.

The motion was adopted by a unanimous vote.

Voted, That five hundred copies of the Constitution and By-Laws, with a list of members, be printed.

Adjourned.

At the close of the business meeting about sixty members sat down and enjoyed the elegant dinner prepared by the proprietor of the Revere House. A general social chat and good time wound up an enjoyable meeting.

SECOND REGULAR MEETING.

LOWELL, MASS., June 19, 1890.

The second regular meeting of the Association was holden by invitation of the Lowell Board of Health at Lakeview Park, the summer resort of the citizens of Lowell.

Upon their arrival the members of the Association became the guests of the Lowell Board of Health, and were taken on a carriage ride through the city, visiting among other points of interest Fort Hill Park, Belvidere and "Little Canada." Upon returning from this ride, special electric cars were taken to Lakeview Park. Before dinner a steamboat ride was taken around the lake. About fifty members sat down to dinner, which was served in the upper hall of the pavilion overlooking the lake. After discussing a delightful ménu the President, Dr. Walcott, rapped the meeting to order, and after cigars had been lighted, Dr. Field, Chairman of the local Board, introduced His Honor, Charles D. Palmer, Mayor of Lowell.

The Mayor welcomed the Association to Lowell in a felicitous address, in which he referred to the importance of sanitary work, and the value to a community of a well-organized Board of Health.

The records of the last meeting were read and approved.

Dr. Field then read a paper on "The Disposal of Garbage," which was listened to with great interest.

The discussion upon the paper was opened by Dr. Charles V. Chapin, Superintendent of Health of Providence, who was followed by Dr. J. Arthur Gage of Lowell, and others, which was hurriedly brought to a close by the necessity of reaching the trains.

THE PRESIDENT — We will now take up the consideration of applicants for membership.

THE SECRETARY — I have the following list of applicants for membership, who have been passed by the Executive Committee, and are recommended to the Association for election : —

F. W. Draper, M.D., Boston, Mass.

Charles V. Chapin, M.D., Supt. of Health, Providence, R.I.

F. W. Jackson, M.D., Weston, Mass.

L. F. Severance, Brockton, Mass.

David E. Baker, M.D., Newtonville, Mass.

The names as submitted were unanimously elected to membership.

THE PRESIDENT — I will appoint as the Committee on Scientific Papers and Publications the following members : —

Samuel H. Durgin, M.D., *ex-officio*, Boston.

David E. Baker, M.D., Newtonville.

Ernest S. Jack, M.D., Melrose.

Voted, To refer the matter of the next meeting to the President and Secretary with full powers.

Voted, To extend the thanks of the Association to the Lowell Board of Health and its Chairman, Dr. Field, for the many courtesies received.

Adjourned.

THIRD REGULAR MEETING.

WORCESTER, MASS., Oct. 15, 1890.

The third regular meeting of the Association was held at Worcester by invitation of the local Board.

The members of the Association met at the office of the Board of Health at 1.30 P.M. Barges were then taken, and a visit made to the city's works for purification of the sewage, the party being in charge of the City Engineer, Chas. A. Allen. After a thorough inspection of the works, the Association were driven back through various parts of the city to the Worcester Polytechnic Institute, where the regular business meeting was held, the visitors first being shown over the building.

In the absence of the President, the first Vice-President, S. H. Durgin, M.D., took the chair.

The records of the last meeting were read and approved.

THE VICE-PRESIDENT — The first business before the meeting will be action on the propositions for membership.

THE SECRETARY — I have the following list of applicants for membership, who have been passed by the Executive Committee, and are recommended to the Association for election : —

Prof. T. M. Drown, Massachusetts Institute of Technology, Boston, Mass.

Prof. W. T. Sedgwick, Massachusetts Institute of Technology, Boston, Mass.

Prof. L. P. Kinnicutt, Worcester Polytechnic Institute, Worcester, Mass.

Charles A. Allen, City Engineer, Worcester, Mass.

Edwin D. Wadsworth, Milton, Mass.

C. L. French, M.D., Clinton, Mass.

T. H. O'Connor, M.D., Clinton, Mass.

T. F. Roche, M.D.,   "   "

P. T. O'Brien, M.D.,   "   "

P. P. Comey, M.D.,   "   "

James Kimball, Agent Board of Health, Springfield, Mass.

By vote of the Association all the foregoing parties were unanimously elected to membership.

Prof. Leonard P. Kinnicutt, of the Worcester Polytechnic Institute, then read a paper on " The Disposal of Sewage, together with an account of the Worcester Sewage Works," which was discussed by Profs. T. M. Drown and W. T. Sedgwick, of the Massachusetts Institute of Technology, Boston, and Mr. Charles A. Allen, City Engineer of Worcester, after which the discussion became general.

A vote of thanks was then passed to Professors Kinnicutt, Drown and Sedgwick and City Engineer Allen, for the interesting and valuable papers and information given ; also to the Worcester Board of Health for the courtesies received from them.

Adjourned at 5.30 P.M. for dinner at the Bay State House, which was attended by about fifty members, several being obliged to leave at the close of the business session.

THE DISPOSAL OF GARBAGE.

BY JAMES B. FIELD, M.D., CHAIRMAN OF LOWELL BOARD OF HEALTH.

(Read at the meeting held at Lowell, June 19, 1890.)

THE consideration of how to properly dispose of the waste materials of a city has given rise to many problems of sanitary science. Under the head of waste products will come a variety of substances which directly or indirectly engage the interest of the sanitarian.

The human body produces several kinds of organic waste. Thus the disposal of urine and fæces, and of the air rendered impure by respiration, leads to the problems of house drainage and ventilation. The disposal of ashes, house-dirt, and street-sweepings also comes within the province of the health officer. Then, again, there are the waste products of manufactures, some of which vitiate the air by their odors, and others of which pollute the streams of water into which they are discharged. Even the subject of disposal of the dead would come under this head.

The present paper does not treat of the disposal of all varieties of waste material, but only of one kind, not as yet mentioned. I refer to the refuse of food-stuffs as found in the household and in the markets, and known as garbage.

Before entering upon a discussion of the disposal of garbage, we ought briefly to consider the methods of its collection. These may be divided as follows : —

1. Collection by private individuals without license or control.
2. Collection by licensed swill-gatherers.
3. Collection by a contractor.
4. Collection by the municipality.

In the small country village nearly every household disposes of its own swill. Perhaps, however, the doctor, the minister, and the postmaster do not keep pigs, but dispose of their table refuse to their neighbors. This may be the first point in the evolution of the swill-collector. As the village grows into a town, with manufacturing interests, the need for gatherers of garbage increases. Enterprising farmers, with cattle and pigs to feed, obtain this refuse matter for little or nothing. They gather it wherever they please, whenever they please, and transport it in any kind of a receptacle or conveyance. This is altogether wrong. Swill should be collected at regular and frequent intervals, and in an inoffensive manner. Fortunately, this can be seen to, even in our smallest towns. The power given by the Public Statutes allows Boards of Health to make such regulations as are necessary for the public health, and under this head would certainly come a rule which should place such restrictions upon the collection of garbage as the following:

1. Each collector of swill should be obliged to obtain permission of the Board of Health before pursuing his calling.

2. The receptacles used to convey the refuse should be water-tight and securely covered, so that no odors could escape.

3. The collector should be obliged to furnish a list of places from which he takes swill, and should be required to visit these places at least every second day.

There is no doubt that every town in the state can thus compel its swill-gatherers to be licensed, and to comply with restrictions similar to the foregoing, or even more rigid. To enforce such measures, fortunately, requires no expenditure of money, but simply an expenditure of energy by members of the Board of Health, and a few prosecutions in the police court.

The licensed collector, thus hemmed in by restrictions, inspections, and fear of prosecution, will do the work much better than the man who is allowed to run wild.

Much more preferable than licensed collectors is the man who does the work by contract, for it is much easier to hold one man responsible than it is to look out for several collectors, each infringing on the other's territory.

The ordinary contractor will bear watching. He collects the city's refuse, not because he is a philanthropic sanitarian, but because he is on the make. To keep down expenses means to do the work in a slovenly manner. The garbage contractor, therefore, should be compelled to live up to a carefully-drawn set of rules. The only satisfactory way, however, to have a city's refuse collected, is to have it done by the health department. It will not do to intrust this work to the street department, the pauper department, or to any other branch of municipal work. It must be under the direction of men who believe the cheapest way to do sanitary work is to do it well. In other words, the ideal way of collecting garbage is to have it done by the employees of the Board of Health.

Far more important than the methods of collecting garbage are the methods of its disposal. We may divide these methods as follows:—

1. Use of garbage as a food for animals.

2. Disposal of garbage upon the land or upon bodies of water.

3. Destruction of its garbage by fire or by extraction of its valuable constituents.

Until recent years the custom was well nigh universal of using swill as a food for cattle and swine. Sanitarians have long recognized the harmfulness of such procedures, but it is only recently that the laity have begun to be aroused on the matter.

The fact that a diet of swill will at times increase the percentage of solids in cow's milk is known not only to the health officer and the chemist, but also to the dairyman. A chemical analysis, however, does not reveal all the qualities of a sample of milk. Whether bacteriological examinations would show that the milk came from swill-fed cows is not known. Two years ago Dr. Abbott, of the State Board, informed the writer that but little had been done in this line of work, and that no definite results had been obtained. Clinical evidence as to the injurious effects of swill milk is very strong. Many farmers assert their ability to distinguish such milk by its odor, and state that fermentative changes occur very rapidly. It is also well known that cows fed on a diet of swill are feverish, restless, and not in a natural state of health. What is of more importance is the fact that the effects of swill milk as an infant diet are extremely injurious. Even if we did not have all this evidence against the use of swill as a food for cows, the mere fact that it is an unnatural food would show that it could not have a favorable effect upon cows or upon the secretion of milk.

Now if a town has to dispose of its swill to outside parties, how can it prevent that abomination of abominations — the use of swill as a food for cows?

Last year, by request of the Lowell Board of Health, a bill was introduced into the Legislature permitting the Board of Health of a city to inspect the premises of all persons whose cow's milk came into the city, and the premises of all persons who obtained swill from the city. A penalty was provided against the owner of the premises on which swill was found being fed to cows.

Several Boards of Health were present at the hearing before the Committee on Public Health, and the testimony introduced went to show that the effects of swill as a food for cows were similar to those just mentioned. All parties at the hearing were of one mind in wishing that some bill similar to the one proposed, should be passed. The committee, feeling that a bill as strict as the one desired would fail of enactment, substituted the following modification, which became a law May 9, 1889 :

[CHAP. 326.]

AN ACT TO PREVENT THE FEEDING OF GARBAGE, REFUSE OR OFFAL TO MILCH COWS.

Be it enacted by the Senate and House of Representatives in General Court assembled, and by the authority of the same, as follows :

Whoever knowingly feeds or has in his possession with intent to feed to any milch cow, any garbage, refuse or offal collected by any city or town, or by any person having authority from any city or town, by contract or otherwise, shall be punished by imprisonment in the jail or house of correction not exceeding sixty days or by fine not exceeding one hundred dollars. [*Approved May 9, 1889.*]

With this law on our Statute Books, the use of swill as a food for cows could be stopped within our state if every town had the will and means to inspect all dairies within its borders, and would prosecute all offenders. Concerted action is what is needed.

Perhaps, however, the Board of Health of some city will say, " What is the use of starting a crusade against swill milk? The surrounding towns are indifferent, and why should we forbid our milkmen to feed swill. when swill milk is brought daily into our city from neighboring towns? "

To such queries we can only reply, that it is far better to partially abate an evil than to make no attempt at all to remedy it.

The Board of Health of a city can, however, obtain the right to inspect dairies in neighboring towns, and thus see that the law is complied with. This right of inspecting dairies in other towns is not given by legislative act, but is acquired in a very simple manner ; that is, by refusing to allow any swill to be taken out of the city, without receiving the privilege of inspecting the farms to which it goes. This method may not be practicable in some communities, but it is certain that the Lowell inspectors are dreaded by the farmers of Dracut, Pelham, Tyngsborough, Chelmsford and Tewksbury.

In some cities the opportunity of feeding swill to cows is reduced to a minimum by the city establishing a piggery to utilize all the city swill. In theory, such a piggery is an intolerable nuisance. The decomposing swill and the presence of large amounts of swine manure, must give rise to an unbearable stench. A practical example of this kind of nuisance and a good warning to all cities contemplating the establishment of a piggery, may be found in one of our Massachusetts cities, in which the pauper department carries the swill to the city farm, where it is fed to nearly six hundred pigs. The process of feeding is carried on partly in an open lot, where the loads of swill are dumped upon the ground. After the pigs have eaten what they desire, the remainder of the garbage is allowed to decompose, thus filling the air with offensive odors. It is but simple justice to the city in question to state that its Board of Health has vigorously fought against the piggery with all its might.

The feeding of swill to hogs is more than a nuisance, for it is dangerous to public health by giving rise to the disease known as trichinosis. This disease in hogs is also propagated to human beings who partake of pork flesh that is not thoroughly cooked. Although epidemics of human trichinosis are much more common in Germany than in this country, yet several cases with a high mortality rate have occurred in our Western states. So far as is known, but few cases are on record in Massachusetts. The interest in the subject of trichinosis has been heightened by the investigations of Dr. Mark, which appeared in the last report of our State Board of Health. He concludes that although hogs may obtain trichinosis from eating trichinous rats, that still by far the greater number of trichinous hogs found in the vicinity of Boston in all probability become trichinous by eating city swill which contained pieces of raw swine-flesh in which trichinæ were imbedded.

Even if there were no danger of trichinosis, yet it is well known that hogs fed upon city swill are not healthy, and that deaths are frequent among them.

Thus step by step do we see that swill is not a suitable food for cows, nor even for hogs. How, then, can we dispose of it?

If garbage is used to fertilize the ground, a large acreage will be required, and it can readily be seen that the process is a nuisance, even if the garbage is plowed into the soil.

To place garbage on a dump is wrong, even if a load of garbage is immediately covered by a load of ashes. A house which has its cellar in a foundation of such material is not fit to live in.

Many communities deposit their refuse matter in some body of water. This method is, however, restricted to towns on the seaboard or on the bank of some swiftly-flowing river. It must be an expensive process to dump all the garbage of a city in the ocean, far away from the channel and from all chances that the refuse matter will be again cast upon the shore.

A town which deposits its garbage in any river or other body of water which is a source of public water supply, by so doing violates the laws of this state. Thus this method of disposing of garbage cannot be availed of.

There is no method which will satisfactorily dispose of garbage without destroying its characteristics. This can be done either by burning the garbage, or else by extracting its valuable constituents.

One solution of the problem of garbage destruction, so far as private families are concerned, is that each family should destroy its own swill. Cook-stoves have been constructed with a receptacle at one side of the fire-box, in which the swill can be subjected to the action of the heat without interfering with the efficiency of the fire. In this way the garbage is gradually dried, and may finally be used as fuel. In the summer, when oil-stoves and gas are largely used for cooking, it would, perhaps, be necessary to saturate the garbage with kerosene before building a temporary fire in the kitchen stove to consume it. Such methods, however, presuppose an amount of intelligence and willingness not found in all our kitchens. This plan must therefore be dismissed as impracticable for universal adoption. Even if this method could be adopted only by the better class of householders, a large saving would be made, not only in the amount of garbage to be destroyed, but also in the expense of collection.

In most cities there is not only house offal, but also the refuse from fruit stores and provision markets. The waste from meats is generally utilized either in soap factories or in fertilizer works. Decayed apples, bananas, oranges, and all other such material should be destroyed in the same manner as swill. There are now very many cities which wholly destroy their garbage. This admirable plan is in force even in some quite small municipalities. In this particular form of sanitary improvement, which is being adopted throughout the country, western and southern cities have led the van. As has already been stated, there are two methods of destroying garbage. One is by burning the waste material; the other is by extracting grease and other useful products from the garbage. This latter method is known as the Merz system.

In this system of garbage extraction the waste material is received in a large iron cylinder, known as the dryer. In this the garbage is thoroughly stirred and mixed by revolving arms of iron tubing. Surrounding this drying cylinder is a jacket cylinder. Between the two cylinders and also into the two hollow arms of the stirrer is forced superheated steam. The garbage remains in the dryer six or eight hours, subjected by this steam to a temperature of from 250° to 300° F. This heat, acting on the liquid portion of the garbage, forces out a vapor containing all the moisture and noxious gases. By suction-fans this vapor is led into a condenser, from which it emerges as a colorless liquid with a slight odor. Nearly, if not quite, two-thirds of the garbage thus passes off as moisture. The remaining third is removed from the dryer and then conveyed to air-tight vats or extractors, in which it is subjected to the action of benzine and other chemicals for ten or eleven hours. Here the oil or grease is extracted, and is collected in barrels as it flows from the bottom of the extractors.

The residue of the garbage is then drawn from the extractors, conveyed to the drying-room, and finally screened, to remove all bones, glass, rubber, etc. The final product is of a dark brown color and comparatively odorless. It is sold as a fertilizer. The following figures were obtained by our city physician, Dr. Gage, after a careful investigation of the Merz plant at Buffalo. There, from ten to thirty tons of swill are disposed of daily. The steam and power is furnished by a sixty horse-power engine, at a cost of about $5 per day. Four men are employed, at wages ranging from $1.50 to $4 daily. There are also three boys to pick out the rags, etc., and the value of the material thus picked out will pay the boys' wages. One hundred per cent of swill yields thirty-three and one-third per cent of product; about thirty per cent is in the form of a fertilizer rich in ammonia (four and one-half per cent), and salable at $9 per ton. Three per cent is fat, and is salable at current prices to soap manufacturers. There is a probable profit of about ten per cent on the investment, aside from the expense of collecting the garbage.

One practical objection to the Merz system is the price demanded for it. The company asks a city to pay something toward the erection of a plant, requires the city to collect the garbage, and also to pay for its extraction. The yearly amount paid by the city is said to pay for the operating expenses and interest on the investment. The amount derived from the sale of soap-grease and fertilizer is all profit, none of which, however, accrues to the benefit of the city. To be free from offence a plant of this character should be well constructed and intelligently operated. Some cities employing the Merz process have from various reasons abandoned it. It is certainly an expensive method for the smaller cities.

Nevertheless, there is something that appeals to all of us in the idea of extracting the valuable constituents from garbage. There is in Providence a method somewhat similar to the Merz process, but less expensive. In it naphtha is used instead of benzine, and of its practical workings the superintendent of health of that city will shortly inform us.

To destroy garbage by cremation in a furnace is a comparatively simple matter. If in addition to burning the material we try to avoid offensive odors, it is by no means a simple problem. If a garbage furnace is to be erected near dwelling-houses, it must not be a nuisance.

To fulfill these requirements a furnace should be of sufficient capacity to receive the garbage as fast as it is brought. There should be no adjacent piles of swill accumulating, and perfuming the air while awaiting cremation. To dump the refuse material into the furnace the garbage wagons should be driven into a shed which can be tightly closed while the dumping is going on. With the furnace should be connected a boiler for steam or hot water with which to thoroughly cleanse the carts after they are emptied. In addition, a garbage furnace should be thoroughly constructed, capable of standing intense heat, and be perfectly tight, to prevent the escape of noxious vapors.

A furnace supplied with all these precautions will be a marked nuisance unless some method is devised for destroying the products of combustion which pour out of the chimney. It is essential that the foul-smelling gases formed by burning the garbage should be themselves consumed. This is done by the use of a secondary fire, over which pass the gases formed by the burning garbage.

This feature of the double fires is an essential part of the Engle Garbage Cremator. In this furnace the garbage is dumped in from above and received on a grating, at both ends of which there is a fire. Below the grating is an evaporating pan to catch the liquid drippings. By an ingenious system of dampers the flame can be made to pass above or below the garbage, and in either direction. After the combustion is once well under way, the resultant gases give forth an intense heat which is of itself a great aid to further combustion. That the second fire thoroughly destroys the odor the members of the Lowell Board of Health can testify from personal observation. There are about twenty-five Engle furnaces already in operation, from New York on the north to Panama on the south. Not only are these furnaces suitable for burning garbage, but they can be utilized for destroying infected clothing, bedding, etc., or even for burning night-soil. The Engle furnace which is the property of the New York Board of Health, is used solely for infected material. The cremators of this pattern used in our southern cities generally destroy night-soil in addition to garbage.

An Engle crematory of suitable capacity for this city could be erected for about $6,000. To run it would require one to one and a half tons of coal a day, and the services of two men. There would be no increase of expense for labor. It would mean for us simply a transferral of men no longer needed at the swill-house and dump. The cost of fuel would be reduced by the sale of ashes, which are rich in materials of a fertilizing value.

Perhaps further investigation will show that the extraction of the valuable products of garbage will be the more advantageous way, but it is certain with present knowledge that cremation is far preferable for cities the size of Lowell. Cremation is cheaper in the first cost of plant, more economical in running expenses, destroys infected clothing, bedding and furniture, and consumes garbage that is mixed with ashes. Extraction of the grease requires an expensive plant, a larger number of employees, treats nothing but garbage free from ashes and other impurities. The profit from the sale of soap-grease and fertilizer does not come to the city. The process, if successful at all, will be so only in our larger cities. Whatever method is adopted, the plant ought to be owned and operated by the city.

To recapitulate, there is only one suitable method by which to dispose of all the garbage of a city. All refuse and waste of food materials should be gathered from the household and markets at frequent intervals. It should be removed in receptacles as nearly air-tight as possible, and conveyed to some locality on the outskirts of the city. Here the swill and other garbage should either be treated so as to extract their valuable constituents, or what is preferable, they should be consumed by fire. The method chosen should be that which gives the least offence to the neighborhood, regardless of the expense it entails. The whole process, from the collection of the garbage to its destruction, should be performed solely by the health department of the city.

Now that the ideal method of garbage disposal has been sketched, perhaps some of you may wonder how far the Lowell Board of Health practises what its chairman preaches.

Because Lowell has, as yet, been unable to adopt the best methods of garbage disposal, it does not propose, therefore, to adopt no method at all. If we cannot have the ideal method, we propose to come as near it as possible. Thus, if we cannot collect all of the garbage, we collect the greater part of it, and require the remainder to be removed in an inoffensive manner. If we cannot cremate our garbage, we can at least prevent its use as a food for cows.

In Lowell all swill from private houses is collected three times a week by the health department, and is conveyed to a swill-house on the outskirts of the city, where it is purchased by farmers at twenty-five cents a barrel. There is seldom any swill left over at night. If any remains, it is conveyed to a farm and buried. Every night the swill-house is thoroughly cleansed, and is kept sweet and clean. Owing to an insufficient force of men and teams the swill from hotels, restaurants and the large mill boarding-houses cannot be collected by the city. It is removed by licensed collectors. To obtain a license, an application, accompanied by five dollars, is made to the Board of Health. On each application is a list of places at which the applicant intends to collect swill. These places are visited by an inspector, to be sure that they are not private houses. The license is revokable at the pleasure of the Board of Health. Among the conditions of the license are the following : that the licensee shall not permit any swill collected by him to be fed to cows, and that he shall permit his premises to be inspected by the Board of Health at all times. The license is never delivered to the applicant until he has brought to the superintendent for approval his swill-wagon, containing a suitable water-tight covered box or barrels. With these precautions, the swill is collected from our hotels and restaurants in a manner almost as unobjectionable as that in which the health department collects it from private residences. The farmers who purchase swill at the swill-depot have to subscribe to the same conditions as do the licensed collectors.

The methods of collecting the swill of Lowell are quite satisfactory, but those of its disposal cannot merit praise. As we have no method of destroying our garbage, it is used as a food for animals, and all the Board of Health can do is to see that the food is reasonably fresh and is not fed to the one animal so necessary to human welfare — the milch cow.

When the present Board of Health of Lowell entered upon its duties a few years ago, there was no penalty against feeding swill to cows, and a farmer could use this kind of diet for his cows, provided the milk was found, as was often the case, above standard. All that could be done was to control the ultimate disposal of our swill by selling it only to farmers who would agree not to feed it to cows and who would permit the Board of Health to inspect their premises. Of course some few men violated this agreement, but were sooner or later found out by our inspectors and thereafter were not allowed to obtain swill in Lowell. As a result of these inspections several farmers had to go out of business, and sold their cows at a loss. Others found such a profit in this disgraceful occupation that they went long distances to other cities for the swill they could not obtain in Lowell.

We have thus restricted the use of swill, but still more remains to be done. We cannot dispose of the refuse from markets. Unfortunately, it is smuggled on to the dumps after dark. We cannot, with all our care, prevent the swill-house from attracting flies and producing some slight odors. Lastly, we cannot prevent the use of swill as a food for pigs.

In order to do away with swill-house garbage on dumps, and feeding to swine, we have twice recommended cremation of garbage to the city government. We hope soon to make a third request, and trust that it may be granted.

Dr. CHARLES V. CHAPIN, Superintendent of Health, Providence, R.I.

I wish to express my satisfaction at this time with the thoroughness with which the subject has been treated by Dr. Field, and I heartily endorse his views, that different towns require different methods for the disposal of garbage. In regard to my own city, Providence, the feeding of garbage to swine and cattle had been in vogue for many years, and I was heartily disgusted with it. The pork from the swill-fed hogs was flatly refused by all local butchers.

Within a few months a new process of garbage disposal has been adopted. It consists not in the destruction of the garbage, but in the utilization of all its valuable ingredients. The process is as follows: The garbage, as soon as discharged from the collecting-wagons, is put at once into the " extractors." These are large wrought-iron tanks, six feet in diameter and eighteen feet long. After they are filled the cover is screwed down, and is not again removed till the process is completed. By means of an arrangement of pipes within the extractor, by which applications of naphtha and steam are made to the garbage, the material is completely dried and the grease extracted at the same time. The details of this operation are its essential features, and the process is a secret one. All the foul odors of the garbage are condensed into a small volume of water, which is, after all, not very offensive, and could readily be discharged into a sewer or small water-course. The only odors which can be a nuisance are those arising from the unloading of the garbage-wagons for the treatment of the garbage itself, which is conducted in perfectly air-tight tanks and pipes.

The grease obtained can be used for any purpose for which dark, cheap grease is applicable. The solid residue, called tankage, is valuable as a fertilizer to mix with phosphate rock.

I am satisfied that both this process and cremation could be conducted without any great nuisance, but neither should be carried on in thickly settled business or resident portions of a town. The trouble is in unloading the swill from the wagons and putting it into the " extractors " in the one case, or the furnaces in the other. The success of either process, so far as freedom from nuisance is concerned, consists in strict attention to details.

As to the pecuniary advantage of the Providence system, it must necessarily depend largely on the local cost of fuel and the value of fertilizers and grease, all of which vary greatly in different places. In most cities, I think the Providence system would prove the best.

SEWAGE AND SEWAGE DISPOSAL,

WITH A DESCRIPTION OF THE SEWAGE WORKS AT WORCES-
TER, MASS.

BY PROF. LEONARD P. KINNICUTT, OF THE WORCESTER POLYTECHNIC
INSTITUTE.

(Read at the meeting held at Worcester, Oct. 15, 1890.)

WHEN six weeks ago your Secretary did me the honor of inviting
me to read a paper before you on the treatment of sewage, I accepted
with many misgivings.

The subject is so large, and so many things might be said, that I
felt I had not the time at my disposal to make a properly condensed
paper, and the paper which I have the pleasure of reading to you this
afternoon, has, I am afraid, many faults of omission and commission.

I have tried, however, to make it merely an outline of the various
methods used for the purification and clarification of sewage.

Sewage, says Professor Drown, is the water supply of a city as it
passes off. A more complete definition is that given by Dr. Tidy,
that sewage is the refuse of communities, their habitations, streets
and factories. A large proportion of the most offensive matter in
sewage is human excrement and urine, but mixed with this, there is
water from kitchens, containing animal and vegetable matter, the
drainage from stables, and further, the drainage of factories, containing all the waste products that are there produced. Sewage is
not, therefore, human excrement diluted with water, but water polluted with a vast variety of matters, some held in solution, some in
suspension.

Sewage is a very variable substance. It differs in composition in
different cities, and in the same city at different times of the year
and day; that flowing at night has fewer solids in it than that flowing by day. The sewage of a manufacturing city is of a very different character from that of a residential town, and its constituents
in a manufacturing city like Lowell, which is chiefly engaged in one
branch of industry, are very different from those in a city like

Worcester, where the industries are varied. We can not, therefore, speak of normal sewage, or say how much organic matter sewage will on the average contain ; roughly speaking, however, sewage of cities or towns contains over sixty grains of solid matter in one United States gallon, a little less than half of which is organic matter. More than one-third of this solid matter is dissolved in the water, the remainder being suspended. Sewage also contains as a rule more than five grains of combined chlorine in a gallon. But each town and city turns out a special type of sewage, whose nature, effect, and proper mode of treatment can only be determined by careful examination and experiment. A method of treatment that might be successful in one place might fail in another.

All sewage, however, contains organic matter rich in nitrogen, and has one common property, that of decomposition. Fresh sewage has very little odor, and gives no more offense than fresh kitchen refuse, but within forty-eight hours decomposition begins, and not only are odors of a most offensive nature given off, but substances are formed which serve as nutriment for those low forms of animal and vegetable life which are considered especially dangerous to human beings. The proper removal and disposal of the refuse of a city is, therefore, a question of the first importance.

This was recognized in very early times, and the sewage works of Rome nearly equalled in magnitude those of its water supply. The most notable example of these ancient sewers is the Cloaca Maxima, built about 600 B.C., which has defied the vicissitudes of more than twenty-four hundred years, and is still used for the purpose for which it was built.

During the wars and political disturbances that followed the fall of the Roman Empire, sanitary science was neglected and allowed to pass into decay, and it was not until the beginning of the present century that the removal of sewage from cities received any serious consideration.

The first method used for the disposal and purification of sewage was, undoubtedly, what may be called the water carrier and purification system. This may be defined as carrying the refuse of towns and cities through drains to a stream, river, arm of the sea, or to the ocean. The theory of the process is, that if sewage is greatly diluted with water the oxygen dissolved in the water will indirectly burn and destroy the organic matter. This method is still the common one everywhere except in England, and its merits and demerits can be ascertained by seeing how it has worked in a large number of cases, under varied conditions.

From investigations that have been made it seems that when the volume of an untidal river is much greater, say thirty to forty times the volume of the sewage, and when the current of the river is over one mile per hour, for a distance of four or five miles from the point where the sewage enters the river, sewage can thus be disposed of without causing any offense.

These conditions, unfortunately, do not occur as often as might at first be supposed. A stream may usually have sufficient water to dilute a sewage discharge, but during the hot summer months it may be found to be insufficient. The current of the river may average over one mile per hour, but have places where there is slack water in which the decomposable matter settles.

As illustrations of this method of disposal, I will cite the following examples: Boston sewage was formerly discharged on its shores at the head of docks; the dilution was very much greater than thirty fold, but there was seldom any current, and solid particles settled in masses, giving off most offensive odors. Now, the sewage of the city is all discharged into a good current in the harbor, and only a very slight nuisance is produced. Providence discharges its refuse into the bay where there is no current, and so much of a nuisance follows that they have decided to purify the sewage by chemical precipitation. Worcester sewage ran into the Blackstone, a stream whose volume is on the average only five times greater than the volume of the sewage, and I do not think it is necessary to dwell on the condition of that stream. The bulk of the sewage of Lawrence is discharged into the Merrimac river where there is plenty of water and a good current, and no trouble has ever been experienced. Sewage discharged into the Mississippi is rapidly oxidized and carried off. The Amazon river might possibly take care of the sewage of the world.

When sewage can properly be emptied into water, this method is generally found to be the best and cheapest. Unfortunately, as we have seen, it can not often be used with safety, and other means must be employed. The small area, great density of population and multiplicity of manufactories in England, combined to produce in that country the most extensive pollution of natural waters, and it was consequently there that public opinion first demanded a solution of the problem of sewage purification, and the various methods which I shall mention, originated there.

THE MIDDEN SYSTEM.

Under the name of the Midden system I include the methods which have been devised to collect human excrement, including urine, separately from the other refuse of a community.

The amount of fœcal matter voided by each person daily, averages a quarter of a pound, twenty-five per cent of which is solid matter. One thousand persons would therefore yield sixty-two and one-half pounds of dry fœcal matter per day. The daily amount of urine per person is in the neighborhood of three pints, containing two and one-half ounces of dry solid matter; for one thousand persons this equals one hundred and fifty pounds per day.

A community containing one thousand persons would void in a year, 77,462 lbs. or 34.6 tons of dry solid matter, of which 58,315 lbs. or 26 tons is organic matter, which undergoes decomposition.

The first method used to prevent this large amount of organic matter from causing a nuisance was to collect it in cesspools. There are so many and such great objections to the cesspool that its use has been prohibited in almost all cities. Among these objections may be mentioned, the obnoxious and dangerous odors given off, the danger of polluting neighboring wells, and the difficulty of removing the contents, as must be done from time to time.

An improvement on the cesspool system is the pail, or what may be called the temporary cesspool system. A simple tub or pail is placed under the seat of the privy, to collect all the excretal matters. These pails are collected every day by contractors and their contents used for manure. This system has been, and is now, used in many large cities to a greater or less extent, as for example Edinburgh, Glasgow, Paris and other continental towns. There is no doubt that this system is more healthy than that of having large cesspools in the vicinity of human habitations.

It necessitates only a pail with or without disinfectants, and a system of carefully regulated collection. The advantage of the plan is that the collection must be carefully looked after, for if the refuse is allowed to remain too long, it immediately makes itself known by offensive odors. I do not think the pail system should ever be introduced into cities ; but for small towns unprovided with sewers, much may be said in its favor.

The Liernur or Pneumatic system is an outgrowth of the pail system. In this, the human excrement and urine are removed from their receptacles and drawn through air-tight iron pipes to a central reservoir, by means of a vacuum, caused by an air-pump, the contents of the reservoir being emptied each day into hermetically closed tanks and carried into the neighboring country to be used as manure.

Two varieties of closets are used in the Liernur system. That for the better classes is flushed by a mechanical device, with a very small amount of water, the quantity being limited to prevent dilution of the fœcal matter ; that for the lower classes has no movable mechanism, and is used without water. The hopper is so arranged that the fæces fall directly into a trap without touching the sides. The trap always remains full and overflows by gravity into the soil-pipe, while the odors arising from the trap are made to pass through a ventilating pipe into the outer air.

The Liernur system is only for the removal of human excrement, and not for the removal of other refuse matter, such as sink drainage and street washings. In Holland, where a general system of sewage like that employed in the large cities of this country can not be introduced except at an enormous cost, on account of the lowness and flatness of the country, the system may possibly be worked to advantage, obviating the trouble and dirt involved in the pail system.

The dry-earth system is another plan that has been adopted for the separation of human excrement from sewage.

The disinfecting power of earth has been known from very early times, but this knowledge took no practical form in Europe as a health measure until 1858. In that year the Rev. Henry Moule, the vicar of Fordington, believing that much of the ill health in his parish was caused by cesspools, experimented on the deodorizing power of earth and invented the earth-closet.

In its simplest form the earth-closet consists of a pail containing a little earth, placed under the seat of the privy, a box of dry earth being kept in the privy, about one and one-half pounds of which is added to the pail after each visit. There is thus formed a consolidated and inoffensive deposit. When the pail is full it is removed, and after being thoroughly dried by being allowed contact with air, in suitably built sheds, can be used again in the closet. The same earth can be used certainly three times without giving offense. Its value is even then very small, being only equal to rich garden soil. The best earth to use for this purpose is clay, and sand is the worst. Ashes can be used, but their deodorizing power is much less than that of earth. Charcoal has also been used; its deodorizing power is much greater than earth, and the amount required is only about a quarter as great, but the original cost is much greater. With the earth-closet, disinfectants can be used when considered necessary.

This system would, I believe, work very well in small villages and towns, when well looked after, and it could be easily introduced. In very small villages, each house-owner could easily be taught the proper method of preparing and taking care of the earth. In large villages, the closets could be taken care of by paid scavengers, who would remove the contents and supply fresh earth. If once introduced, it would certainly be a great improvement over the common method of cesspools, which is, as we all know, a constant source of danger.

The advantage of the various forms of the Midden system is, as we have seen, that a large quantity of organic matter, of a kind which is believed to be most injurious to health, is kept out of sewage by excluding human excrement from it.

I know that high authorities state that the sewage of towns in which the Midden system is used is almost identical with that of water-closet towns; but this, I think, rests on very doubtful experiments, and I believe that a much less dangerous sewage would result if human excrement were excluded. Still it would be a very brave man, who would at the present time advise a city to provide itself both with a Midden and a water-carriage system.

WATER—CARRIED SEWAGE.

There are three methods now in use for the purification of water-carried sewage:

Surface or broad irrigation.

Intermittent downward filtration.

Chemical precipitation.

You may notice that I do not mention any form of straining the sewage, as a method of purification. Sewage cannot be purified in this way.

A great number of processes have been tried, using a variety of substances for the straining material, among which may be mentioned hay, charcoal, ashes, dry earth, sand, and iron slag, and all have been failures. For if the straining material be of too fine a texture it soon clogs, while if it is too coarse, the organic suspended matter is not removed. Any process that depends merely upon straining as a means of purification, is to be condemned.

SURFACE IRRIGATION.

This method was based on the assumption that all the offensive and decomposable substances held in suspension and solution would be absorbed by the soil and taken up by the growing plants, while the effluent sufficiently purified, would pass away into drains, and could be allowed to enter streams and rivers without fear of pollution.

That such a purifying process does take place, may be seen by the simple experiment of pouring a little sewage on a flower-pot filled with earth : the water which oozes out, if not too great a quantity of sewage has been used, will be found to be freed to a great extent of its disagreeable odor.

This system is known under the name of the Sewage Farm system. The sewage is brought to the highest points of the land to be irrigated, conveyed by carriers of a more or less permanent character into some form of sewer channels. These open carriers or surface channels can be mere trenches, and the land more or less flooded by the carriers being dammed up at certain points. The land must of course be so levelled and drained that the sewage will flow over different portions of the ground, and not into hollows, where it would soon become stagnant, or pass away without undergoing the needful purification.

The advocates of this system claimed that the process not only purified the sewage, but that the plants would absorb and assimilate the organic matter of the sewage. Or in other words, here was a process by which the land would be so enriched that the crops obtained from the land would more than pay the expense of purifying the sewage. Enthusiasts full of faith were found to embark in private sewage farms, but it was not long before an unpleasant awakening occurred ; it was found that sewage farms were commercially a failure.

The failure can be easily understood, if, as Dr. Tidy well puts it, we consider that the sewage farmer was compelled, if the sewage was to be purified, to take it at all times, day and night, Sunday and week-days, winter and summer; to take it whether his crops needed it or not; to take it in seed-time and harvest, in wet weather and in dry. Nay, just when the rain is most plentiful, and moisture the least needed, the sewers pour out an increased volume, which must be admitted to the land.

Without going further into details I will only say that it is now universally conceded that no profit can be expected from the cultivation of crops on a sewage farm.

Allowing this, can the system of broad irrigation be used successfully for the purification of sewage? I believe that there is very little question that under favorable conditions, and with certain kinds of sewage, this method of purification is very efficacious. Let us consider for a moment what the favorable conditions are. The first essential is a large plot of land. If, in the experiment with the flower-pot, too much sewage had been added, the water draining out at the bottom would be as impure as the sewage itself. So on a large scale, if too much sewage be added to a plot of land, the sewage will not be purified. Experiments have shown that the smallest amount of land allowable is one acre to one hundred persons, or for a city of the size of Worcester eight hundred acres would be necessary. The land must be at some distance from the city supplying the sewage, and should not border on any populous district, for I do not suppose there was ever any irrigation field which did not in summer give off a loathsome odor. The kind of soil is also a consideration; if it is too open and porous, the sewage passes quickly through it, and emerges scarcely, if at all, purified. If, on the other hand, it is too compact, the water cannot escape, and the soil is rendered swampy. Finally, it must be remembered that all kinds of sewage are not fit to be applied to cultivated land. If there is a large proportion of industrial refuse, such as acids, metallic salts, dye and tan liquors, the sewage will injure or destroy the crops, and may completely sterilize the land.

These difficulties, and the expense of obtaining large areas of efficient land, suitably situated, soon showed that the method was not a practical one for the majority of large cities. The land difficulty must, at least, be overcome, if the system was to be universally employed. The outcome was the development of the intermittent downward filtration.

This system is due to experiments made by Dr. Frankland, of England. It differed from the irrigation system in having the land deeply under-drained, and by applying the sewage intermittently. The soil being drained at a depth of six feet or more, allowed a considerable distance for percolation, and this constituted filtration as opposed to irrigation. The land becomes an indirect oxidizing instrument to burn the impurities, and so transform them into harmless gases, rather than a mere separating or filtering machine.

To obtain the best effects of oxidation, and to keep the land in the most effective condition, the sewage was to be applied intermittently; i.e., with regular intervals of rest, to give time for the air to go into the ground as the water runs out, thus fitting it for a fresh dose of sewage. This constituted the intermittent filtration.

This intermittent action, it was claimed, would avoid clogging the soil and secure its frequent aeration. By such means, it was stated that the sewage of 3,300 persons could be applied to one acre of ground, and perfect purification of the sewage would result. To illustrate the working of the intermittent filtration system, let us imagine a population of 9,900, with three acres of suitable land drained to a depth of six feet. Each acre is sub-divided into four parts, for the purpose of the work; the sewage of 3,300 persons being placed successively on each quarter acre for a period of six hours, eighteen hours being allowed for aeration before it receives another dose. It was allowed that this process involved the sacrifice of the manurial value of the sewage.

This system has received most careful consideration from sanitary men, and it is with this system that extended experiments have been made by the Massachusetts Board of Health at Lawrence. Their report on the subject is now in press, and will appear before many months. Therefore it is not yet time to discuss the method at any length. From what I know concerning the work, however, I believe their experiments will show that domestic sewage — sewage that does not contain refuse from manufactories — can be sufficiently purified to enter a river not used as a water supply, by intermittent downward filtration through carefully prepared beds of sand, and that the sewage of about 1,500 persons can be thus purified on one acre of coarse mortar sand. Their report will also show that the purification does not depend in any way on the removal of organic matter by what we call filtration; that is, mechanical separation, but is due to living organisms called bacteria, which require free oxygen for their growth. That if the bacteria are not present the purification ceases. The sand filter must therefore be continually supplied with air, and the filtration must be intermittent, so as to allow the air to run in as the water runs out.

The filter beds of sand have now been used for over three years, and their action is as good, if not better, than during the first year; or, in other words, there appears to be no filling up of the air spaces between the sand. With domestic sewage, their experiments have been most successful. These experiments, however, have been made only with domestic sewage, and do not prove anything as to what would take place with sewage containing acid liquors, iron salts, wool waste, and the refuse from tanneries and other manufacturing processes. Could the bacteria live in such sewage and do their work? Would there not be great danger of the spaces between the sand particles becoming filled up, which would not only make the sewage penetrate the ground less readily, but would also retard the entrance of air; and the work of the bacteria depends on their being supplied with oxygen that is in the air.

I have now considered the two systems of purification of sewage by earth treatment, but before I speak of chemical precipitation, I would like to say something as to the hygienic effect of such treatment. The discussion of this question would, however, occupy too much of your time, and I therefore pass directly to the consideration of the next process — chemical precipitation.

Chemical precipitation means the addition of certain chemicals to the sewage, whereby the solid suspended matter and part of the matter in solution is precipitated, and a more or less general deodorization of the offensive constituents, — both those precipitated and those remaining in solution, — is brought about. In this process the sewage from which the grosser matters have been removed is treated with certain chemicals, either suspended in water, or, if soluble, dissolved in water. After such treatment the sewage is run into subsidence tanks, where it is either allowed perfect rest for a few hours, or is passed slowly through a series of tanks. In both cases the precipitation takes place, and the clear liquid, or the effluent, as it is called, is then either allowed to run directly into a water-course, or over a small area of land. The precipitate, known under the name of sludge, is removed from the tanks, and is treated and disposed of in various ways.

The processes for the chemical treatment of sewage are so numerous — I believe that about four hundred and fifty patents have already been obtained — that even a casual mention of each is clearly impossible in the time I have at my disposal, and as the processes differ from each other mainly in the kind of chemicals used, I will restrict myself to mentioning two of the best-known processes, and then point out certain details of treatment essential for the success of any precipitation process.

When lime is added to raw sewage, if the sewage is acid, which is often the case in manufacturing towns, the lime neutralizes the acid, and then carbonate of lime is formed. This salt is insoluble and is heavy, and if the opportunity is offered, the light, flocculent suspended matter in the sewage will be carried down with the precipitated carbonate. In addition to this a certain amount of dissolved organic matter is also precipitated, the lime forming with the organic matter a compound of varying chemical composition.

Salts of aluminium, as alum, have what is called a great affinity for organic matter, and it is on this account that these salts are used as mordants in dyeing. When they are applied to cloth fabrics, they unite with the coloring matter of the dye, which is in solution, and form insoluble compounds on the cloth. This property holds good for the organic matter in the sewage, as it does for ordinary colors used by the dyer or printer. If a solution of crude alum is thrown into a slightly alkaline sewage it is decomposed, a basic sulphate of aluminium is formed which combines with the greater part of the organic impurities, forming insoluble compounds which are precipitated. Aluminium salts, it is believed, have not only the property of precipitating dead organic matter, but also that of removing to a great extent the germs of disease.

The combination of these two salts, lime and alum, was first suggested by Anderson, of Coventry, England, and the process in which they are used is known as the Coventry process. In my opinion this is the best and simplest of all the precipitation processes. It is the one which is used in Worcester, and I shall refer to it again when I speak of Worcester sewage.

The second process is the A. B. C., which consists in adding charcoal mixed with clay and a little blood or other glutinous substance capable of coagulation, and then sulphate of aluminium. No lime is added unless the sewage is decidedly acid. The addition of the charcoal and clay, it is claimed, arrests all offensive odors, no matter how foul they may be, and the aluminium sulphate acts in the way I have already mentioned.

This process is more expensive than the Coventry, and for the treatment of manufacturing sewage I do not believe it is as successful.

In all precipitation processes, as I have already said, certain details of treatment are essential. The most important of these are the following : —

It is necessary that sewage should be treated when fresh. By fresh sewage is meant that in which active fermentation has not taken place. Speaking generally, the sewage should not be more than forty-eight hours old for effective precipitation, and undoubtedly better results could be obtained with a smaller amount of chemicals when the sewage is only twenty-four hours old.

It is essential that a sufficient amount of chemicals should be used to effect complete precipitation. No greater mistake can be made than to try to save expense on the chemicals, and because this has often been done, the failure of the precipitation process has followed.

One most important essential for the success of the process is sufficient tank accommodation. This is necessary for two reasons: First, that the precipitate may subside perfectly, leaving a clear effluent. If the tanks are too small the sewage will be forced too quickly through them, and this would mean imperfect subsidence of the precipitate. Second, sufficient tank room is necessary, so that the precipitate or sludge may be frequently removed, otherwise the freshly precipitated sewage may be contaminated by the decomposing materials of a previous precipitation. Many a good effluent has been spoiled by foul materials being allowed to remain in the tanks. These materials undergo decomposition, and the gases given off contaminate the effluent.

Using these precautions, what kind of an effluent can be obtained?

My own opinion is that it depends greatly on the character of the sewage treated. If the sewage contains large amounts of metallic salts, with more or less free acid — sewage, for instance, like that of Worcester or any other large manufacturing town — I believe that by using the Coventry process, a clear, odorless effluent can be obtained ; that the effluent will contain no suspended matter, and less soluble organic matter than the sewage, and that the organic matter it does contain in solution will, when allowed to flow into a stream whose volume is from five to ten times greater than the effluent, or allowed to flow on a very small area of sand, be quickly oxidized and destroyed without causing any nuisance.

But before we can decide on the success of the process we must remember that we have the sludge containing the organic decomposable matter of the sewage, still left on our hands. Can the sludge be disposed of so that it will not become a nuisance?

The sludge, as it can be obtained from the tanks, is a slimy mass containing more than ninety per cent of water. It has no commercial value, and I believe the only proper method of treatment at the present time is by fire. This is not so difficult as might be supposed. The sludge can be taken from the tanks to a filter press, where the amount of water can easily be reduced to fifty per cent, and the slimy mass be changed to a solid cake, without odor, and easily handled. Furnaces have been constructed for burning these cakes, and the amount of fuel necessary for the complete destruction of the organic matter is very small. A furnace similar to the one which all cities should own for the destruction of city garbage can be employed, or one and the same furnace can be used for both purposes.

We have seen that a clear effluent can be obtained, and that the sludge can be disposed of without any nuisance being caused ; then it may be asked why chemical precipitation has sometimes been a failure. I believe this not to be the fault of the system, but the fault of the way the process has been worked. We have here a process which needs constant, intelligent oversight, just as much as a process of chemical manufacture, and instead of being a process of manufacture it is one of destruction, where in place of money being gained by the improvement of the article manufactured, there is a gain by lowering the standard of the work done. Consequently there is a constant temptation to do poor work, to save chemicals, to neglect looking after the tanks, which, when yielded to, results as all such work must, in making the process a failure instead of a success.

Until a year ago the three processes which I have mentioned were the only ones which had received any attention from sanitary engineers. Last summer a new process was brought to their attention by Dr. William Webster, of England, and though it has not as yet been tried on any very large scale, still on account of its novelty and theoretical correctness, it deserves mention. This process is known as electrical decomposition of sewage. It depends on the fact that the water and salts, like chlorides and sulphates, which occur in the sewage of all manufacturing towns, are decomposed by a current of electricity. The oxygen, chlorine and sulphur trioxide, which are formed by this decomposition, are given off at the positive pole, and being just liberated from their combinations, are in their most active state, and rapidly oxidize and burn up the organic matter which is in the sewage, odorless and harmless gases being formed. The beauty of the process will be recognized if we remember that the three strongest reagents that the chemist can use in his laboratory for destroying organic matter, are just the three that are here produced in the sewage itself; that we are not obliged to add any chemicals to the sewage, and that the amount of sludge is reduced to a minimum.

The process has, however, not been carefully enough investigated to allow an opinion to be formed as to its practicability on a large scale.

This completes my classification of the methods used for the disposal of sewage, and I venture to submit my own conclusions regarding the various methods; but not wishing you to think for a moment that my opinion is the settled opinion of sanitary engineers,— for the purification of sewage is still in an experimental state, and experts disagree widely as to the value of the various processes.

THE WATER PURIFICATION SYSTEM. For cities situated on the sea or on large and rapid rivers, this method affords the most economical and efficient means of dealing with their sewage.

CESSPOOL SYSTEM. Cesspools should not be allowed in any city, town or village.

PAIL SYSTEM. The pail system affords an efficient means for the disposal of the worst organic substances, in villages or towns which have no sewage system.

THE LIERNUR SYSTEM. This system can not be recommended for any New England city.

THE EARTH-CLOSET. This I consider preferable to the pail system, and should strongly advocate its use in small villages and towns.

BROAD IRRIGATION. — SEWAGE FARMING. This method for the purification of sewage can not be recommended for the great majority of cities. I admit that in certain places it may be successful, as in Berlin, where there is a large sandy area of twenty-six square miles, not more than twelve miles from the city; but I believe that purification of sewage by the sewage-farm system as carried out in England, should not be introduced into this country.

INTERMITTENT DOWNWARD FILTRATION. The system as first proposed by Dr. Frankland, can not be recommended, but it seems probable that, using carefully prepared filter beds, this system may be considered in the future as the best method of treating the sewage of towns and cities whose sewage is of a residential rather than of a manufacturing character. For sewage which contains large quantities of manufacturing refuse, it certainly can not be recommended at the present time.

CHEMICAL PRECIPITATION. This method is, at the present time, the most satisfactory known way for the disposal of sewage containing large amounts of acid, mineral salts, and refuse from factories. A sufficiently pure effluent can be obtained to run into a stream not used as a water supply, or to be run over a very small area of land. The sludge obtained can be pressed and burnt without causing offense.

ELECTRICAL DECOMPOSITION. At the present time no opinion can be formed in regard to its practicability.

In conclusion, I wish to say a few words about Worcester sewage. When Worcester was at last compelled to take the sewage question into serious consideration, Mr. Allen, our most efficient City Engineer, was requested to study the question and make a report. He made a careful examination of the various methods, visiting England and the Continent for this purpose, and after consultation with experts both in this country and in Europe, reported, as I think, correctly, that the best system for Worcester was the chemical precipitation process.

As regards the plans and the work done, full details may be of interest. All the sewers of the city enter Mill Brook, which empties into the Blackstone at Quinsigamond village. The minimum flow of Mill Brook is about 2,000,000 gallons, and its maximum flow at least 50,000,000 per day, while the normal flow of Worcester sewage is between three and four million gallons per day. For any system of sewage purification, therefore, some means will have to be devised to carry the sewage to the purification works without allowing it to mix with the water of Mill Brook. After a careful study of the problem, Mr. Allen has recommended the building of a separate conduit for the waters of Mill Brook, and working plans are now being made.

At the present time three or four million gallons of the sewage and water of Mill Brook are diverted from their course by a gate-way at

Quinsigamond village, and carried to the precipitation works. In this way, in the hot summer months, when the brook is in its most offensive state, over two-thirds of its total flow is subjected to chemical treatment, while in wet weather, when the brook is in a much better state, only one-tenth of the flow is taken to the works.

The works consist of a boiler and engine house, a mixing-room for the chemicals, precipitation tanks, sludge well, etc., so arranged that their capacity can be easily doubled.

Reference to the drawings I have placed before you may make the arrangement more easily understood.

The sewage is brought by the outfall sewer A to the gate-house B, which is divided into two parts, each part containing an iron screen. The gross matters in the sewage are thus removed, and by means of gates the sewage can be carried through either part, allowing a continuous flow while the screens are being cleaned. From the gate-house the sewage runs through the channel C to the tanks. From this channel, by means of a small pipe, a little of the sewage is carried into the mixing-room D, where there are four mixing tanks, two for the lime and two for the alum. The mixing and dissolving of the chemicals is aided by mechanical stirrers run by steam, and the lime and alum, which after this treatment are partly in suspension, partly in solution, are carried back by pipes into the channel C. This channel is furnished with baffle plates made of wood, and the fall being about one foot, the chemicals become thoroughly mixed with the sewage.

The sewage then enters the precipitating tanks ; these are six in number, made of brick, with concrete floors one foot in thickness. They are each 66 feet long, 100 feet wide, and 6 feet in depth, — the total capacity being 1,500,000 gallons. They are so arranged that they can be used intermittently or continuously, and for the purpose of removing the sludge and cleaning the tanks, any one can be shut off from all the others.

The sewage enters the tank marked 1, and from there flows to 2, 3, 4, 5, 6, the flow, however, being so slow that on looking at the tanks when filled, very little movement of the water is noticed. The time required for any given volume of water to pass through the six tanks will be about six hours, thus allowing full time for complete precipitation.

The clear effluent passes over a weir at the end of tank 6, and falls

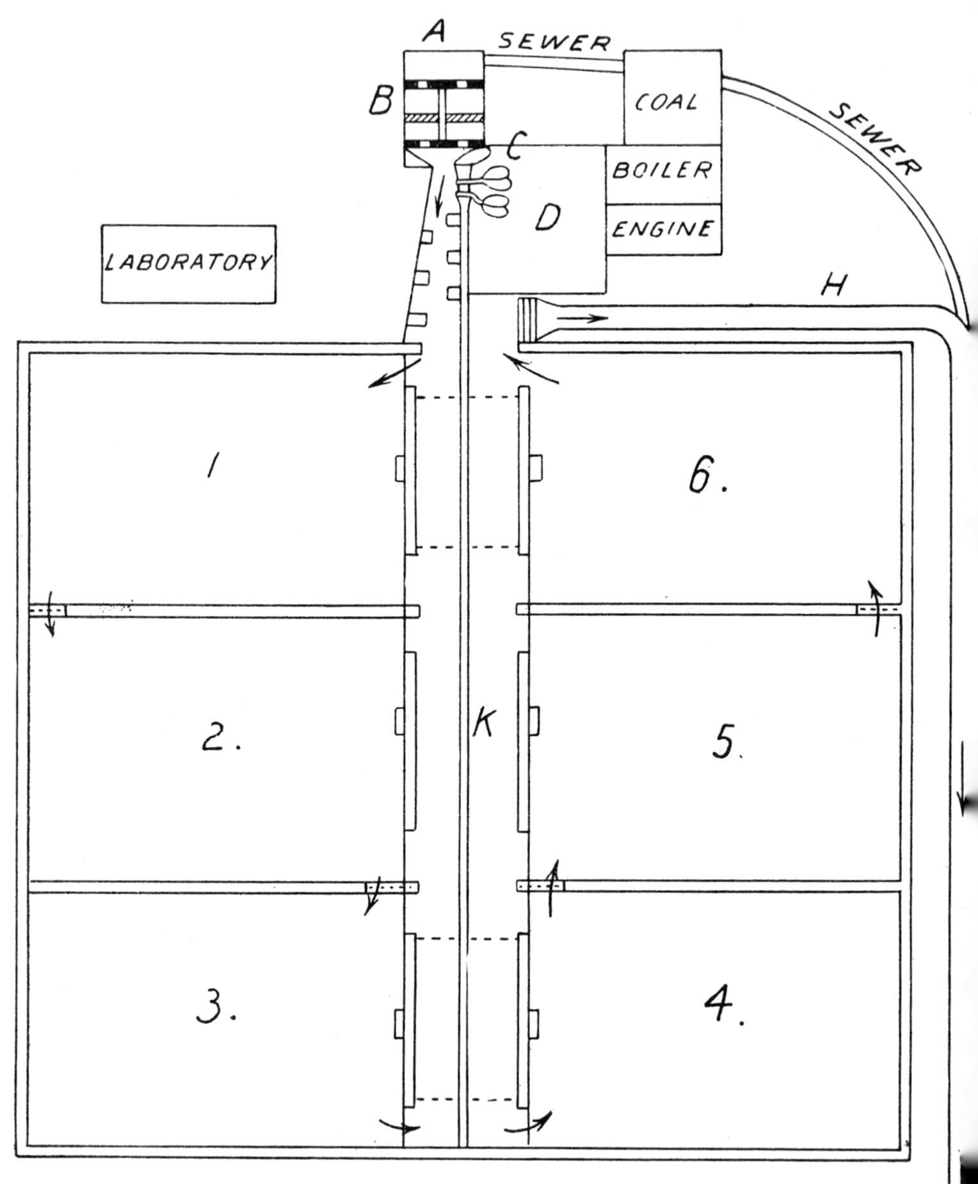

SCALE 50 FEET TO 1 INCH.

over stone steps into the effluent channel H, which conducts it to the Blackstone River. Provision is also made, however, for removing the clear effluent from any one of the tanks. The concrete bottom of each tank inclines to the centre, where there is an opened drain ; these drains are connected with the sludge-pipe K, which carries the sludge to the sludge-well L. Here the sludge is raised fifteen to twenty feet by means of a pump, and is conducted by a pipe to a sandy plot of land having an area of about twelve acres. For the present the sludge will be placed upon this land, and from time to time is to be covered with sand. This will answer for the present, but a time will soon come when it must be pressed into cakes and burned.

The sewage as it now comes to the works varies greatly from hour to hour, sometimes containing large amounts of acid liquors and iron salts, and at other times being nearly neutral, and containing very little mineral matter. Tests are made every five minutes during the day and night to determine roughly the amount of acid liquors and iron salts present, and by these tests Mr. Arthur Forbes, who is in charge of the works, and to whose intelligent oversight their successful operation is due, decides the amount of lime and sulphate of aluminium that is to be used. At times it is necessary to add 120 grains of lime to a gallon of sewage ; at other times the amount is reduced to two or three grains. On the average, about two tons of lime are used each day. The amount of sulphate of aluminium added also varies very greatly, depending on the amount of iron salts present in the sewage. Very often the amount of iron sulphate present renders the addition of aluminium sulphate unnecessary. The average amount of aluminium sulphate used each day is about two hundred pounds.

As is to be expected, most of the sludge is found in the first basins ; the first and second basins are cleaned every thirty hours, the third every three days, the last basin every two weeks. As has been explained, this sludge, which at present contains over 98 per cent of water, is carried from the sludge-well by a pipe-line to the large sludge basins. The water gradually sinks into the sand, and at the end of eight days the sludge contains only about 80 per cent of water, and can be easily removed by shovelling. No odor is to be perceived at the sludge basins, which is undoubtedly due to the amount of free lime contained in the sludge.

As regards the sewage, effluent and sludge I cannot at the present time present any tabulated analytical results, but the analyses I have made show that, with Worcester sewage, chemical precipitation does much more than simply precipitate out the suspended matter.

The total amount of soluble matter in the effluent is twenty per cent less than in the raw sewage, and the volatile matter is reduced from about sixteen parts in 100,000 to nine parts, and the albuminoid ammonia from eight-tenths of one part to about three-tenths. The effluent has, I think, been brought to such a state of purification, that while it would not be allowable to run it into a stream used as a water supply, it is sufficiently pure so that the organic matter which it still contains will be easily destroyed without causing any nuisance, when it is run into the Blackstone River.

Remarks of T. M. DROWN, on Professor Kinnicutt's paper.

Mr. Chairman and Gentlemen: — I have listened with great pleasure and interest to Professor Kinnicutt's paper, which has presented the subject of sewage purification, both from the standpoint of historical development and of adaptation to special needs, in a most admirable way.

The idea once prevalent that it was an economic duty to utilize the manurial value of sewage on the land is now giving place to the more sensible notion, that it is a sanitary duty to get rid of sewage as quickly as possible.

There is no doubt that the simplest method of disposing of sewage is to pour it into the nearest water-course, or into the sea, and this is also the best method where it can be done safely.

In the case of a stream two considerations enter the problem: First, Is the water of the stream used for drinking below the point at which the sewage enters? Second, Is the volume of sewage entering the stream large enough in proportion to the volume of the stream, to make the water offensive to the sight or smell, or to injure the water for manufacturing purposes?

That the water of a sewage-polluted stream is not fit to drink may be assumed at the outset. It is true that in the case of large rivers, like the Mississippi, the Hudson, the Merrimac, sewage-polluted water does form the supply of some large cities. Immunity from harm is supposed to be obtained in such cases by the very great dilution of the sewage, and also in consequence of the " self-purification of streams " — a consoling expression which had its origin in the days before we knew anything of micro-organisms and their power of producing disease.

But when a stream is not used for drinking water it may properly receive the drainage of the towns on its borders to an extent that will not make the stream a nuisance, or prevent its use in boilers, or for manufacturing purposes.

In Worcester this limit has been far overpassed, and the water of its river resembles sewage much more than the water of the lakes in which it had its origin. The question here in Worcester was not to take the sewage out of the river that its waters might be used for drinking, but simply to prevent a nuisance. And any process that will do this most cheaply and simply is clearly the one to adopt. It seems to me that the process of chemical precipitation selected will, when the system of sewerage is complete, and all the city sewage is treated by chemicals, do what is expected of it.

As most of you know, the State Board of Health has been carrying on experiments at Lawrence for the last three years in the purification of sewage by intermittent filtration. The purifying power of porous soil on organic matter, whereby it is completely oxidized, has long been known, and the sewage farms so general throughout Europe for the combined purification and utilization of sewage are instances of the application of this well-known principle.

But it is safe to say that never has there been a systematic and comprehensive series of experiments on the purification of sewage by intermittent filtration that can compare with those which have been in progress in Lawrence under the direction of Mr. Hiram F. Mills, the engineer member of the Board of Health. The report of the work of the Lawrence Experiment Station is now in press and the results obtained will shortly be available to all. I will merely say in this connection that it has been shown that sewage may be continuously purified by simple filtration through sand at the rate of 100,000 gallons per acre a day (and even higher rates have been obtained), and yield an effluent that is purer, organically speaking, than many well-waters in general use.

But this statement does not convey the idea of the real importance of the Lawrence work, which is mainly directed to determining the conditions of successful purification of sewage by its disposal on land. For this purpose it is necessary to determine by actual experiment the unfavorable conditions, that money may not be wasted in installing plants for sewage purification on land unsuited for the purpose.

There have also been carried out at Lawrence by Mr. Allen Hazen a very thorough series of experiments on the chemical precipitation of sewage, which exceed in accuracy anything heretofore attempted.

I would in conclusion like to express my thanks to Professor Kinnicutt for his instructive paper, and to Mr. Allen for the description of the very complete works which he has designed and built for the city of Worcester.

Prof. W. T. SEDGWICK, of the Massachusetts Institute of Technology, Boston, spoke substantially as follows : —

Mr. Chairman and Gentlemen : — It seems to me to be a matter for congratulation that the City of Worcester has had the courage to introduce a method of sewage disposal entirely new to this vicinity, thus enabling us to observe the actual working of sewage disposal by chemical precipitation. It seems to me, furthermore, that Worcester has shown commendable enterprise in sending her engineer, Mr. Allen, to Europe and elsewhere, and in giving him afterwards the means to mature and carry out his plans. I desire to express my own personal pleasure in having been allowed to-day to witness the outcome of Mr. Allen's work. Hitherto, sewage problems have not given us very great solicitude, but as our country grows older and the density of population increases, we are bound to be confronted with new and more difficult problems of water supply and sewage disposal. And here I desire to express my thanks to Professor Kinnicutt for his full and interesting treatment of the subject before us to-day,— a subject which concerns vitally every officer of the public health and every intelligent citizen of the Commonwealth.

Among the numerous important questions arising out of this subject to which one might well address himself, I feel impelled to take up, for a moment, that in which I am personally most interested, namely, the question of the effect of the several methods of disposal upon the living organisms or " germs " in sewage. It must be distinctly understood that sewage is a decomposing fluid, and is crowded with the germs of putrefaction. These are wholly invisible to the naked eye, although so abundant that the sewage of Lawrence, for example, contains usually more than half a million to the cubic centimeter (about a cubic — one-third of an inch). European sewage, being usually more concentrated, contains sometimes as many as five to fifteen millions of organisms to the cubic centimeter. I do not know of any bacterial analyses of Worcester sewage, and it may be that the acid which appears to be so abundant at times, may tend to diminish the number. Most of these "germs" are undoubtedly merely putrefactive and not pathogenic; but among them there may be some — like those of typhoid fever — which are dangerous disease germs. It becomes, then, an interesting question to inquire, What, precisely, is the influence of chemical precipitation upon the organisms of sewage?

For, while this question may seem comparatively unimportant if the effluent is not to be used for drinking and the end sought for is clarification rather than purification, it is quite otherwise in those cases in which the effluent is to be turned into a stream that may possibly be used at some point for drinking purposes. But even if clarification be all that is desired and purification is deemed unnecessary, there is still required a knowledge of the sewage organisms that survive in the effluent, since, if these be added to an ordinary stream, it is possible that in the presence of the residues of sewage precipitation, they may produce new and unlooked-for consequences in the main stream further on. Now it seems to me that it is this biological aspect of the question that most concerns an association like this, especially if we inquire, in the next place, What is the effect of any particular method of sewage disposal upon the disease-producing germs which must frequently occur in sewage?

At the Lawrence Experiment.Station of the State Board of Health studies have been made of the two principal methods of sewage disposal, in respect to their influence upon the organisms of sewage.

The first method is that known as intermittent filtration, or the disposal of sewage upon sandy land. The second is chemical precipitation. In both methods the sewage organisms are materially reduced in numbers, but in chemical precipitation far less completely than in intermittent filtration. Very considerable concentration of the chemicals used is required if the results are to compare at all, bacteriologically, with the results obtained by simply pouring the sewage upon finely sandy land. Now, if the object of a particular system of sewage disposal be clarification to prevent a nuisance, chemical precipitation will often suffice ; but if purification, in the biological sense, be desired, it is infinitely less satisfactory. From the point of view of the public health, there can be little question that ordinary chemical precipitation leaves much to be desired. In the absence of careful experiments in this direction with specific disease germs, the question must, however, remain an open one. It would be especially interesting to experiment here at Worcester, since, according to Professor Kinnicutt, the sewage of Worcester is made acid by receiving waste from the manufacturing establishments, and it might appear upon investigation that this directly favors or hinders the life of the sewage organisms.

It may interest the association to know that it is possible by means of only five feet in depth of finely sandy soil to purify sewage so that all organisms are removed from it. I have frequently drunk of the effluent of such a sewage filter without observing any ill effects whatsoever, and others have done the same. This probably explains why so many wells that, from their surroundings, ought to be dangerous, really produce for a time no bad effect.

But, after all, a great volume of sewage, as we find it in cities like Worcester, seldom has to be purified to this extent. It will generally suffice if it be freed from offensiveness, and here chemical precipitation is probably, at present, most useful. Some experiments at the Lawrence Experiment Station, however, indicate that the proper use of small pebbles or coarse gravel stones as rapid filters, may hereafter prove to be cheaper and equally effective.

CHARLES A. ALLEN, City Engineer of Worcester.

Mr. President and Gentlemen: — I have not a great deal to say. You have visited our works and seen the result. It might be interesting for you to know what the practical result has been upon the river. Of course when I say the practical result I mean what the effect has been as the ordinary observer notices it. We have made no analyses of what the result below Worcester has been so far, but it is a common thing for people to come into my office who live, say, down at Saundersville or Whitinsville, and say something like this: "Have you been down the river lately?" "No," I reply, "I have not." " Well, are you aware that the river is in a much better condition today than it has ever been before? " I generally expressed surprise ; and I really am surprised. But we are told by people below that the river is very much cleaner than it has been for ten years.

I would like to explain further as to the amount of sewage we are treating, and also what we propose to do. We have the combined system of sewers, which care for surface water as well as for sewage proper. Nearly all of our sewers are planned in this way ; a few of them, in outlying districts, are designed to care for domestic sewage only. We treat from three to four million gallons per day of polluted brook water ; and, until we can take all the sewage to be treated, we don't expect and don't claim that the river will receive the full benefit of the process. I am now at work on the plans for the separating of brook water from the sewage, and in a year, or two years, we will convey all the sewage to the works and treat it.

The question has been asked today, several times, about the disposing of the solids, and whether our process is to be a permanent method, and I have answered the questions a number of times. I'll take the risk of explaining again. The land on which we dispose of the sludge is owned by the city and is some twenty acres in extent. We have the river on the east and the Providence and Worcester Railroad on the west. There is no possible way of getting on to that land except through our grounds and the right of way across the railroad, owned by us, so that it is entirely isolated. The ultimate disposal of the sludge will be by burning it ; we first decided to see what could be done by storing it. We also wanted to see whether there was any chance of the sludge becoming a nuisance, so we have let it lie there all summer without covering it up. We have never had the least trouble from it, so that, as far as that question is concerned, it is safe to say that the sludge can be run into basins and dried, without any danger of becoming a nuisance, and it can be afterwards burned. My own opinion is that, in the course of a few years, we shall burn the sludge. The present method is not a permanent one, and ought not to be so considered. It was simply a matter of convenience. The works were not entirely completed when operations were begun ; there were many things that we had to hasten to construct, and the disposal of the sludge was one of them.

Now we have found out that, after all, we know very little about

Worcester sewage; that is, about how it is made up. In the first place it is very much more acid than we expected. When we began to treat the sewage we had a good deal of difficulty in obtaining an effluent that would not be more or less discolored. When we took it and put it into a glass it looked very much like amber. But we very soon found, thanks to some experiments by the State Board of Health, that the trouble was that we did not neutralize all the acid. We experimented every five minutes during the day, neutralizing the acids with lime, and there was no further difficulty in getting a good effluent. The tendency at first was to use more lime than was necessary I think the amount now used is one-half that used at first. and the result is equally as good.

We find that it is not always necessary to treat the sewage with chemicals as it flows into the tanks. That is where we take advantage of the acid in the sewage. Perhaps I can best illustrate what I mean by explaining our method of operating the tanks. Number one is emptied in season to receive the extremely acid sewage, the flow generally lasting about an hour and a half. This sewage is thoroughly treated with lime, and the tank is filled with it; the machinery is then stopped and crude sewage is run through the tank. and is thoroughly treated by the excess of chemical matter in the sewage just preceding it. We can frequently run four or five hours in this way with good results. It is very largely a question of manipulation, where a uniform effluent is desired.

Something has been said in relation to mechanical filters in place of intermittent filtration. If your cities and towns have the same experience that we have had, when they come to the point of disposing of their sewage, you will undoubtedly have an immense number of advisers in favor of mechanical filtration. I think, however, it may be said that sewage is very little improved by mechanical filtration.

[Mr. Allen at this point passed round several samples of the sewage that had been operated upon at the Worcester sewage works.]

Professor FULLER — Is it not quite possible that that is owing to the growth of bacteria?

Mr. ALLEN — I think it is quite likely, Professor Fuller. I am not an expert upon that point. There is one statement I wish to correct that Professor Kinnicutt made, inadvertently, perhaps, and that is about the difference in the quantity of water running into the river and in the sewer. He said, as I understood, that there was five times the water running in the river as in the sewer. I think he must have meant the flow of Mill Brook. Judging by the water-sheds there would be about seven times the flow of water.

The tanks are similar in design to those at Leeds, England, and are of sufficient capacity to treat a greater amount of sewage then we now have.

When we first began to treat the sewage it was in this way: Tank number one was filled and then cut out, tank two filled and cut out, and so on through the series. In that way each tank would have from six to seven hours in which to rest, and the effluent obtained was very fine, indeed. It is a very much more expensive way of doing than the present method. It takes more men, and the difference in the effluent is not such as to seem to warrant the additional expense.

I entirely agree with Professor Drown that there is no one system of sewage treatment that is to be adopted in all cases. I think, however, it has resolved itself down into two systems, because I don't imagine that irrigation will be very extensively used. When I was in England I saw Mr. James Mansergh, who was the engineer of a very large number of important works, and who is now consulting engineer for the Metropolitan Board of Health in London, and he told me that in ten years, irrigation, as a means of disposing of sewage, would be entirely done away with. So that really we have but two ways — chemical precipitation, which is the method in use in Worcester, and downward intermittent filtration.

Now, just one more point I wish to touch upon, and that is, the liability of sewage-disposal works becoming a nuisance. Undoubtedly, some of you today were looking for more or less odor at our works. It is very natural that you should. I have visited many works abroad where the odor was anything but pleasant. It is simply a matter of manipulation and care, and keeping the works in the best possible condition. It does not matter whether the works are chemical precipitation or intermittent filtration, if they are properly looked after there need be no nuisance and no trouble. Therefore I say, keep your disposal-works out of politics. [Laughter and applause.]

Mr. FRENCH (of Newton) — I wish Mr. Allen would give us a few items in regard to the cost of maintenance

Mr. ALLEN — I have said nothing about the cost for the reason that we are continually changing and reducing the amount of chemical matter that we use. At the time the works were decided upon we calculated to deal with three million gallons a day at a cost of $22,500 a year, and we have been able to keep the cost considerably inside of that. We have only been running three months, and that is the reason why we have not given you the cost and a chemical analysis — simply because we are just beginning operations here.

Mr. French — Does that include the cost of the plant?

Mr. Allen — No, sir, it does not; simply the operating expenses. In London the price is something like a shilling a head. It will probably be more here, for labor is higher and chemicals are dearer.

Mr. French — What has been the actual cost of the plant?

Mr. Allen — The outfall sewer cost $75,000 and the tanks and machinery about $47,000. With some additional expenses for grading and the like, the total cost will be a round sum of something like $150,000 or $175,000.

Dr. Baker — I think the gentlemen of the Association are greatly indebted to the city of Worcester for the interesting and instructive afternoon we have had here, and far more to the gentlemen who have given us such able and instructive addresses, and I, therefore, wish to move a vote of thanks to Professors Kinnicutt, Drown and Sedgwick, and Mr. Allen. I hope that some of this will reach print. I think the Society should have in permanent form the result of this report. [Applause.]

MASSACHUSETTS ASSOCIATION BOARDS OF HEALTH.

MEMBERSHIP ROLL

JAN. 1, 1891.

Note.—The Secretary requests to be advised of existing errors or changes of address from that which appears in the following list.

MASSACHUSETTS STATE BOARD OF HEALTH.

Henry P. Walcott, M.D., of Cambridge, *Chairman*.
Samuel W. Abbott, M.D., of Wakefield, *Secretary*.
F. W. Draper, M.D., of Boston.

BELMONT.

H. A. Yenetchi, M.D.

BOSTON.

Samuel H. Durgin, M.D., Board of Health, *Chairman*.
George F. Babbitt, Board of Health.
Edwin L. Pilsbury, Board of Health.
Charles E. Davis, Jr., Board of Health, *Clerk*.
John H. McCollom, M.D., City Physician.
F. W. Draper, M.D., State Board of Health.
Prof. T. M. Drown, Massachusetts Institute of Technology.
Prof. W. T. Sedgwick, Massachusetts Institute of Technology.

BROCKTON.

Charles H. Carey.
C. O. Batchelder.
L. F. Severance.

BROOKLINE.

Albert L. Lincoln, Jr.

CAMBRIDGE.

D. H. Thurston.
H. P. Walcott, M.D., also State Board of Health.
W. H. Whitney.
Edwin Farnham, M.D.

CLINTON.

Charles L. French, M.D.
T. H. O'Connor, M.D.
Thomas F. Roche, M.D.
Philip T. O'Brien, M.D.
P. P. Comey, M.D.

DEDHAM.

A. W. Cheever, State Cattle Commissioner, *Secretary*.

EVERETT.

W. K. Knowles, M.D., Board of Health.
E. Cazneau Newton, M.D., Board of Health, *Secretary*.
William Goodhue, Board of Health.

FITCHBURG.

Charles H. Rice, M.D.
John D. Kielty, M.D.
Charles Smith.

GARDNER.

Edward A. Sawyer, M.D.
Charles D. Burrage.

GEORGETOWN.

Ralph C. Huse, M.D.

GLOUCESTER.

Charles H. Morrow, M.D.

HAVERHILL.

John F. Croston, M.D.
Chester Bryant.
Perley E. Goodhue, M.D.   (Deceased.)
G. Colburn Clement, M.D.

LANCASTER.

George L. Tobey, M.D.

LOWELL.

James B. Field, M.D., Board of Health, *Chairman*.
Charles R. Costello, Board of Health.
J. Arthur Gage, M.D., Board of Health.
Frederick A. Bates, Board of Health, *Agent*.

LYNN.

M. R. Donovan, M.D.
F. F. Brigham, M.D.
M. S. Foye.
W. C. Lamphier.
Henry Farrell.

MALDEN.

A. G. Griffin, M D.

MEDFORD.

J. E. Clark, M.D., Board of Health.
John W. Cosden, Board of Health.

MELROSE.

Ernest S. Jack, M.D.
George W. Burke.
Frank L. Washburn.

MILTON.

M. V. Pierce, M.D.
H. P. Jaques, M.D.
Edwin D. Wadsworth.

NATICK.

W. H. Sylvester, M.D.

NEW BEDFORD.

Nathaniel Hathaway, Board of Health, *Chairman*.
William N. Swift, M.D., Board of Health.
Thomas W. Cook, Board of Health.
Louis H. Richardson, Board of Health, *Agent*.

NEWTON.

Otis Pettee, Board of Health, *President.*
Edmund T. Wiswall, Board of Health.
David E. Baker, M.D., Board of Health.
William S. French, Board of Health, *Clerk and Agent.*

PLYMOUTH.

Henry Harlow.

PROVIDENCE, R.I.

Charles V. Chapin, M.D., City Registrar and Superintendent
of Health.

SHARON.

James W. Hemenway.

SPRINGFIELD.

Walter H. Chapin, City Physician.
James Kimball, Board of Health, *Agent.*

WAKEFIELD.

Samuel W. Abbott, Board of Health; also Secretary State
Board of Health.

WALTHAM.

E. R. Cutler, M.D., Board of Health.
I. S. Hall, M.D., Board of Health.
R. B. Foster, Board of Health.
Edward N. Quinn, Board of Health, *Agent.*

WARE.

D. W. Miner, M.D.
D. M. Ryan, M.D.
William Metcalf.

WARREN.

J. W. Hastings, M.D.

WATERTOWN.

E. True Aldrich, M.D.
James R. Harrison.

WESTBORO.

B. C. Hathaway.

WESTON.

F. W. Jackson, M.D.

WINCHESTER.

B. F. Church, M.D.

WORCESTER.

Lemuel F. Woodward, M.D., Board of Health, *Chairman*.
George E. Batchelder. Board of Health.
James C. Coffey, Board of Health.
Charles A. Allen, City Engineer.
Prof. Leonard P. Kinnicutt, Worcester Polytechnic Institute.

PROGRESS
IN VENTILATING
SCHOOL-HOUSES

Frederic Tudor

PROGRESS IN VENTILATING SCHOOL-HOUSES.

BY FREDERIC TUDOR, ENGINEER, OF BOSTON.

(Read at the meeting held at Boston, Jan. 21, 1891.)

It is characteristic of the human mind to seek an explanation of everything. The astronomer and the novel-reader, the chemist and the explorer of continents are all impelled by the same motive — curiosity. All wish to know what there is, where it is, how it is, and why it is. But it is only in recent times that the question has been asked, What is the cause of disease? It is not so long ago but that all who are present can remember it, that the inquirer was told that the cause of disease and premature death was the anger of the Creator; by their infliction the wicked were punished, the righteous chastened. Christianity has long cherished this belief, which is so strongly set forth in the Old Testament, especially in the Book of Jeremiah; nor have later priests quite given it up, though, fortunately for human progress, especially in the domain of hygiene, the generation is passing away which was content with this cruel faith.

The world is coming into the hands of another race, one which is in quest of truth and light, and, impressed with the belief that like causes assure like effects, is inclined to reject the supernatural and to rely upon facts yet to be discovered, though comprehensible, to reveal the explanation of every mystery. This is especially so in sanitary science; there is beginning to be a readiness to accept its discoveries and follow its teachings which promises great developments and is very encouraging to those who believe that the best way to promote health is to prevent disease.

Just now there is some interest in the sanitation of school-houses, which will certainly be greatly increased by proof of some actual progress. Interest and progress react upon and sustain each other; without evidence of success, interest will be discouraged and will abate. If nothing of real value is accomplished now, the whole thing may be dropped in disgust for another twenty years, as happened when an impetus was given to the subject by Franklin in the last century, and in this by the writings and efforts of Dr. Reid and our own Dr. Wyman, who still flourishes in Cambridge, and whose treatise on Ventilation, written many years ago, has long been regarded as a classic work. It would be well therefore to take account of stock, as it were, and see what we have to offer to an inquiring public in search of information. The time allowed limits us to a hasty review of the subject, treating only the leading points without much discussion or demonstration, and stating chiefly established facts and methods.

In the first place, what are the requirements of good ventilation? Before going in search of anything it is important to know exactly what is to be looked for. This rule has not always been observed, consequently some things have been found and applied which seemed very promising, yet were after all disappointing when made use of, because they were not exactly what was wanted; or, while they might have been a part, and a very important part, of it, yet were not the whole thing. Let me dwell upon this tendency to accept a part instead of the whole. It has been the chief cause of all the failures in practical work. These have been due not so much to error as to incompleteness. One swallow does not make a spring, nor does one law of nature, however carefully applied, make the art of ventilation; yet many schemes have been carried out by people who had acquired only one or two facts or knew only one or two laws, perhaps equally as wonderful and beautiful in their action as essential to any scheme, yet because less so than the many others which had been overlooked or neglected, they did not win success. A few years ago an expert in this mysterious art used to entrap victims by means of a well-known experiment with a glass bottle, with which I suppose many of you must be familiar. Placing the bottle upright, he lowered into it a lighted candle, whose burning speedily exhausted the oxygen to the point at which combustion is arrested. This happens, as you know, when only one-tenth of the oxygen is consumed. At this stage, when the flickering flame seemed on the verge of extinction, he slipped a strip of tin into the neck of the bottle, dividing it into two channels, through one of which fresh air poured in, driving the hot burned air out of the other and instantly reviving the almost extinct flame with a new supply of oxygen. The experiment is very pretty and instructive, and, as a flickering candle in a bottle bears some analogy to a breathing man in a house, especially when one considers that the open mouth of the bottle is well represented by the chimney of the house, it was not very difficult to effect a sale of a patent ventilator to the delighted witness of the experiment. If a natural law would condescend to work with such promptness and certainty in the case of a common glass bottle, it would be hardly necessary to guarantee it to operate with equal certainty in ventilating the building where the patent ventilator should be applied. It is very evident that this is a phenomenon whereby a space containing hot spent air is replenished continuously with new fresh air, but it is not the whole art of ventilation, nor can it be applied except in extremely rare instances. The construction, use and arrangement of modern buildings are such that the process described cannot come into action at all. Yet the ventilators are still on sale, and are to be seen in every town in Massachusetts on buildings which deserve better treatment. So in regard to heating apparatus, it is some unduly magnified trifle or catch-penny device which decides the choice in most cases. Buyers are apt to prefer a plate steel furnace with a row of big handsome rivets round the top, which attract the eye and prevent it from detecting the open and loosely fastened joint round the bottom through which unlimited dust and carbonic dioxide are sure to pass directly into the fresh warmed air, and to reject the far preferable cast iron heater, with its extended, convoluted and gilled surfaces and with its apparently loosely fitted but practically gas-tight joints, well designed to withstand the effects of unequal expansion. A leading physician of Boston was chiefly instrumental in establishing the worthless and wasteful plate iron furnace in its present place of favor. He wrote a book based upon a mistake, and which is of course worse than a waste of paper, for it tends to perpetuate error. It is dangerous to speculate upon imaginary facts. Again, to show the undue influence of type or feature, how many times we hear it said that '' hot water '' is the right system to use, as if it carried with it everything that was needful and desirable in heating and ventilation. Good enough in itself, it is only a part of an apparatus from which a combined heating and ventilation may be obtained. It has been adopted for the most important building in Boston, the new Suffolk County Court House, where, instead of being subservient to the ventilation, the ventilation is made subservient to it — is but an incident of the heating. This is a case where, next to a hospital, the greatest sacrifices should be made for the sake of ventilation ; everything else should give way to it, architecture and all, yet the commissioners were so captivated by the merits and advantages of hot-water heating (which I, personally, do not concede, at least in this case,) that they quite overlooked every other detail. They accepted a part in lieu of the whole. When buyers don't really know what they want and turn to a salesman for advice, he is not very capable unless he can show them that he only has just what they need. If they have got plenty of money, so much the better for him; he has goods to suit all purses. This sort of thing is going on all the time; commissioners, boards of trustees and building committees, charged with the responsibility of getting the best for institutions in their care, are constantly adopting schemes of ventilation, because one or two things which they understand, or think they understand, seem to be plausible, but do not, because they cannot, give due consideration to other, perhaps more important, elements, to the great discouragement of competent and conscientious designers. Pardon this digression, but I could not otherwise show you the damage which is done by half-knowledge in this matter and by the disposition to overlook essential elements in the presence of one or two striking details. It is as if one bought a ship on the sole question of her ability to float, and neglected all the considerations of speed and sailing qualities in all winds and weathers.

At first thought it appears simple enough, this question of ventilation; it is only to find a means of allowing the close air to escape. It is only a question of opening a window where the cold draft will blow on some one else; or of making a hole in the ceiling to let the heat out; for most people do not distinguish between foul air and an uncomfortably high temperature. Today the average man believes that the open window or a hole in the ceiling is all that is necessary. With such an imperfect knowledge of the real demands of ventilation, really satisfactory means could scarcely be chosen. Fortunately scientific men have thoroughly investigated the laws of physics and hygiene which affect the question, and careful observers have accurately reported the results of well-considered experiments, in which they have shown how desirable conditions may be reproduced and what must be done to maintain them. The facts which they have collected form an immense fund which is accessible to every student, but whose volume is so great that I can here neither recount their steps nor repeat their demonstrations, but only their undisputed conclusions.

It is shown that efficient ventilation demands a continuous supply of a volume of fresh air equal to fifty cubic feet a minute to each adult occupant of an apartment, which implies the removal reciprocally of the same volume of vitiated air.   It is shown (I am quoting de Chaumont, Pettenkofer, Angus Smith, Parkes) that although each man actually breathes only one-quarter of a cubic foot a minute, that this small volume combined with other bodily exhalations is sufficient to vitiate fifty cubic feet of the surrounding air to the extent of not being able to bear further vitiation without becoming noticeably tainted.   The conditions are such that the supply of fresh air is to be poured into and become mingled with the already somewhat vitiated air contained in the room, and it is shown both demonstratively and experimentally that the vitiation can only be kept down to the limit imposed by considerations of health by the continuous supply of fifty cubic feet per minute to each occupant.   It is obvious that if the air could be distributed to each person, a much smaller quantity would suffice, and that it could also be somewhat diminished in case the occupants are children.   On the basis of fifty cubic feet to each adult man, thirty-three cubic feet would be the right quantity for the grammar school pupil, or two thousand cubic feet per hour, if the fresh air is pure and not already contaminated by being taken from a polluted source.   Parkes says that the diminished consumption of air by young persons is balanced by the importance of favoring their healthy development by securing to them the best conditions, and advises that the standard of fifty cubic feet per minute per person be adhered to as the lowest limit.   Moreover, the imperfections of apparatus must be allowed for.   It is not practically possible to cause a perfect diffusion of the fresh air, thus preventing a disproportionate accumulation of vitiated air locally, nor to prevent some premature escape of the former by way of the ventilating outlets before its work is done.   Experience shows that thirty, or even thirty-five, cubic feet a minute per occupant is not enough for school-rooms, and it is probable that the standard of fifty is too low unless the method of distribution is much improved over what prevails today.

It is a curious fact that the earlier theorists decided that five cubic feet per minute per person would be adequate ventilation.   It is a very bad condition of things where scholars do not get more than this, and such cases are promptly condemned by the state inspectors. When Moody and Sankey's Boston Tabernacle was in use, it was experimentally found by careful tests, the audience numbering about six thousand persons, that when the air supply was as low as five cubic feet per head per minute, fainting of a number of persons was certain to ensue, but that it was prevented altogether by increasing the supply to seven cubic feet. The fainting was confined to one locality remote from the fresh-air inlets; I am confident that with a better distribution than there was in some parts of this great hall, five cubic feet would have been adequate to prevent fainting altogether, if uniformly distributed to each person, although far from being adequate in the sense of proper ventilation. This fact is interesting because it shows that what was at first believed as a theoretical deduction would be sufficient for good ventilation, is proved by trial on a large scale to be the very least that will support life without distress. When this quantity was fixed upon, it appears to have been taken for granted that the five cubic feet of air would reach the individual for whom it was provided without any taint; in other words, the important element of distribution was overlooked. Later writers have taken this into account with a result showing that the quantity of the early investigators was ten times too small. This is a remarkable illustration of the uncertainty of purely theoretical deductions, or rather, of the importance of bringing every element into the question which may have any influence, and this cannot be done without thorough practical trial under all possible conditions. Weighed against a few facts obtained by actual trial, pages of discussion on paper are of no real value, except as mental gymnastics for mathematicians.

Accepting, then, the fifty feet per minute standard and applying it to the modern class-room of the graded school in the larger towns of this state, we find this is arranged for about fifty occupants; it has a space of about ten thousand cubic feet, or two hundred to each occupant. Great importance is attached to this matter of space, but it is apt to be overlooked that aside from questions of convenience of arrangement, it is the rate of ventilation, the time required for a complete change of the air, which determines the space. Thus, for a two-hours' session with no ventilation, the factors of the space are fifty cubic feet vitiated each minute by each one of fifty people, or $50 \times 120 \times 50 = 300,000$ cubic feet, which is thirty times larger than what is usually provided; with complete change of air each hour, one-third of this space will suffice, or ten times as much as is found in the most liberally equipped school-houses; and if the space be limited to ten thousand cubic feet, the capacity of the standard room, the change should be clearly ten times more rapid. This means that the flow of air should be so abundant as to equal in volume the entire contents of the room in six minutes, effecting a change ten times in an hour. This is only part of the problem, but one which without the complication of other elements, demands some well-studied engineering. Let us suppose that we may neglect both temperature and drafts, and that the air is already at the proper temperature; how can it be moved at such a rate as is shown to be needful? It is important to adhere to this rate, on the one hand not to give less air than good sanitary conditions call for; on the other, not to give more, because that will entail excess of power in the apparatus and excess of fuel to operate it.

Now it is alleged that there is such a thing as natural ventilation. By this expression is meant a ventilation which results without the aid of artifice. Since there can be no motion without force, even natural ventilation must depend upon some form of it. One form of force in natural ventilation is difference of temperature between the air within and the air without the building; but this being extremely variable the force and the effects derived from it must be correspondingly uncertain. Another form is the pressure exerted by the wind; but this not only varies in force, but in direction, and is therefore unreliable in both respects, whose value can be most effectively illustrated by putting it into the shape of a mathematical statement.

If a is a variable quantity indicating the force of the wind, and b another variable representing its direction, then we have x the resultant of their combination, not equal to $a + b$, but to $a \times b$, a quantity which may have any value from nothing to infinity. Now bring the effect of fluctuating temperature into consideration, and the impossibility of obtaining any exact or even approximately satisfactory result will be apparent. There is no choice between these Protean forces. In order to make natural ventilation effective, we must be prepared to utilize either of them wherever found or however fluctuating between the extremes of maximum effect on one hand and almost total restraint on the other, in any of its possible moods, or both of them together in any of the infinite combinations of both their possible moods. This kind of ventilation should be

called accidental ventilation, since by its aid there can be no certainty
of effect except by accident, and it is evident that the chance of the
accident happening is infinitely remote.

Thus is accounted for and explained the undeviating regularity
of failure of all schemes which depend upon accidental conditions
for their operation. In fact it should be said that failure is the only
element of certainty which they possess.

It would seem as if nothing more need be said to prove the futility
of depending upon such uncertain forces as wind and temperature
as sources of power to do the work of ventilation. To make the
proof overwhelming it is only necessary to show that these forces
are not only variable and uncertain, but lacking in quantity. It is
extremely seldom that sufficient power can be obtained from them
to do this work, which, it would be well to understand, is no small
matter. The work of ventilation involves mainly two things to be
done which consume power: they are overcoming the inertia of mass
and the resistances of friction and change of direction and discharge.
I cannot at this time go into any demonstration of the extent of
these resistances; it is enough to indicate them by pointing out the
weight alone of the air to be moved. In the case of an eight-room
school-house the weight of the air supplied for ventilation at the
standard rate in one hour would amount to forty-six net tons.
Besides overcoming the inertia of this mass in putting it into rapid
motion, the sum of the frictional and other resistances acting continuously against its movement may amount to the weight of a
column of water one-half inch in height, which is equal to a pressure
of about two and a half pounds per square foot. It is usually less
than this when the ducts are very large, but even when they are so,
the saving by this is more than offset by the devices used to secure
thorough diffusion of the fresh air in the rooms if at all efficient.
As a rule, the diffusion is very imperfect, causing draughts and local
accumulations of foul air which I think can only be remedied by
means which will consume additional power. I intend to revert
to the importance of uniform distribution later on; I only mention
it at this stage because it represents work to be done, and we are
considering how extensive this is, how regularly it has to be carried
on, and how unfitted for it are the uncertain forces to be obtained
from the accidental conditions of wind and weather. It can readily
be shown that if the air-ducts are of the usual dimensions and do

not occupy a disproportionate space that sufficient power to move the air can only be obtained from these conditions when the air-inlets happen to face the direction from which a high wind is blowing, or when the external temperature is extremely low. You will observe that when the latter condition exists it is the very time, if ever there is any, when the use of air ought to be economized, for it is then that the consumption of fuel is greatest. It has already been made evident that there can be no systematic ventilation effected by wind power, but since an extremely low temperature may persist for some time, the force derived from it may be temporarily utilized, but it appears that this can only happen when the heating apparatus is loaded up to its full capacity. Consequently natural forces are useful only at times when we are in the worst position to avail of them, and when a liberal supply of fresh air can be least afforded. It ought to be just the other way, because the days of severest cold are proportionately few, and to restrict the ventilation on those days is the only time when, if ever, it ought to be restricted. Moreover, while these accidental forces might be of some aid on the coldest blustering days in winter they are not actually so, because ventilating apparatus is not really designed to utilize them, nor are heating appliances usually sufficiently powerful to stand the strain of heating so much extremely cold air.

To sum up this branch of the subject it is shown that no certainty of effect can be obtained from reliance upon natural conditions, because the forces derived from them are uncertain, irregular, and inadequate, besides which, it is an obvious fact that apparatus cannot be designed to act under such a variety of conditions as must be anticipated without such an excessive complication of construction and management as to overload and obstruct its practical usefulness, to say nothing of its great cost and expense of maintenance and operation. I do not believe the attempt has ever been made to design such an apparatus by any person of scientific training who had by experience acquired practical familiarity with the question. Outside of the tropics natural ventilation exists only as a hypothesis. It is a sort of scientific fetich whose charm has a potency only for the careless and superficial student. So much for the so-called natural ventilation. In these days of systematic and orderly procedure people do not expect regularity of result where the means employed to secure it are accidental and unreliable.

It is now perfectly clear that we can accept this point as settled, and that to assure a regular, quantitative ventilation we must employ some force artificially applied and adapted to the work to be done; that is, it is solely a question of engineering. I have treated this branch of the subject with rather more fulness than it merits, but I cannot neglect the present opportunity to attempt some proselyting with a view to breaking down the superstition which is strangely prevalent in this state regarding the supposed efficacy of natural ventilation, and which I feel it my duty to say seems to be an article of faith of many medical men, even of some who have the reputation of being skilful hygienists.

If, then, artificial force is an essential element of ventilation, what should be its form? This is as much a question of practical economics as of engineering; it depends upon the conditions. The simplest is the heated shaft; one type of it has the heat applied to each extraction-flue separately, or to a chamber in the upper part of a building, to which several flues are connected. This is a convenient method when steam heating is used. But the best type is that in which all the extraction-flues are carried downwards and led to the base of a capacious and lofty aspirating shaft provided with a fire-place at the bottom, a common open grate being as economical and efficient as any source of heat. Sometimes the smoke-pipe of the boilers or furnaces can be made to take the place of the grate; but this should only be done with the advice of a skilful engineer. I know of one hospital where the iron pipe was put in place in such a way that the building was completed before it was found that the extraction-ducts could not be connected to the shaft. I know of another hospital where the iron flue was so chilled by the current of outflowing air which surrounded it in the shaft that the man whose duty it was to keep up the steam pressure, finding he could not do so with a cold chimney, closed the opening into the shaft and thus cut off the whole ventilating movement. The consequences were endured for a long time, but the cause was only revealed after a painstaking investigation, and the difficulty was not an easy one to remedy.

Other forms make use of blowing fans which propel the fresh, or extract the foul, air, or have both in operation at the same time, the power being obtained from various types of motors, in which water, steam, gas, electricity, or compressed air may be the moving force. Sometimes an aspirating shaft supplements a propelling fan. Still another type utilizes compressed air, delivered in jets in the flues, and so inducing a regular flow. What may actually be the best type for use depends upon the circumstances of the case. The choice must be left to good judgment. As to economy, if fuel were the only consideration, the fan and steam-engine system is preferable, but there are often other considerations which outweigh the question of fuel, such as competent attendance, the form of heating used, etc. For example, where furnaces are used for heat, the appropriate motive power to operate the ventilation is the heated extraction-shaft, although less regular and effective, and as respects fuel, more expensive than the fan. This is the type best adapted to small school-houses, with few rooms, especially in the country districts.

We have seen that the volume of air in ventilation is large, and that force artificially applied is essential to its regular and necessarily rapid movement. There remain to be taken up the questions of temperature and humidity, avoidance of draughts, and thoroughness of distribution. Next to the wind the most uncertain thing is temperature. We can successfully evade the former by refusing to have anything to do with it, but the latter we must be prepared to deal with and bring to a fixed and regular standard no matter where we find it nor how quickly it changes its state. The heating apparatus must be capable of effects as variable as the temperature itself. It is needless to say that this is an embarrassing problem, which as yet has found no solution which is commendable as a simple and practical one for common use. I hazard the opinion that the regulation of temperature in schemes of ventilation, such as that of school-rooms, is the most difficult branch of the subject, yet it is quite ignored or superficially touched upon in all of the treatises with which I am familiar and which investigate almost all the other branches with great thoroughness. Morin, the distinguished, but I must say unpractical, engineer, did not appreciate it at all until after he had published his great work on ventilation, and the failures of apparatus, based on his elegant and abstruse calculations, began to come home to him. By the way, let me throw out the hint that you will find Morin to be a first-rate example of the scientific snob. Admire his book, it is the fashion; but if you want information go to good, honest, unpretentious, and reliable Peclet, who all his life was kept in the background by the undue influence of Morin's army and social prestige.

There are other people like Morin, perfectly sane on all other subjects, who become victims of an hallucination that they have a call to attack the problem of ventilation. Intelligent men usually recognize the necessity of special study to fit themselves for any line of work; but when ventilation is the question there is no lack of people who will take hold of it as unreflectingly as the greenhorn who, when asked if he could play on the violin, replied: "I guess so; I never tried." Ventilation, as a practical art, has been sadly discredited by educated men who have undertaken it without proper preparation. The chief stumbling-block which overthrows these over-confident venturers is the management of the heating, the regulation of the temperature, which always has been, and still is, the most difficult element of the problem. It is unfortunate that this fact is not appreciated by writers on the subject. I have the best of reasons for knowing that whatever measure of success in actual results has been obtained by "professors" or "doctors" whose title may have been fairly earned by faithful work in their legitimate occupation, but who were lacking experience in this work, has been due in all cases to some silent partner, whom you will find to have been a man who united to a thorough practical knowledge of heating a skill quite analogous to the *main d'œuvre* of the artist, which is acquired only by diligent practice and patient observation.

When a furnace or hot-water apparatus is the source of heat a heating effect may be obtained which is approximated to the demands of temperature. It is found practically, however, that the approximation is not near enough to depend upon, and it is necessary to use the device known as a mixing-valve, which by admitting a greater or less portion of cold air directly to the flue conducting the warm air to the room from the heater gives control over the temperature, providing it is attended to.

This device seems very simple and attractive, especially in a neat drawing on paper. In fact, it is but a make-shift contrivance, well enough if only one or two of it are used in one building, but applied to every flue it becomes a mechanical nuisance, yet a nuisance which in many systems we cannot get along without for want of something to take its place. In my own work I make considerable sacrifices to avoid using it.

Steam apparatus is ill adapted to variations in temperature, but the facility and economy of the distribution of heat in any direction by its aid, even from remote sources, greatly recommend its use ; and since by the aid of the mixing-valve the same result may be obtained as with a furnace or hot water, I think it preferable for large buildings. Some method of automatically controlling the temperature is urgently needed, but nothing has yet been evolved which is cheap and simple in operation. There is, however, an electric contrivance in the market which is in successful use, but which is too complicated and expensive for general application. The need of such a thing has not been felt long enough, nor is it widely enough recognized to attract the attention of inventors. This is mainly because it is only when the air is changed rapidly that it is important to regulate the temperature very closely. Before I leave this question, which I think in its present state is the most unsatisfactory of all, I wish to emphasize the fact that the less such devices are resorted to the better the result will be. If they cannot be avoided it is well to use as few of them as possible, and one way of effecting this is to concentrate the control. If the temperature can be regulated at a central point for the whole building, it is manifestly better than separate mixing-valves for each flue and each room, because it is a way to concentrate and simplify the management, which, it does not need any argument to show, contributes more to successful operation than any other feature. I beg you will weigh this statement carefully. The shortcomings of ventilating apparatus are not always so much owing to omissions in the design as to the neglect of the attendants to make the proper adjustments at the proper time and in the right way, or their inability to care for a vast number of confusing details. The careless and stupid we have always with us, and besides the careless and stupid, the shirking janitor must be included in the design as an unavoidable part of it. Woe to the designing engineer who leaves him out of account! I do not mean that these men are careless or stupid except as regards their duties ; in one direction, that of saving themselves trouble, they are assiduous and intelligent in a high degree. Their work, even if arduous, should be so laid out for them that circumstances will exact it and forbid neglect of it in spite of them ; they should not be required to do any reflecting or to exercise any judgment, but be furnished with the means of producing required effects with simplicity and certainty and without possibility of evasion.

I must refrain from discussing the question of humidity. It is a moot question, and I think, being the least important part of the subject, we can afford to put it aside until the more essential elements have been definitely settled. Some misapprehensions concerning it, however, are very prevalent, and I think a word or two tending to remove them may not be a waste of time. Natural air contains the vapor of water at all temperatures, but its capacity for absorbing it increases rapidly with the temperature. For example, at thirty-two degrees a cubic foot of it can hold two grains of water, but at seventy degrees it can hold eight grains, though it weighs less because expanded by heat. In nature it is only at times saturated, the mean in this climate being seventy-one per cent of saturation or seventy-one per cent relative humidity, while it varies between the low limit of thirty per cent when it is extremely dry and one hundred per cent when it either rains or snows. If we take air from out of doors at thirty-two degrees and at seventy per cent relative humidity and heat it to seventy degrees without adding water, the 1.4 grain by weight which at first represented seventy.per cent, in the new temperature represents only seventeen per cent relative humidity, which is an abnormally low proportion. This is not because the heating process has dried it, as commonly supposed, but because, by the rise of temperature the capacity to absorb water and the avidity for it are enormously increased. Air as dry as this is very disagreeable to many people, but I am inclined to think it is apt to be so when there is a preponderance of foulness along with the dryness. If the air is fresh, it may perhaps be dry without harmfulness; at any rate it is not proved to be hurtful in that condition. On the other hand, if we moisten somewhat the air which we heat, we shall be imitating nature, a safe guide.

The next step to be taken is to provide against the movement of the air being felt by the occupants. The volume to be poured into the room is so large that unless the inlet is judiciously placed and carefully proportioned, drafts will be felt by some of the occupants. The difficulty is increased in proportion as the space is diminished, and is obviated by adding to the number as well as the size of the inlets. The common registers are not suitable for inlets; the openings should be so constructed as to cause the air to flow at a moderate velocity and to reach every part of the room without motion in the vicinity of the occupants greater than two or three feet a second.

The location of the inlets is consequently a matter of prime importance. In the early days of ventilation, their proper location was thought to be susceptible to theoretical demonstration ; Morin, heading the theorists, advocated placing them at the top of the room, but the practical men insisted on having them at the bottom. The difficulty with purely theoretical deductions is that they cannot deal with more than one or two elements at a time if they are variable ; that is, a certainty cannot be deduced from a variety of conditions unless the number of them is very small, and it is in fact impossible to take all of them into account even if every one is anticipated and recognized. But when you come to a trial, something of importance is almost sure to turn up which was wholly overlooked, yet capable of influencing the result. The first case which was submitted to me for practical solution was Sever Hall of Harvard University in 1878. Accepting the method of practical men in bringing the air in at a low level, I was confronted with the questions of drafts and distribution, to avoid one and insure the other. After balancing together theoretical considerations and such experience as I had personally the advantage to have gained, I concluded to place the inlets as low as possible, which location was in fact high, for it was above the level of the occupants' heads, about half way between floor and ceiling. They were placed on the warm side of the room, and the outlets near them in plan, but at the level of the floor. The arrangement worked well, though not without some complaints of drafts. I used the common registers to cover the openings, which I said above are not well adapted to a real ventilation such as this was, for it was the first educational building to be ventilated by a fan. This arrangement of inlets and outlets was shortly after adopted in the Bridgeport, Ct , High School, and has now come to be the standard method, being used by the two largest firms engaged in school-house ventilation as a specialty, and advocated by experts. I do not consider that the provision is complete for removing the air without an additional outlet at an upper level, which may be opened in case the room gets too warm, and be kept permanently open in summer. To omit it is in the direction of simplicity, which is no small advantage ; but I have not yet seen sufficient reason to sacrifice its benefits on that account.

Finally, let us take up the question of distribution. This involves the means of assuring to each occupant his share of the fresh air.

The problem is complicated by the importance of not wasting the heat which has been imparted to the air by the apparatus in the cellar, to be transferred and given up to the room by it before it escapes, for in all types of apparatus, except that which is peculiarly my own, the fresh air is required to do double duty; it is a carrier of heat as well as a diluent and displacer of vitiated air. From this it follows that the entering air must be warmer than the air contained by the room, consequently it rises. Now it is perfectly established that the bodily exhalations, carbonic acid and all, rise also, and that at the top of the room, if occupied by a number of people, the foulest air is to be found. Therefore the first thing that happens to the entering fresh air is its mixture with these exhalations at the upper levels, and the compound has to be cooled by walls and windows before it can descend to the breathing line. Does it not seem desirable that some way should be found to cause this air to be diffused at a low level and follow the exhalations rather than meet them when already on their way out, thus rising through the breathing line before it has required any taint? Moreover, in a sanitary point of view, is it not of paramount importance that the exhalations from each person should be swept directly away altogether if possible, rather than that they should be brought back to another, bearing perhaps some specific contagion? For it must be borne in mind that though dilution by fresh air diminishes the chances of infection by foul air, it is not a perfect safeguard against it. How is it that the school becomes so often a focus of disease of the greatest danger to the health of the community? If an infectious disease breaks out in one home, it can easily be held in check by isolation; but if it breaks out in a school, there is no way to check it short of closing the school and suspending its work. This is not only because it is dreaded as a possible focus of disease, but as a focus whose effect the school-house itself may greatly magnify by its imperfections. These considerations make it evident both that perfection is not yet reached in the matter of the introduction and diffusion of the air, and that improvement in the method would be highly advantageous.

As the result of experience in trials on a large scale I have found that thorough diffusion, or rather a quantitative distribution to each occupant, permits an enormous reduction in the standard amount of air, which it has been observed should not be less than fifty cubic feet per minute. You will remember how this standard was fixed; it was with the assumption that the fresh air acts as a diluent to keep down the accumulation of exhalations, and that owing to imperfections of apparatus and consequent bad diffusion it is a low requirement, it ought to be somewhat higher. Beginning with thirty cubic feet per person per minute, that is, distributed to each one, and working downwards, I have found that the quantity may be reduced to fifteen cubic feet; that this is ample, and can be supplied readily without producing drafts, a great advantage, more than compensating the reduction in volume, which, however, is not so much a loss as a superfluity, since what is not needful is superfluous. Possibly it may be still further reduced, even reaching the standard of ten feet recommended by Dr. Reid, or the five cubic feet of the early speculators on the subject. This, in my opinion, is the direction in which economy and efficiency should be sought; I mean that the diffusion system, which is suitable for ordinary inhabited rooms and inclosures subject to a variety of uses, should be abandoned in the case of rooms where numbers of people meet, and that the distribution system should be adopted.

We have now been over most of the important ground relating to this subject, but only superficially; as I said at the outset we would have to be content with a brief examination of the leading points, and many of the statements made will have to be taken on trust. Before concluding, it may not be out of place for me to describe here some of my own methods of meeting the difficulties which I have called your attention to, particularly the regulation of temperature and the diffusion of the air. Where steam or hot water is used, it is the feature of my method of treating such buildings as school-houses, that the heating and ventilating are entirely separated. The rooms are all heated by local concealed radiators which have no connection with and no relation to the ventilation. The air is abundantly supplied, but only during the hours of occupation; that is for twenty-five hours a week. Notice what a saving there is in this; using only fresh air at the times when it is needed. It is warmed uniformly to seventy degrees as a standard, never any higher nor any lower, and it is all treated at a central point by efficient and positive but simple means. This reduces the entire management to the lowest terms, and it is obvious that it cannot be surpassed for economy of fuel. As to the temperature in the rooms, variation must be expected in the case of the local radiators, but the effect of neglecting to watch and regulate them is vastly different from what it is with any other system, because variations in either direction are modified by the constant flood of air which is poured in at seventy degrees, entirely changing the contained air every five or six minutes. This steady flow of air at seventy degrees is the balance-wheel of the system, and prevents local fluctuations quite effectively, even if the radiators are not strictly proportioned in heating power to the exposure, and the steam pressure is not quite suited to the weather for the time being.

As to diffusion, let it be understood that the room and all it contains are warm, thanks to the direct radiators. The temperature is apt to be higher than seventy degrees, influenced in part by them and in part by the occupants. The fresh air from the central apparatus is cooler than the contained air and tends to fall rather than to rise, which is evidently preferable to what was pointed out to be the usual, and, under the conditions, necessary, course. The logical deduction is, that with this system the escape of air should be by way of the upper openings. I am not yet able to state whether this is practically correct in the case of a school-room, but before many months it can be tested exhaustively. I would say that at the new building of the Institute of Technology, for which I designed the system of ventilation in 1883, the upper outlets are never used, but it is important to add that there is no direct radiation, and that the building has no interior finish to protect the cold from penetrating the thin, bare brick walls.

This building is well known as possessing the most thorough ventilation of any in the world; the air never reaches a degree of vitiation which is more than nominal, and the temperature is manageable throughout within close limits, though the construction presents great difficulties in heating. This case is one in which the system of local radiators which I have described would have been most appropriate, but it was the one thing that the Institute authorities objected to, as they preferred what is called indirect radiation, on general principles.

Our review of the progress in school-house ventilation will not be complete without a notice of what is being done in that other department of sanitation, the construction of water-closets and urinals. A new system, that is, new in this locality, has met with great favor, the dry-closet and urinal system introduced by the Smead Ventilating Company. The credit (and I think it is very great) of introducing this system into school-house construction belongs, I believe, entirely to that Company. There are also the systems of the Fuller and Warren Company and of others who have been quick to appreciate the advantages of the Smead system, and by improving upon it, or by slightly changing the construction, have been able to gather part of the harvest which the latter sowed the seed of. There can be no doubt that the system is efficient and safe, besides being simple to construct and maintain. I regard it as safer than the water-carriage system, because with the latter, careless construction and neglect to detect defects positively insure sickness sooner or later, the drain-pipes and their moist contents favoring fermentation and the generation of noxious gases and disease germs.

With the dry system, the moisture essential to the propagation of these dangerous things is absent, so that the consequences of suspended action or occasional back draft are of trifling importance; and if we must expect imperfections, I should say they would cause vastly less injury to health in the dry than in the water-carriage system. Besides, with the former not only are the consequences of bad work likely to be less dangerous, but the chances of the work being bad are much diminished; and still another advantage is the immunity from frost, disarrangement, stoppage of traps and pipes, and repairs. I believe the system is perfectly safe, practical and commendable, especially where there is no system of sewerage.

On the other hand, it is not probable that the water-carriage system is to be displaced by it. The tendency in all departments of building construction is to elaborate and refine, to increase comforts and conveniences, and not to be governed by practical and economical considerations alone. We are getting farther and farther from simplicity every day, and are adopting complex and costly expedients, provided they offer substantial advantages. We have constant evidence of this on every hand, and it is probable that this question will be controlled by the same tendency, and that while we may install the dry-closet system in particular cases, it will be because it is better than the horrible privy rather than because it is preferable on practical grounds to the water-closet system, which has established itself too strongly to be ever overthrown, as being the highest type for comfort, cleanliness, and convenience. I cannot leave this topic without saying a word upon the importance of exacting the utmost care and cleanliness in the use of this apparatus on the part of every occupant of the building.

In this state, the descendants of the old colonial settlers are being rapidly driven out and replaced by the children of ignorant and degraded foreigners, coarse in their ideas and filthy in their habits. It is of great importance that these young savages should be taught not only those things which will make them useful as citizens and producers of wealth, but those things upon which the health and comfort of the community depend; and the first step in doing this is to teach them to be personally clean and cleanly in their habits. The teachers should personally supervise the sanitary arrangements, and exact from their pupils the most careful use of them.

Let us not flatter ourselves in the face of the social conditions which seem to be changing for the worse rather than for the better in our state of Massachusetts, that our civilization is assured; this cannot be while ignorance and degradation are so disproportionately large. The process of refining the crude elements of society must go on continuously, for without refinement the sentiment is absent which appreciates the true value of the ounce of prevention, and lends a willing aid to the enforcement of the laws of hygiene. (Applause.)

RABIES

Harold C. Ernst

RABIES,

WITH AN ACCOUNT OF PASTEUR'S WORK AND METHODS.

BY HAROLD C. ERNST, M.D.

Mr. President and Gentlemen: — It is hardly a courteous thing, I fear, for me to be here this afternoon at all, because through some misunderstanding I was unaware that to-day was the day upon which I was expected to speak, until yesterday. Even with this amount of time, under ordinary circumstances, I might have been able to offer something which would be a little more connected than what I have to say. but circumstances with me just now are extraordinary, and in addition to an enormous amount of experimental work that I am endeavoring to conduct properly, I am suffering anxiety in regard to a member of my family. As I told Dr. Durgin yesterday afternoon, from Thursday morning last until Monday night, I have not had my clothes off at all; therefore, I beg your indulgence, if what I have to say is a little disconnected, and if it is not as full as I should like to make it.

In regard to this question of rabies, of course it is entirely unnecessary for me to say that there has been and is a very great diversity of opinion among men, perfectly competent to judge, in regard to the existence even of such a disease. But the advances in our knowledge of pathological processes that have been made within the last few years will enable us, I think, to look at the question from a little clearer point of view than it has been possible to do in the past, and I hope I shall be able to show you that there is distinctly such a disease as rabies, that it is a specific disease. and that it depends upon a special virus which, whilst not isolated as to its identity, has certainly been traced to its place of most common occurrence. Now in considering such a point, the descriptions of the older books are distinctly at fault. The descriptions of the disease that was called rabies are almost diametrically opposite, — if different authors are consulted. The reason for that, I think, is shown by the result

of the experimental work that has been done. One of the main
points to be remembered is that it has been distinctly shown that the
especial seat of the virus of this disease is in the spinal cord, not
in any particular part, but in any portion of it from the lumbar region
up to and including the brain. It is perfectly evident that any one
portion of the central nervous system being affected, it is the portion
of the muscular system governed by that nervous system that is
particularly disturbed, and it is the symptoms shown by the muscular
system that are especially noticeable to the eye of the ordinary observer; therefore, the clinical symptoms as recorded of rabies, it is
easy to conceive, may be anything that may result from the irritation
of any portion of the central nervous system, and that is the reason
for the descriptions we have of furious rabies, dumb rabies, paralytic
rabies. That is a point which, it seems to me, has not been sufficiently made clear, that by all the laboratory experiments that have
been carried on, it is distinctly shown that the seat of this disease
is in the spinal cord and in the medulla, — in the central nervous
system; and therefore any symptoms described in the books may be
from a case of true rabies, but there is no one picture to be given
of the disease that will enable the ordinary clinical observer to make
a proper diagnosis.

Now that there is such a disease, as it seems to me there is, and
that it is produced by a virus introduced into the central nervous
canal, and possessing a pretty definite period of incubation, with no
very definite symptoms excepting any that may result from the irritation of the central nervous system; that this disease may be produced
by the inoculation of healthy animals with portions of the cord or
brain of diseased animals; that it may be carried on through a long
series of years, it seems to me that there is no question at all; that
it can be the result of but one form of virus also, it seems to me
there can be no question. It is not possible to dispute the assertion
that the introduction of various materials under the meninges, as
Pasteur has done in carrying on experiments in rabies, may produce
similar symptoms to those of rabies in the first animal experimented
upon, but it has been shown by no one and at no time that long
series of inoculations can be carried on from one animal to another
week after week, month after month and year after year, with the
production of precisely the same symptoms in every case, excepting
in this one instance of the work done in Pasteur's laboratory; and

therefore, it seems proper to me to consider the disease that Pasteur has been handling, and that was derived from the saliva of a child dying, after the bite of a dog, as a specific disease named rabies. It is from that point of view that I spoke in a discussion upon this subject last fall in New York. Dr. Spitzka made the assertion (his remarks are in print, so that it is not too soon to announce them,) Dr. Spitzka made the assertion that he was carrying on in his laboratory experiments with an organism which would produce precisely the same symptoms as are produced by Pasteur's virus; and he also said that this organism carried on through animal after animal would continue to produce the same thing. If that be true, it does not, to my mind, vitiate Pasteur's experiments at all; it merely indicates that we have two viruses that may produce the same clinical symptoms, precisely as it is already shown that we have more than one specific organism which will in medicine produce croupous-pneumonia, and yet many medical men to-day will deny the possibility of there being more than one form of croupous-pneumonia, while it is distinctly proven there are several. Therefore, in the same way we may be on the verge of the discovery of a second virus producing symptoms similar to that of Pasteur; but this is merely a preliminary announcement, and is not yet proven.

But even if it should be proven, it seems to me quite distinctly proper that the term rabies should continue to be applied to this disease that Pasteur has been handling. It was derived by him originally from a child bitten by a dog supposed to be rabid. It has again been derived by him from dogs affected by what is known as street rabies. I have myself obtained it in the same way, this similar disease, in rabbits and guinea-pigs, and many other observers have done the same thing; and that there is this virus to be obtained from animals dying in the way that is supposed to be the way in which animals affected with rabies die; and that it can be made to do all that Pasteur has said that it can be made to do, there is no question, if one can believe the evidence of one's own eyes; and so, again, it seems to me distinctly shown that we have to do with a specific disease, that there is such a disease, and that it does produce all of the symptoms that are spoken of in our text-books; but no text-book yet written has given the proper description of the disease as it may exist, because such a description would include all symptoms that might arise from the irritation of the central nervous system.

Now it has been shown certainly that the virus is present most prominently in the brain, and in the spinal cord to a less degree. It is also present in the organs of the body, in the lymphatic glands, and in the saliva. That has been shown by experimental work in the laboratory, carrying out a similar series of experiments to those that have shown its existence in the spinal cord. The special point which is to be made from this fact, and from what I have already stated in regard to the special position of the virus in the brain and cord, is that no absolute diagnosis, to my mind, of rabies can possibly be made except by the experimental method; that in order to be absolutely certain that one is dealing with a case of rabies, either in man or in the lower animals, it is necessary that the experimental evidence in regard to the disease should be carried out; and certainly the corollary from this is, that before the evidence is obtained, startling the public should be avoided with all the strength which one has at hand.

Another point that can be readily deduced from these facts is that the disease is transferred only by inoculation, that the virus either in the cord or the brain loses its strength after a certain length of time; in other words, if it be a bacterium that produces the disease, that bacterium is distinctly parasitic in nature, and not saphrophytic.. It cannot develop outside of the living organism, and therefore this disease can be carried, and carried only, by inoculation, and the inoculation usually occurs, of course, by a bite and introduction of the saliva from a rabid dog.

Then the question arises, naturally, inoculation having occurred, what should be done? The ready method, the one with which everyone should be familiar who runs any danger of coming in contact with rabid dogs, is, if the bite be upon the extremities, upon the finger, upon the hand, upon the arm, or upon the lower extremities, in some way ligation should be practised as speedily as possible, and then very vigorous sucking of the wound. Cauterization, it seems to me, is a relic of the dark ages. I do not believe it does any more good than to ease the patient's mind, on the one hand, and on the other, perhaps, to create a local irritation that may be of service in carrying out the same thing, — the easing of the patient's mind; but beyond that it has not anything to do, and rarely has done any good, and it sometimes produces a very bad ulceration. The same thing, as far as possible, should be practised in the case of bites upon the body, although in such cases the safety of the patient is much greater than is usually supposed, because in the clothed portion of the body the teeth of the animal inflicting the bite are partially cleaned in passing through the clothing, and the danger of inoculation is greatly diminished. That is the immediate step — ligation, if possible, and sucking of the wound immediately. There is no danger at all in taking this virus into the mouth, if the mouth be in a properly healthy condition, and therefore sucking is the one thing to be depended upon, aided, if possible, by ligation.

Then comes the next point as to the advisability or not of protection by inoculations as suggested by Pasteur; and there has been so much discussion in regard to the effectiveness of his methods, of the way in which he has carried them out, that the controversy has become almost classical, so that it seemed to me it would be of interest to you if I gave simply the details of the various articles in which he introduced the subject of experimental rabies to the world. The first one was published in the "Comptes Rendus de l'Academie des Sciences," in Paris, upon the 24th of January, 1881. The title of it was "On a new malady produced by the saliva of a child dead of rabies." That certainly is an extremely modest beginning. The point that I wish to make in this part of what I have to say, and in all of it, in fact, is to insist upon the perfect frankness and simplicity of Pasteur and his work. He has been accused of all sorts of quackery, and with no justification whatever, so much so that in a discussion in which I took part at one time, the gentleman who led off in the discussion — there were three of them who preceded me — and who meant to give a fair view, I believe, of the subject, was ignorant of the fact of the existence of the magazine called "Annales de l'Institute Pasteur," in which for four years there have been monthly records of every case that he has had; they did not know that that was in existence, and yet accused him of keeping his results secret.

Now the second article published in the "Comptes Rendus" was upon the 11th of December, 1882, nearly two years afterward, and that was merely a continued study of this same disease, the title being, "A continued study of a malady produced by the saliva of a child dead of rabies." On the 25th of February, 1884, he published an article emphasizing the occurrence of the paralytic form of rabies resulting from his experiments with this saliva, this paralytic form occurring entirely in animals in the laboratory, the so-called furious form being a very rare manifestation. Then on the 19th of May, 1884, he first called attention to the attenuation of the virus, and the possibility of so changing the strength of this virus that instead of producing death, as it had certainly done before, it could be introduced without producing more than very mild symptoms of paralysis, from which the animal would recover.

Then again on the 11th of August, 1884, at the International Medical Congress in London, he emphasized this possibility of the attenuation of the virus, and from it drew a number of interesting conclusions in regard to the possibility of preparing viruses for the prevention of other diseases besides rabies, others that are more common, making this the text for throwing out broad lines of investigation that certainly will bear fruit as the years go on. And upon the 26th of October, in 1885, came the announcement of a method for the prevention of rabies after the bite of a rabid animal. Then on the 1st of March, 1886, and on the 12th of April, 1886, and again on the 1st of February, he published results, the preliminary results of the application of this method to human beings, and ever since that time, as I said a moment agó, there has been a monthly publication and tabulation of every case that has come under his care, so that he who runs may read, if he chooses to look at the tables. And it has been perfectly extraordinary to me that gentlemen who have been interested in this question have not known even of the existence of those tables. One of the great neurologists in this country less than a year ago in speaking of something I was doing said, " Don't follow Pasteur's method, because he doesn't publish his results," and I asked him if he had ever seen these tables. He said he had never heard of them. Now that is not fair. As far as any man can be frank, I think Pasteur has been upon this question, and in discussing his results, it is only fair to look over what he has to say. In these results he claims a lessened mortality, and the figures bear him out; he has certainly reduced the mortality from rabies to less than one per cent, which is very much less than the mortality from such cases, as appears by all the records we have had before. It is impossible to give it exactly, but certainly it was very much larger. Every author who has written on this subject puts it above fifty per cent. Those older statistics were made up when it was impossible to separate the cases where the bite was from an animal truly affected with rabies from those that were not. They included also those that any passer-by happened to say had rabies, therefore it seems to me if anything is done by the French work, this diminution in mortality is certainly shown by Pasteur's statistics.

Now in regard to the method of attenuation of this virus and its application to human beings. A few words, I think, will make it very plain to you. By a series of experiments it was shown that the cords of animals dead of rabies, if they were removed at once and placed in a dry atmosphere at an even temperature, in fourteen days would lose absolutely their power of producing any symptom whatever of rabies when inoculated, and this loss of virulence was progressive. It went on at the rate of about one-fourteenth on each day, so that at the end of eight days it was about four-sevenths gone, and so on. By experiments upon animals, the introduction of a portion of this cord in an emulsion, a sterilized fluid of a few drops introduced under the skin of an animal of the weakest, and on the following day an emulsion of the cord of the next strongest virus, produced immunity in the animal experimented on, — to an emulsion of the cord from an animal that had died of rabies. And it was because that fact had been well established in the laboratory, and because it had got out, not because of the public announcement of it, that Pasteur was first forced to make his experiments upon human beings. Patients were brought to him, and it was practically impossible for him to avoid trying this experiment upon human beings; and so far as can be seen by a conscientious examination of the statistics, if they be true, which I certainly have not had time to make, but from what I have made within a year, no death can be laid to the door of this method, as has been asserted in a number of quarters, no death at all; and as I have tried to emphasize, if it is possible to believe anything, the mortality from rabies has been distinctly lowered by the introduction of this means of prevention.

One more fact that has been pretty fairly well established by all that has been found in this experimental study is that the period of incubation of rabies is brought somewhere within proper bounds; that in the case of a bite from a rabid animal upon the exposed parts, the face or hands, the danger period is fairly well passed at the end of six weeks. The treatment, if treatment be decided upon in this way of the preventive protective inoculation, should be begun as soon as possible after the bite, but there is practically no danger if it be delayed for ten days or a fortnight. The cases of so-called rabies resulting seven, eight or ten months after a known bite, are either not true rabies at all, or else they are the result of a fresh inoculation, not the result of a bite that was known ; the inoculation probably comes from some source that the patient knows nothing about.

In regard to pathological appearances, a few words may be of interest. They are very few in gross, only the appearance of congestion of the internal organs. The distention of the external vessels of the membranes of the cord and brain is about all that strikes one, and of course this has nothing very peculiar about it, and even under the microscope thus far substantially nothing distinctive has been made out. But in two cases in human beings which came under the observation of Dr. Fitz some ten years ago, and which were very perfectly described by him at that time, the same changes were seen that it has been my fortune to see in two cases occurring in human beings within the last year. They consist, in the first place, of a very marked engorgement of the smaller vessels, of an apparent forcing through the walls of the vessels in certain places, of collections of round cells looking almost like localized hemorrhages, and the occurrence of a few miliary abscesses, in other words, the presentation of the appearance of a bulbitis. The results show there is a certain amount of swelling and infiltration, which would indicate an acute miliary bulbitis, but beyond that there has been nothing. At the same time, these appearances have been seen in cases that have come under observation, so far as I know, in this city and abroad ; in animals experimented upon, those appearances are carried out always.

In regard to the occurrence of the disease itself : some five years ago I carried out a series of experiments to see whether Pasteur's assertions were true or not, and I became thoroughly convinced that whatever he had hold of, he certainly had a specific virus. Since then it has been my fortune to have a number of cases of so-called street rabies submitted to me for diagnosis, and I have carried on experiments so as to convince myself that the so-called rabid dog of the streets may be the origin of this poison or virus with which he (Pasteur) is dealing. But at that time I tried very hard to find or to hear of a case of true rabies outside of my own laboratory, and I utterly failed. Since I was a medical student when I knew of these cases of Dr. Fitz of which I have spoken, I have never been brought in contact with a case of true rabies either in man or the lower animals until a year ago last June. At that time through the kindness of Dr. Peters, a dog which had been under his care was brought to me, and we proved the existence of true rabies in that dog; and from that time until I went away last fall, I cannot say exactly how many cases I have seen, but the number has been pretty large. The largest number was during last spring, beginning at about January and running through to May. I heard of a great many others where the symptoms corresponded precisely with those in the animals which were submitted to me, but those of which I speak were only those that I saw and tested. This limited personal experience indicates what has been the experience drawn from all the statistics that Pasteur has collected; that this disease is distinctly not a disease of summer or hot weather; that its time of greatest intensity is in cold weather, in the winter, and that it diminishes along during the spring months through into August and September, when the curve of its occurrence is at its lowest height; therefore, the common notion of its having anything to do with the sexual organs of the dog is a mistaken one; this reason alone is not sufficient for saying so, but it is with everything else we know in regard to the disease.

I have had the misfortune to see one case of true rabies in man. It is the most dreadful thing that one, I think, can be compelled to watch. After the disease has once started, it is absolutely hopeless. It was a true case, because I proved it by the experimental method. Two other cases came to me, where I proved the diagnosis in the same way, and I know of a fourth. Here are four cases occurring in human beings where the disease was certainly true rabies within the last year. It should be said, however, that for the last six months I know of absolutely no case of rabies, excepting in one suspected case which was brought to me during my absence in Berlin, that I have not yet tested. The disease has been distinctly an epizootic among animals and among dogs during the spring of a year ago. As I told Dr. Durgin yesterday, I am not prepared to say what it is now, for the reason that I have been away for two or three months. I have hardly seen a newspaper. I do not know anything that has been going on in regard to the disease in this locality since last October, but certainly for two or three months before that time it had died out of my observation almost entirely.*

* (NOTE.—Since the meeting, up to date [May 14. 1891], there have come to my knowledge two cases of rabies in man, both occurring at the Massachusetts General Hospital, and four cases in dogs. — *H. C. E.*)

An interesting fact in regard to the occurrence of the disease was communicated to me through Dr. Peters, from a gentleman living in the Berkshires who had some friends coming to stay with him who had been there two or three years before, who went out shooting, and upon their first visit they had found practically no partridges, but upon their second they found a great many, and on inquiring the reason, they were informed that all the foxes had died off of rabies. Now whether that has any connection with what has gone on here the last two years, or two and a half, of course it is impossible to say.

I am extremely sorry that I have not been able to present my thoughts in better shape. (Applause.)

RABIES

Austin Peters

RABIES: ITS PREVALENCE AND SUP-PRESSION.

BY AUSTIN PETERS, M.R.C.V.S.

Mr. Chairman and Gentlemen : — I supposed this afternoon that Dr. Lyman, of the Harvard Veterinary School, would first address you on the subject of Rabies, and that he would be followed by Dr. Ernst, but Dr. Lyman being unable to be here, the only person that has spoken on it is Dr. Ernst, and that leaves me second instead of third, as I thought I should be. I expected that Dr. Lyman would speak to you on this disease in its clinical aspects, the symptoms in dogs and other animals, the mode of extension, etc., and I thought Dr. Ernst would speak to you very much as he has, looking at it from a scientific standpoint, and telling you of Pasteur's work, his methods, and his successes, so that there would be little left for me to say ; but what I had to say, I thought I would write out, for I can always write my thoughts, and read them, more readily than I can speak off-hand, and I had written this paper, assuming that there were to be two preceding me, and I started by telling the following story : —

My position is, I am afraid, like the embryo statesman who had never made a speech. He was asked to go out of town a little way and speak at a political meeting ; at first he did not want to go, as he had never made a speech, but some one told him it was easy enough to speak in public, — all one has to do is to tell a few good stories connected together by a little conversation (much as epithelial cells are connected by a little homogeneous cement substance). Upon learning what an easy and simple matter it was he consented to go ; he selected three excellent stories to illustrate what he intended to say, and set out full of courage. Upon arriving at the meeting he learned that there were to be two other speakers beside himself, and that he was to speak last. He felt a little grieved when the first speaker told his best story, but still congratulated himself that he had two pretty good ones left. But when the second speaker told his next best story his dismay can better be imagined than described, as he only had one miserable anecdote left which fell flat when not supported by the first two, and he retired from the political arena a sadder and a wiser man.

. Now, I fear that I am in much the same plight as this young man, and after the eminent gentlemen who have preceded me there is little for me to say except to reiterate and corroborate their remarks. Nevertheless, I am glad to have an opportunity to add my quota to the evidence of the prevalence of rabies the past two years, and can best do so, perhaps, by detailing my own experiences with this disease.

I began practice as a veterinarian in 1885 ; and never met with a case of rabies in my practice until May 8, 1889, when I was called to see a bull terrier belonging to a client, and made a diagnosis of probable rabies. I did not make a positive diagnosis, because I had not seen a case of rabies around Boston, and therefore was not quite sure.

The dog was securely chained, and I left word that he was on no account to be unloosed, and that I would call and see him the next day. The next day I called again, and found that the owner had shot the dog, as he had become so violent that morning that he became alarmed for fear he would break away.

I carried the carcass of the animal in town to the Harvard Medical School, and Dr. Ernst inoculated two rabbits with an emulsion made from the dog's cerebrum and sterilized veal broth,— the cerebellum and medulla were destroyed by the charge of shot, the owner having shot him in the back of the head and neck, so these could not be used, as is usual. One of the rabbits died that night from the operation ; the other showed symptoms of rabies May 22, and died the night of May 26, confirming the diagnosis.

I also learned from the owner of the dog, that two or three weeks previous to his dog's showing symptoms a stray dog appeared in the neighborhood acting strangely. He ran into the yard and bit the dog that was shot, and then ran out and bit — or snapped at — two dogs owned by neighbors ; the waif then ran off in a southerly direction. How many other dogs he bit in his course, nobody knows.

I reported the matter to the Boston Board of Health when the dog was shot, as the law requires, and my duty too, I thought, and also wrote that I would report the result of the inoculations on the rabbits, which I believe I did.

Since then I have had in my practice nine cases of rabies, all in dogs ; — three more in 1889, five in 1890, and one so far this year. Most of these cases occurred in my immediate neighborhood at Jamaica Plain, but I have seen one each in Brookline, Newton, Milton, and Pembroke. The one at Pembroke I think was bitten at Jamaica Plain before being taken away by his owner for the summer.

I have also had one or two dogs killed that were bitten by rabid ones, and have known of a good many cases coming under the notice of other veterinarians, but have reported no more cases to Boards of Health, as it did not seem to me that the one I reported was sufficiently appreciated.

Rabies, like all epizootic diseases, is at times very prevalent, and then after a varying duration becomes very much less frequent, and finally is seldom or never heard of until a fresh outbreak occurs.

When prevalent among dogs, cases are constantly occurring in the human, and as the malady subsides among the canines, fewer or no cases of death from this cause are reported in man.

From Jan. 1, 1842, the beginning of a systematic registration of human deaths in Massachusetts, until Jan. 1, 1890, there were eighty-eight deaths of people with rabies in this state, and the varying number in the last few years make an interesting study.

In 1876 there were four deaths from this cause, then fourteen in 1877; fifteen in 1878, then it ·gradually subsides, there being five in 1879, three in 1880, three in 1881, and then none until 1888, when there were two; then it increases rapidly, there being fourteen in 1889. The vital statistics for 1890 are not made up yet, but it is likely there will be more cases reported than in 1889, as probably there have been more cases in dogs. Previous to 1876 there were no cases in humans after 1870, when two deaths occurred.

The cases of human rabies occurring in 1889 were by months as follows : —

January	1
April	2
July	1
August	3
October	3
November	3
December	1
	14

It may be seen that it occurs in cool as well as in hot weather, and it also increased very greatly in the last half of the year.

By counties the following is the arrangement : —

Bristol	3
Essex	6
Middlesex	1
Norfolk	2
Plymouth	1
Suffolk	1
	14

For 1890 I think that instead of being confined to the eastern end of the state it will have extended to the central and western portions as well.

There were twelve persons from Massachusetts, who were bitten by rabid dogs, inoculated at the Institute Pasteur in New York City, between Feb. 18, 1890, when it was first opened, and Oct. 15, besides 118 others from different parts of the country, — sixty-four of these coming from New York State. If the present outbreak acts as the previous one, there should be fewer cases this year, gradually decreasing for three or four years, until a period arrives when here are none for several years, when a fresh outbreak may occur.

It is an excellent idea for the Cattle Commissioners to have at last called the attention of local Boards of Health to the prevalence of rabies, and it is to be hoped that the result of the discussion here to-day may lead to active and concerted measures being taken for its abatement.

If action is to be taken for the suppression of this terrible disorder, only the local authorities can properly and thoroughly enforce the law, but they must co-operate with each other.

For example, last summer the town of Framingham ordered that all dogs within its limits must be muzzled. Now the town of Brookline orders all dogs muzzled or chained for sixty days, while most of our cities and towns take no action whatever in regard to the matter ; but it is very doubtful if such erratic and independent action has any marked influence upon the prevalence of the disease.

In order to obtain the best results every city and town in the commonwealth should act together ; an order should go into effect on the same day in every township and municipality that every dog found at large, without being properly muzzled, would be instantly shot, whether accompanied by his owner or otherwise; and the order should be thoroughly carried out by the authorities. At the expiration of sixty or ninety days this regulation should go out of effect in every community upon the same day, and should not cease in one until it ceased in all.

If such a step had been taken two years ago this spring when it was at first apparent that we were about to have an epizootic of rabies, thirty or forty human lives might have been saved to the State of Massachusetts. If proper measures are taken at once all over the state many more lives can be saved and this outbreak of rabies brought to a speedier termination. Even then there would be danger of outside infection again unless contiguous states could arrange to act at the same time that Massachusetts did.

Rabies can be spread very widely by an affected dog, and it is not infrequent for a rabid canine to run forty miles, biting many others in his path; it would spread to a much greater extent if it were not for the fact that a very large proportion of dogs attacked with the malady are not seized with the desire to run off and bite all obstacles in their way, but are noticed to be acting peculiarly by their owners, and are secured, and finally are killed or die without doing any damage.

Most of the contagious animal diseases with which our Cattle Commission now has to deal are of as great interest to the sanitarian as to the breeder or owner of live-stock, because so many are common to both man and animals; and it has been a question in my mind lately whether it would not be better to transfer the powers now vested in the Cattle Commission, to the State Board of Health. This idea occurred to me with particular force after reading that portion of the Governor's message in which he refers to the great number of commissions we have, and asks if something cannot be done to simplify matters.

I say this in a perfectly friendly spirit to the Cattle Commission, recognizing the good work they have done in the past, but I merely offer the suggestion, would it not be better to merge matters pertaining to the public health in one bureau, this board not only to do what the present Cattle Commission does, but also to act in a broader scope, considering contagious animal diseases in their relation to the public health, as well as a menace to our live-stock interests.

In such a case the State Board of Health should be made up of the best experts on human and animal diseases and sanitary engineering, to act as an advisory body to local Boards of Health, — the latter to enforce and carry out the laws. The State Board might also require power to stimulate and direct local boards when they were inefficient or lethargic. In addition I believe it would be an excellent plan to have a National Board of Health to secure co-operation between the State Boards of Health.

Because animals have and transmit to man such fatal and loathsome disorders as rabies, glanders and tuberculosis, it does not follow that they are less important than leprosy and typhoid fever, or that it detracts from a man's dignity, knowledge or usefulness, to do what he can to prevent the ravages of the former as well as the latter.

Before we can ever have a system of protection to the public health approaching perfection, it will be necessary to place the contagious and infectious diseases of animals in the same category with those of man, and have the same authorities exercise a supervision over both.

I believe it would be a matter of great utility if veterinarians (that is, qualified veterinarians) were required to make returns of the contagious diseases that occur in their practice among animals. These returns could be tabulated, and although they would not be complete, yet they would show to some extent the relative frequency of the same diseases among man and animals in certain localities, and for this reason would prove of great interest and value.

The law requiring all persons having knowledge of or suspecting any contagious animal disease to report the same to local Boards of Health is a good one and should be lived up to, although I am sorry to say I rarely practice what I preach; for if I can carry out the proper regulations alone I do not report the case, as the owner is generally averse to having it done. I therefore obey only the spirit, but not the letter of the law. But I think that this regulation should be enforced, and that an attempt should be made to tabulate the contagious animal diseases in the same manner contagious human diseases are tabulated, and then valuable tables of comparison could be drawn.

When legislative hearings are to be granted upon any subject of sanitary importance, experts in human or animal diseases, as the case may be, should be called upon for an opinion, and their evidence should be given the consideration it deserves. Because officers of anti-cruelty societies and professional dog fanciers do not believe in the existence of rabies, or think that muzzling dogs is cruel, it is no reason that such a disease does not exist; and what they have to say on the subject should be taken for just what it is worth,— that is, nothing.

If a man is going to law he has to employ a lawyer; if he has a piece of land to be surveyed he employs a civil engineer; or if he wants a piece of electrical engineering performed he engages an electrician; yet when it comes to questions that more nearly affect our lives and health, then the most foolish and ignorant presume to advance their opinions, and they are accepted as though their mouths were the openings of the profoundest oracles.

A dog should be a luxury and not a necessity, and I am in favor of any measures which will tend towards a limitation of their number and the responsibility of owners, and lead to the destruction of a horde of valueless mongrels and curs belonging to careless and irresponsible individuals. There is too much puerile sentimentality about the "poor man's dog;" and he is too cruel towards sheep, poultry, and other animals to command a great deal of compassion when we consider the property he destroys and the ravages of rabies.

I commenced this discourse without a text; permit me to conclude by announcing that I might have preached from either of the following scriptural passages : —

Psalms XXII. : 20. "Deliver my soul from the sword; my darling from the power of the dog."

Or

St. Paul's Epistle to the Philippians, III. : 2. "Beware of dogs."

I give you your choice of either or both. (Applause.)

OBSERVATIONS ON THE SUPPRESSION OF INFECTIOUS DISEASES

J. H. McCollom

OBSERVATIONS ON THE SUPPRESSION OF INFECTIOUS DISEASES.

BY J. H. McCOLLOM, M.D., OF BOSTON.

IN this paper an attempt will be made to show what has been done in Boston during the past ten years in the suppression of the three principal infectious diseases, small-pox, scarlet fever, and diphtheria, and also to offer a few suggestions regarding the best methods to be employed for this purpose.

At first your attention will be asked to the subject of small-pox, a disease much more dreaded in the community than any of the other infectious diseases, and without reason, for in no other disease do we have the protective power of vaccination.

When we read the accounts of the fearful havoc that this disease caused before the discovery of vaccination, it is difficult to understand how any sane person can be in doubt for a moment regarding the advantage to be gained by this operation. It is painful to witness a severe case of scarlet fever; an attack of diphtheria is distressing alike to the patient and his friends; but an attack of unmodified small-pox in the amount of actual suffering, in the repulsiveness, in the intolerable odor, and in the subsequent disfigurement, far exceeds any of the other infectious diseases. One argument used by the anti-vaccinationists is that small-pox is not so prevalent now as it was formerly, and therefore the necessity of vaccination is not so great. This is the very best argument in favor of vaccination, and it proves, without a shadow of a doubt, the beneficial effects of the operation. Again, the statement is frequently made that vaccination does not protect; this remark is so erroneous, and so entirely without foundation, that it seems hardly necessary to attempt to refute it. No man of any experience in the treatment of small-pox has any doubt of the protecting and modifying power of vaccination.

I speak thus warmly in regard to this subject because I know the immense amount of harm the anti-vaccinationists are doing, not only in England but also in this country. It therefore becomes us as officers of sanitary commissions, with the public health in our charge, to take a firm and steadfast position in regard to this matter. An argument frequently used by the anti-vaccinationists is, that the vaccine disease is not small-pox modified by its passage through the bovine species, but that it is a separate and distinct disease, and therefore it cannot be protective. The whole theory of the protective power of vaccination, which has been proved by innumerable experiments, is based upon the very fact that it is one and the same disease. An account of the latest experiments bearing on this subject is published in *La Semaine Médicale* of Dec. 31, 1890. The investigators, Professor Elternod, of the University of Geneva, and Charles Haccius, the Director of the Vaccine Institute at Lancy, are men eminently well fitted to pursue these investigations. Their conclusions are :

"1. Small-pox is inoculable on the bovine species when the method of operation is good and when the virus is taken at the proper time.

"2. Inoculation of the calf with small-pox forms a valuable source, in a new direction, of animal vaccine. This is of great practical value, not only for the vaccine institutions of Europe, but also for those of warm climates, where variola is frequently endemic, and where vaccine rapidly deteriorates.

"3. Variola inoculated on the calf is transformed after several transmissions into vaccine by its passage through this animal. This is not duality.

"4. Our practical conclusions confirm the ideas set forth by Depaul in 1863, at the Academy of Medicine of Paris."

Dr. Fischer, Director of the Vaccine Institute at Karlsruhe in Germany, performed at about the same time a series of similar experiments and he arrived at practically the same conclusions. This refutes the argument of the duality of these diseases.

The history of the great epidemic of 1872–73, in Boston, and the comparative freedom of the city from this disease since that time are most convincing arguments in favor of vaccination.

The operation of compulsory vaccination was suspended in Zürick, Switzerland, in obedience to popular clamor in 1883. The deaths from small-pox, per 1,000 deaths from all causes for the two previous years and that year had been in 1881, 7 ; 1882, 0 ; in 1883, 8.   They rose, after compulsion had ceased to be used, to 11.45 in 1884 ; to 52 in 1885, and in the first eight months of 1886. to 85 per 1,000.

Without wearying you with an immense amount of statistics, it may be of interest to state that for the past ten years the percentage of deaths from small-pox in the unvaccinated at the hospital in Boston has been 75, while of the vaccinated it has been only three.   This, however, does not give a perfectly clear idea of the situation, for many of those who had been vaccinated did not have typical scars, and also in many instances the operation had been done a very long time previous to the attack of. variola.   There is no fatal case on record at the hospital in which vaccination was done within five years of the attack of the disease, except in those instances in which the patient was vaccinated at the time of exposure, and even then, if the operation was done within five days of the exposure the disease was always modified, to a remarkable degree.

The effect of one vaccination does not always last for a lifetime, and therefore the importance of re-vaccination is perfectly evident. For the ordinary exposure, in the routine of daily life, two or three vaccinations, at intervals of ten years, are sufficient ; but after any extraordinary exposure a person should always be vaccinated.

In regard to the kind of virus to be used, I would say that my predilections are decidedly for animal lymph ; because the protection is greater ; because you can always be sure of an adequate supply for any emergency ; because there is no danger of communicating syphilis.   The possibility of communicating any other disease than this is so slight that no mention need be made of it.   That certain eruptions do follow vaccination, and, owing to some inherent vice in the individual constitution are, in a measure, dependent on the operation no one with any experience will pretend to doubt ; but these eruptions are acute in their nature and yield readily to treatment.   A very common example of this condition is an eruption of urticaria following the ingestion of lobsters, or of strawberries, yet no one for a moment thinks of considering lobsters and strawberries unwholesome food.   It is an interesting fact that young adults, and more particularly young immigrants, are liable to have these eruptions.   In order to illustrate how frequently vaccination is unjustly blamed for the appearance of an eruption, I wish to relate the following case which occurred in my practice some few years ago.   A perfectly healthy child, five months old, was vaccinated with fresh calf lymph ; at the end of eight days the vesicle was perfectly typical in appearance, and there was the usual amount of constitutional disturbance. At this time the mother of the child, who had never been vaccinated, expressed a wish to be vaccinated with lymph from the child's arm. This was done. At the end of four or five days the mother had a most extensive and general eruption of vaccinal urticaria, with marked constitutional disturbance. If, in this case, the mother had not seen the lymph taken directly from her child's arm, no amount of argument would have convinced her or her friends that the lymph was not impure. These vaccinal eruptions, which are comparatively frequent, and which can be easily explained, serve as a never-failing source of argument against vaccination.

Let us now pass to the consideration of the measures to be adopted for the suppression of small-pox. In Boston, as soon as a case is reported, the patient is visited and the diagnosis verified. If the disease proves to be small-pox the patient, in suitable cases, is removed to the hospital, with as many of the family as the circumstances seem to demand. The hospital is always ready to receive any number of patients. When the premises are vacated disinfection is immediately commenced. All persons in the vicinity, who have been exposed to the disease are vaccinated. There is a careful medical supervision of the infected locality until all danger of an outbreak of the disease has passed. Every inducement is offered for vaccination, which is free. The question of diagnosis is a very important one, and while it may be simple in a severe case, in a mild and modified form of the disease it is very often most difficult and perplexing. To give some idea of the difficulty of arriving at a positive diagnosis in these cases it is enough to say that during the past eight years there have been reported to the Board of Health as variola, about five hundred cases of eruptive disease, of which only forty-four were found to be small-pox.

In former years this disease was much more prevalent in Boston than it has been of late ; but this comparative immunity cannot be explained by the wave theory of epidemics, and must, therefore, be due to the management of the outbreaks of small-pox that have occurred. Chart A represents the number of deaths from this disease in Boston for two decades ; 1862 to 1871, and 1881 to 1890, inclusive. The years of the great epidemic, 1872 and 1873, have

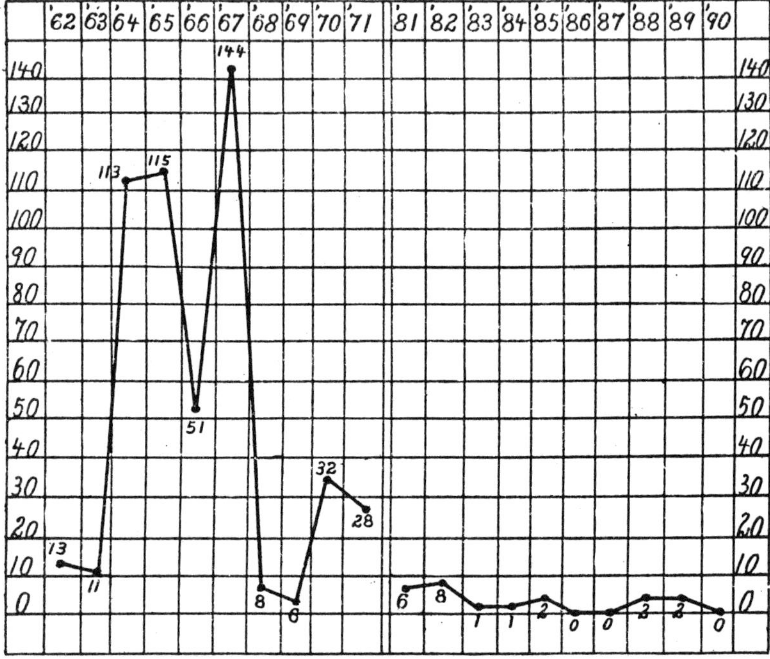

CHART A.

Deaths from Variola for Twenty Years—1862-71 and 1881-90.

Deaths 521, p. 211,865.   Deaths 22, p. 425,250.

been purposely omitted; because, as this was an exceptional time,
correct deductions could not be made from them. It can be seen
at a glance that from 1862 to 1871, with a population of 211,865,
Boston had 521 deaths from this disease, while from 1881 to 1890,
inclusive, with a population of 425,250 there were only 22 deaths.
It is of interest to note that during the last decade immigration was
very much larger than during the first. It must also be borne in
mind that during the last ten years Baltimore, Philadelphia and
Montreal have had moderately severe epidemics of this disease.

SCARLATINA.

Satisfactory as the result has been in the suppression of small-pox
there is no such favorable showing in the case of scarlet fever,
although much has been done, and with improved methods still more

may be done. As this disease is pre-eminently one of childhood it is evident that the removal to a hospital cannot be so easily accomplished as in the case of small-pox, which attacks the unvaccinated of all ages alike, and rarely, if ever, attacks a vaccinated child. The existence of mild cases of the disease in the community; cases that are not recognized, and therefore are not reported, and in which there is no attempt at isolation, is one of the most potent factors in causing the prevalence of this disease. Notwithstanding the great amount of good done by the isolation of reported cases, to expect that this disease can be stamped out when in the schools and in the public conveyances, there are so many mild cases which serve as centres of ever widely extending waves of infection, is to expect an impossibility. The difference of opinion among physicians regarding the time when a case ceases to be infectious, is also a source of great danger to the public. Children are frequently permitted, on the certificate of a physician, to return to school, while they are passing through the stage of desquamation, and are therefore particularly liable to communicate the disease.

In Boston, a child living in a house where there has been a case of infectious disease, before he can return to school must bring a certificate from a physician stating that two weeks have elapsed since the death, removal or recovery of the last case reported. This regulation is a wise one so far as it goes; but, while the period of two weeks is long enough in the case of death or removal, the time of recovery is so vague and indefinite that it would be much better to require the lapse of six weeks from the commencement of the last case.

The isolation of a patient at his house is a difficult thing, but by the liberal use of disinfectants, and with the most careful and painstaking attention to detail, it can be accomplished, if the house is large enough and is occupied by only one family In the ordinary tenement-house it is impossible.

The *British Medical Journal* of June 11, 1887, contains a paper entitled "Observations on a Method of Prophylaxis and an Investigation into the Nature of the Contagium of Scarlet Fever," by Drs. W. Allen Jamieson and Alexander Edington, in which are found some very important and interesting facts. Without quoting at length, it will be sufficient to give a few extracts:

"The method recommended was to disinfect the throat by painting it frequently with a strong solution of boracic acid in glycerine. In dealing with the skin more exact methods were available. These consisted in the employment of warm baths every night from the very first, and in the application to the entire surface of the body, including the head, of an ointment composed of thirty grains of carbolic acid, ten grains of thymol, one drachm of vaseline, and one ounce of simple ointment. . . . Seven cases were selected; the baths and anointing were persevered in from the second day of the disease till the eighth day of desquamation, the seventeenth or eighteenth day of the disease. An ointment for inunction containing carbolic acid in the proportion of one in sixteen, had formerly been employed. Now and again slight evidences of absorption of carbolic acid had taken place, and therefore in these seven cases an ointment of only one in thirty-two was made use of. On the eighth day of desquamation one leg was once more carefully anointed, enveloped in a thick layer of sterilized cotton-wool, bandaged and covered with a stocking, and allowed to remain undisturbed till the thirtieth day. The wool was then removed by Dr. Edington, with the same precautions as in the other cases, and the scales transferred to sterilized tubes for cultivation. It will be seen that the wool was put on at a period of the disease before the bacillus had been obtained from the scales, in cases where no disinfectants had been applied to the skin. This method subjected the procedure, therefore, to a rather severe test. In cultivations of scales from five of the seven cases no bacillus was found. In two it appeared in the cultivating medium; but, whereas under ordinary circumstances the bacillary pellicle is formed in thirty-six hours it took six days to develop any evidence of its presence in the jelly. In five, therefore, the powers of reproduction of the bacillus had been checked by the method adopted, while in the two others a remarkable retardation of the virus had resulted. We submit, therefore, that proof, clinical and experimental, has been furnished that by such simple methods one can neutralize the contagiousness of scarlet fever, so far as that arises from the desquamating flakes of cuticle."

The importance of the facts brought out by these experiments is so great that the account of them has been quoted somewhat at length.

DIPHTHERIA.

The difficulties of dealing with an epidemic of scarlet fever, great as they may be, are much increased in the case of diphtheria. In the first place one attack of scarlet fever, in the majority of cases, protects the person from subsequent attacks; in diphtheria just the reverse is true; the first attack predisposes to a second. In the second place, perplexing as the diagnosis may be in a mild case of scarlet fever, it is still more embarrassing in a mild case of diphtheria. In the third place, the erroneous opinion that true croup and diphtheria are separate and distinct diseases, and that important as isolation may be in the latter, it is unnecessary in the former, renders the stamping out of this disease an impossibility.

The investigations of Klebs and Loeffler, and the confirmatory experiments of Roux and Yersin show conclusively that the diphtheritic germ is not absorbed by the healthy mucous membrane, and that the frequence of this disease during an attack of tonsilitis or during the course of scarlet fever and measles is due to this fact. In these experiments it was found that simply painting the mucous membrane of animals with the culture fluid was not sufficient to cause the disease, but if the mucous membrane was wounded by a platinum wire charged with the culture, diphtheria was invariably produced. This fact also explains to a certain extent the prevalence of this disease in New England, for it is apparent to the most casual observer that disease of the respiratory passages are more common here than elsewhere.

The degree of infectiousness of diphtheria has an important bearing on the subject of isolation. A very considerable amount of exposure is necessary to contract diphtheria, and therefore a degree of isolation that would be useless in scarlet fever would be effectual in diphtheria.

One very important measure for the suppression of these diseases is the disinfection of school-books, but advisable as this is there seems to be at present no safe and reliable method for accomplishing it. Sulphurous acid gas will not do this; heat, although it may kill the germs of disease, also destroys the books, and the same may be said of chlorine, and of a solution of corrosive sublimate. A series of very interesting experiments bearing on this point was made some little time ago by two German observers, who found that, if the tips of the fingers were dry when turning leaves of books there was no deposit of microbes on them, but if the tips were wet with water or with the saliva a large deposit was found.

Another and still more important expedient for the suppression of these diseases is a careful medical supervision of the schools, not only for the purpose of ensuring good ventilation, but more particularly for the detection of mild cases.

There can be no doubt that many epidemics are caused by the presence of these mild cases in the schools. Chart B shows the total number of cases of diphtheria and scarlet fever, by months, for five years in Boston, comprising an aggregate of 11,794 cases, certainly a number from which reliable deductions can be made. It will be

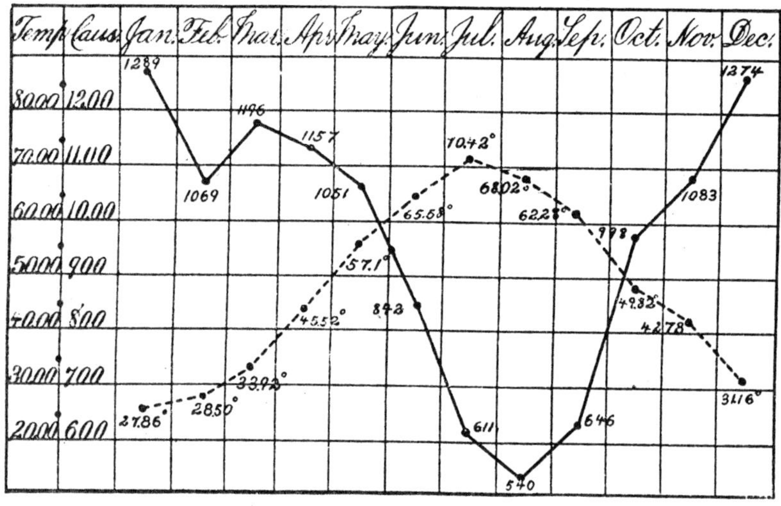

CHART B.

Cases of Diphtheria and Scarlatina, by Months for Five Years, with the Average Mean
Temperature—1886-90.

Temp......... Cases———

seen at a glance that the largest number of cases occurred during the months of January, February, March, April, May, June, September, October, November and December, or during the time the schools were in session, while during July and August, or in vacation time, the cases diminished more than one-half. It is true that during the month of June there is quite a marked diminution; but this can be explained by the fact that at this time there is better ventilation in the school-rooms. It is very significant that during August, with an average mean temperature of 68.02°, when the schools are closed, the number of cases is 540, while in June, with an average mean temperature of 65.58°, there are 842, and also that in May, with an average mean temperature of 57.10°, the number of cases reaches 1,087, more than twice as many as are reported in August. As the difference in the mean temperature between June and August is only 2.44°, being 65.58° in the former and 68.02° in the latter, it is not to be supposed that this slight difference can account for an increase of 300 cases, or in round numbers a fall of one degree in the temperature is responsible for an increase of 100 in the number of cases. If a low temperature has such a remarkable influence on the prevalence of these diseases as has been claimed by some, we ought, on general principles, to have instead of 1,289 cases in January, 4,000. Again, as is well known, the schools open in Boston on the first Wednesday of September, and during this month the increase is 100 as compared with the number of cases in August; but there is a still greater increase from September to October, November and December. By following the broken line which indicates the average mean temperature, it is evident that the temperature has no direct influence on the number of cases. This certainly refutes the argument that the low temperature of the winter months is responsible for the increase in the number of cases.

The method adopted in Boston for the suppression of these diseases is: First, a report of the case by the physician in attendance; second, posting of a card on the house notifying the public of the existence of the disease; and in the case of diphtheria examination of the drainage; third, investigation of the case by one of the medical officers for the purpose of giving advice regarding isolation, and the importance of removal to hospital when the case occurs in a tenement-house; fourth, the sending a notice of the case to the school committee and also to the public library; fifth, the sending of a printed circular to the house of the patient, containing plain and explicit directions regarding isolation and the best methods of disinfection of the clothing and discharges of the patient; sixth, the visitation of the house by the disinfector, who leaves a postal card addressed to the Board of Health, on which is to be stated when, in the opinion of the attending physician, the premises will be ready for disinfection. In the case of a death, as soon as the death certificate is received at the office of the Board of Health arrangements are immediately made for disinfection. It is, of course, understood that public funerals in these cases are prohibited.

The method of disinfection adopted at present consists in the use of a solution of corrosive sublimate one part to five hundred for washing the wood-work of the apartment, and walls, if painted ; in some instances of sponging the mattresses and carpets with a similar solution. The apartment in which the patient has been ill is then tightly closed and four pounds of sulphur to every 1,000 cubic feet of space is burned in it. In addition to this there is an apparatus

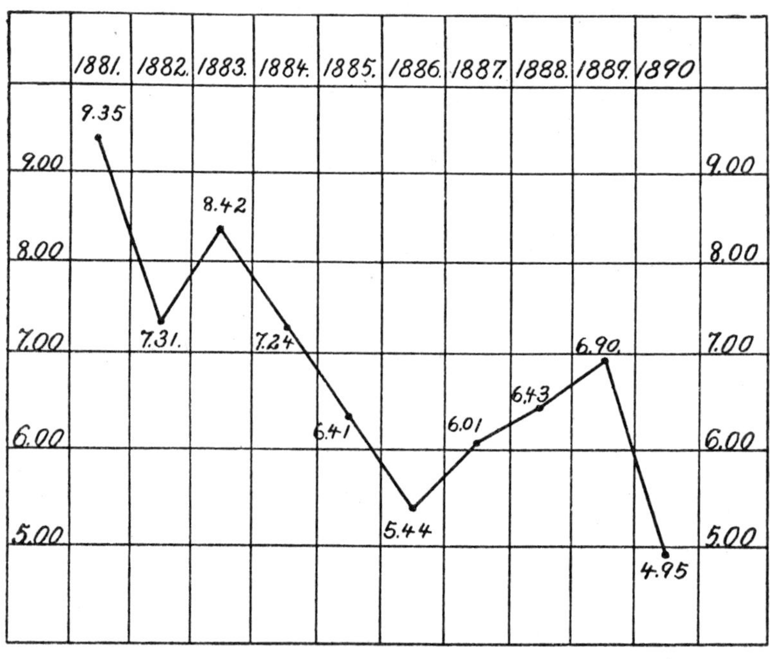

CHART C.

Percentage of Deaths from Croup, Diphtheria. Scarlatina and Variola to the Total Mortality for Ten Years—1881-90.

for the generation of a certain amount of steam, for it has been proved by many experiments that the disinfecting power of sulphurous acid is much increased by the presence of watery vapor. Without, at the present time, stating the arguments for and against the use of this substance as a disinfecting agent, it is sufficient to say that during the past five years only two per cent, or 236 of the cases of scarlet fever and diphtheria of the 11,794 reported, could by any possibility oe traced to infection from rooms or clothing that had been disinfected in the manner just described. So far as small-pox is concerned, in the 112 cases during the past ten years, where sulphurous acid gas has been the only disinfectant used, there is not a single instance of infection from an apartment in which there had been a previous case.

A study of Chart C, which indicates the percentage of deaths from croup, diphtheria, scarlet fever, and small-pox to the total mortality in Boston for ten years shows that in 1881 the percentage was 9.35; in 1882 it fell to 7.31; in 1883 it rose to 8.42; from 1884 to 1886 there was a gradual decline until the rate was 5.44; from 1886 to 1889, a somewhat exceptional period, in which these three diseases were quite prevalent throughout the whole country, the percentage gradually increased until it reached in 1889, 6.90; during the year 1890 it fell to 4.95; a diminution of nearly two per cent in a year, and of nearly five per cent in ten years. But it might be said by some that although the number of deaths from these diseases may have diminished, the number of deaths from other zymotic diseases has increased. The answer to this is the fact that in 1881 the percentage of deaths from all zymotic diseases was 26.67, and that the rate has gradually fallen to 16.47 in 1890, a diminution of nearly ten per cent. This certainly is a remarkable record, which cannot be explained by any of the so-called wave theories of disease, and it proves, if it proves anything, the beneficial effect of sanitary regulations.

DISINFECTION.

The whole subject of disinfection has such an important bearing on the suppression of infectious diseases that a few words regarding it may not be out of place at the present time. It is generally conceded that steam under pressure is the best disinfectant known. The arguments for and against sulphur dioxide are so many and so convincing that one is left somewhat in doubt regarding this agent. Dr. L. H. Thoinot, an eminent hygienist of France, published a very interesting and instructive paper in the *Annales d' Hygiène Publique* of October, 1890, on "Disinfection by Sulphur." After giving in detail the various arguments for and against the use of this substance he gave an account of a series of very carefully conducted experiments with the germs of septicæmia, malignant pustule, erysipelas, glanders, tubercle, typhoid fever, Asiatic cholera and diphtheria.

He found that the germs of septicæmia, malignant pustule and erysipelas resisted absolutely the action of sulphurous acid, although it was used in large doses and with a prolonged exposure ; while the microbes of glanders, tubercle, typhoid fever and diphtheria were absolutely destroyed. This observer in speaking of the use of sulphur as a disinfectant in variola, says : " Former experiments, also, which have recently been criticised, teach us that sulphur is a good disinfectant for vaccine, and by analogy the conclusion has been reached that it is also an efficient disinfectant in variola. Its empirical use in epidemics of this disease has given satisfactory results." This writer recommends the use of sixty to seventy grammes of sulphur to the cubic metre of space, a quantity somewhat larger than is generally used in this country, and twenty-four hours' exposure. Finally this investigator gives as his opinion, based upon actual experiments, that disinfection by sulphurous acid should not be laid aside until we have a more perfect apparatus at our disposal, such as the stove for the generation of steam under pressure. In the meantime its scientific value should not be called in question in certain cases ; nor the signal service it can render in the time of an epidemic, such as an epidemic of cholera, where it can be easily and promptly instituted at slight expense as a most efficient prophylactic agent.

Disinfection by a current of steam without pressure, which, until the year 1887, was used to such an extent on the Continent, is being gradually abandoned because of its unreliability and lack of penetrating power, and steam under pressure is being substituted. There are many different forms of the disinfecting stove, but the principle is the same in each. This consists in having an iron receiver capable of standing a pressure of thirty pounds to the square inch, and in which the temperature can be raised to 250° F., an iron truck on which to place the articles to be disinfected, a pipe for the admission of steam and one for the escape, a pressure gauge, and a thermometer. In the system of Rohrbeck there is a stage preliminary to that of disinfection which is said to increase the penetration, make the pressure uniform, and causes even saturation. This is done by partially exhausting the air in the stove before admitting the steam. The time required for disinfection by steam under pressure is fifteen minutes for articles not specially contaminated. In the case of special infection, an exposure of from thirty minutes to an hour is required.

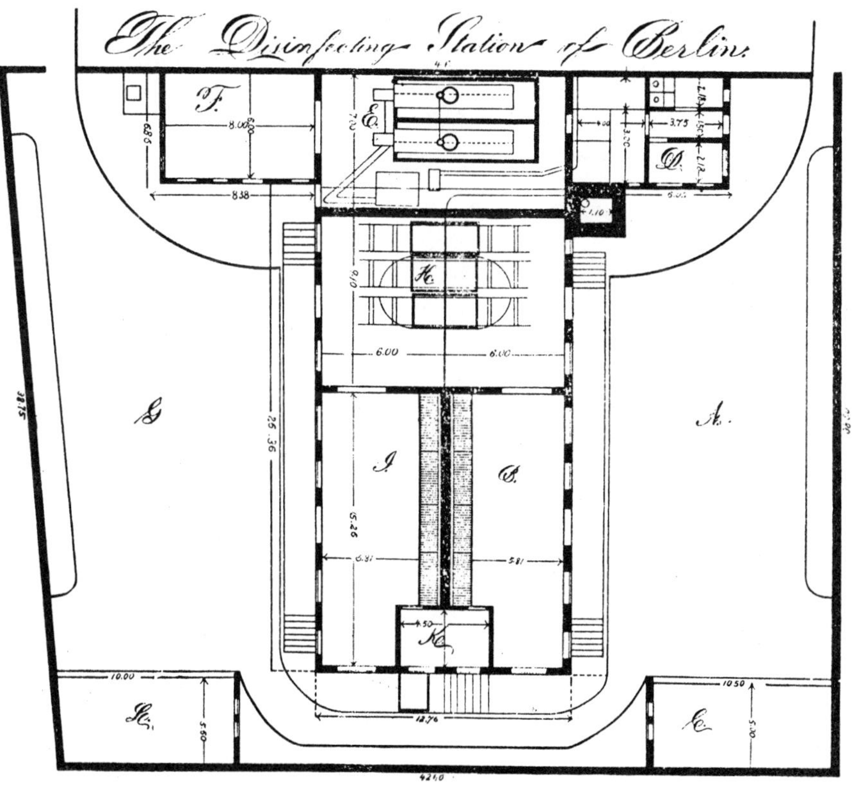
The Disinfecting Station of Berlin.

The importance of a permanent disinfecting station in a large city cannot be overestimated. In Germany, and also in France and in England, hygienic measures, of which this is a very important factor, receive a much more liberal support from the Government than it is possible to obtain in this country. The disinfecting stations of Berlin, of Vienna and of Paris, are apt illustrations of this fact.

Plan D* represents the public disinfecting station of Berlin, opened in the year 1886. This station occupies a lot of land about 126 feet deep, 149 feet wide at one end, and 137 at the other ; a central building divides this plot into two nearly equal courts, one for the reception of articles to be disinfected, the other for the delivery of articles after disinfection ; a narrow passage connects these two courts. In each court is a wagon-house about 16 feet by 32, for the reception of the disinfecting wagons. At one end of the central building is the boiler-house, with two boilers ; on one side of this is the coal-shed ; on the other, bath-rooms, water-closets, and a place for the storage of chemicals. Immediately adjoining the boiler-house is the disinfecting apparatus, which consists of two rooms divided by a perfectly tight wall, and in which are the disinfecting stoves. Connected with the disinfecting chambers are two storage-rooms, each about 50 feet by 19, one for infected articles, the other for the disinfected. On the dividing wall are racks for articles disinfected or to be disinfected. At the end and between these two storage-rooms is the administration chamber, which can be entered only from the courts, and in which are two tightly closed windows having an outlook on the storage-rooms. The disinfecting stoves, made by Schimmel & Co., are three double-walled, iron chests, each about eight feet high, five feet wide and nine feet long. Each stove has a manometer to indicate the degree of pressure. A, represents the court for infected articles ; B, the storage-room ; C, the wagon-shed ; D, the water-closets and bath-rooms ; E, the boiler-house ; F, the coal-shed ; G, the court for disinfected articles ; H, the disinfecting stoves ; I, the storage-room for disinfected articles ; K, the administration-room ; L, the wagon-shed. The different parts of the station are connected by telephone. The utmost care is taken to prevent the contamination of disinfected articles either by the wagons or by the clothing of the disinfectors.

---

* Die Öffentliche Gesundheits, und Krankenpflege der Stadt, Berlin. Berlin, 1890, p. 98, et seq.

While the reliability of disinfection by steam cannot be disputed, it must be acknowledged that in certain conditions this process cannot be used, as, for example, in the disinfection of the walls of houses. For this purpose some gaseous disinfectant, therefore, is imperatively demanded. A painted wall can be disinfected by washing with a solution of corrosive sublimate, it is true, but for the cracked walls, covered with soiled paper, of the ordinary tenement-house, and for upholstered furniture, sulphurous acid seems to be the best agent to use, notwithstanding the fact that its disinfecting power has been disputed. Carefully conducted experiments prove, it is true, that when cultures of many microbes are placed on cloth and subjected to the fumes of sulphurous acid they are not sterilized; but the conditions are entirely different in the case of the microbes on the walls and floating in the air, for in the latter the germs are exposed directly to the action of the gas and are therefore more easily killed, while in the former the fibre of the cloth protects them to a certain extent.

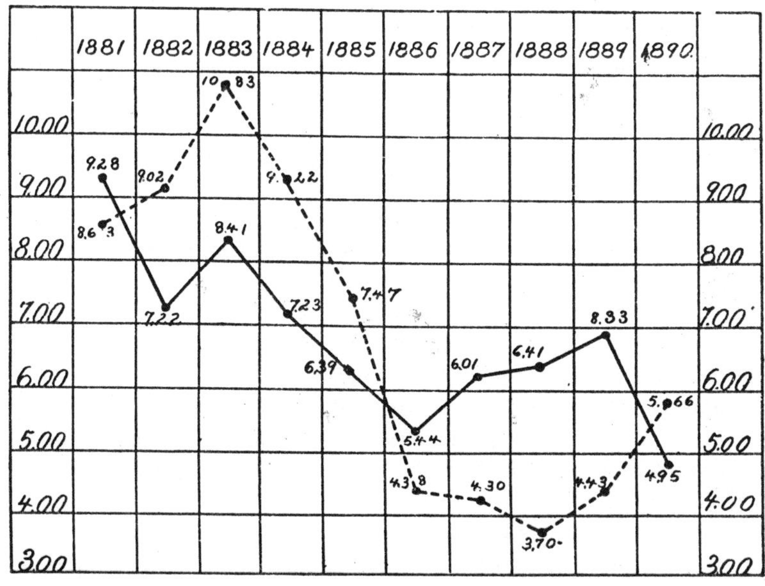

CHART E.

Percentage of Deaths from Croup, Diphtheria and Scarlatina to the Total Mortality in Berlin and Boston for Ten Years—1881-90.

Berlin........   Boston———-

A study of Chart E, which shows the percentage of deaths from croup, diphtheria and scarlet fever to the total mortality for ten years, 1881–90, indicates that in Boston, where sulphur is used, the rate has fallen from 9.28 to 4.95, a diminution of 4.33. In Berlin, where the steam process is used, the rate has fallen from 8.63 to 5.66, a diminution of 2.97 ; 1.36 in favor of Boston. The municipal disinfecting station in Berlin, just described, was opened in 1886 ; for that year the rate was 4.38, and by following the broken line it will be seen that the percentage varied slightly during the subsequent years, but that in 1890 it reached 5.66, an increase of 1.28. In Boston, on the other hand, it will be seen by following the full line that in 1886 the rate was 5.44, and that in 1890 it was 4.95, a diminution of .49. It is of interest to note that the average percentage for ten years in Berlin is 6.76, and that in Boston it is 6.82. So far as the advantages to be gained from different methods of disinfection are concerned, the foregoing statistics show that the sulphur process, although it may be open to severe criticism, has been an important factor in causing a diminution in the number of cases of scarlet fever and diphtheria ; and, on the other hand, that the steam process, although its scientific value cannot be denied, has not been such a potent agent for this purpose as might have been expected.

In conclusion, I would suggest the adoption of the following plan for the suppression of infectious diseases : —

1. The prompt report of cases.

2. The removal to hospital of suitable cases, and the isolation of others.

3. The establishment of private hospitals, in which the patients can be under the care of their family physicians.

4. The posting of cards on houses where cases of disease exist.

5. The careful medical supervision of the public schools, not only for the purpose of detecting mild cases of disease, but also to prevent the return of children who have been ill, until all danger of infection from them has passed.

6. The prohibition of public funerals.

7. The establishment of a disinfecting station and sanitary laundry.

8. The disinfection of the houses in which these diseases have occurred.

9. The establishment of a house of refuge for families during the disinfection of their homes.

In closing, let me add that I have no such Utopian ideas as to suppose, that even with the most elaborate system of disinfection; that with the most careful medical supervision of the schools; and that with the best arranged hospitals it will ever be possible to absolutely stamp out diphtheria and scarlet fever, but it is evident from the history of the course of these diseases in Boston during the past ten years that a very considerable progress has been made towards their suppression.

DISCUSSION.

Dr. Chapin, of Springfield — The most important cause of the spread of contagious disease is the neglect of mild cases by both the family and the physician.

We have had in Springfield an epidemic spreading through the entire city, which originated from a single case of scarlet fever.

Public schools also are an important factor, and I am in favor of a medical supervisor. I would also include tonsilitis as among the contagious diseases, as I do not think a differential diagnosis possible between this and diphtheria. I have had good success with disinfection by sulphur dioxide, using moist fumes. I consider the dust accumulating in the cracks of a school-house floor a source of danger, and I.think the floors should be scrubbed with corrosive sublimate quite often.

Dr. Comey, of Clinton — I have had more or less scarlet fever for the past ten years. For the year ending March, 1891, there were two hundred and eighteen cases, forty in the month of October.

As my town has a dense population and many school children, the disease spreads through the schools. It is difficult to enforce school quarantine, as the mild cases do not call a physician, and often returns to school before they have recovered. I am in favor of educating the people in any way possible in regard to these diseases, and the strict enforcement of school quarantine.

I am also in favor of placarding all houses where there are infectious diseases.

Dr. Cutler, of Waltham — There are some diseases which though contagious are so mild that it is hardly worth while to attempt to control them ; for example, whooping-cough, measles and chicken-pox.

They are very contagious, but so rarely fatal that a physician is only called exceptionally ; hence are hard to manage by a Board of Health, even if it seems worth while.

The diseases which the Board should devote itself to are, in my opinion, diphtheria, typhoid fever, cholera infantum, entero-colitis, small-pox, scarlet fever, tuberculosis, and hydrophobia.

Small-pox can be controlled by vaccination and isolation. Every child should be vaccinated in the first year. Formerly it was the custom for the family physician to attend to this; now it has been thrown upon the Boards of Health. There should be a stricter inspection of all children entering school as regards vaccination.

Scarlet fever and diphtheria should be treated by isolation, disinfection and school quarantine. In typhoid fever the milk and water supply should be inspected by the health officer, and special instruction should be given by him as to the care of the dejections. A case was cited where the germs may have been brought into the house on the person or clothing of a servant.

Hydrophobia. — All dogs should be restrained from running at large in the public streets. Tuberculosis should be considered among the preventable diseases, and stringent measures should be taken to stamp it out. The sputa from phthisical patients should be disinfected and the officers of the Boards of Health should inspect carefully the milk and meat supplies of the town with reference to this disease. Koch and Pasteur's views may be a step in the right direction for all contagious diseases. I favor hospitals for all contagious diseases, and would allow any respectable physician to send patients to such hospitals and retain the care of the case himself. The time will come when all epidemics of contagious disease will be considered an opprobrium to the Board of Health.

Dr. Morrow of Gloucester — I believe that we should take a high stand in relation to contagious diseases, and while it may be that they *will* not be exterminated, yet I believe they *can* be if the right measures are applied. Carelessness is responsible for their spread, and it should be the aim of health officials to awaken a sentiment which will demand absolute quarantine of each case as it arises, for each case may be the cause of a widespread epidemic. Mild cases are the most dangerous as far as the propagation of these diseases is concerned, for they are allowed greater freedom of movement than the severe cases, which are confined to one room and to their beds. Take the history of small-pox for example, and in this disease I would give due credit to vaccination as a protective, yet each case is seized by the authorities and absolutely quarantined while the germs are destroyed in the room where they were originated. To this isolation and quarantine I believe we should give more credit than we do for our comparative immunity from small-pox, which has not been seen in my city for many years, although we have considerable foreign trade. If the same principles were applied to scarlet-fever, diphtheria and other contagious diseases, it would be reasonable to expect the same results. With others who have spoken this afternoon I believe that the schools are responsible for their spread, or more definitely, the attendance of infected children at the schools; for some cases are so mild that being overlooked the children are not taken from school at all, while other children who are exposed to infection manage to retain their places by various promises or explanations; many also return to school before they are through with the scaling process in scarlet-fever, and I am inclined to believe that many of these cases are not free from this scaling for six weeks, which, there is some reason to believe, would be a better period of exclusion from schools than four weeks; then again, disinfection by thorough washing of the person should be as rigidly done as disinfection of the house or apartments.

We have recently begun the placarding of houses in our city for diphtheria and scarlet fever, and I am much pleased with the way in which the people have received the innovation; and judging from this, I believe the people could be educated to receive other and more rigid methods of quarantine.

Dr. Abbott, of State Board of Health — Hydrophobia runs in waves. In 1890 there were seventeen cases, in 1889 there were fourteen, in 1888 there were only three, while for several years previous to 1888 there were none. Among dogs most cases occur in mongrel curs which run from town to town. I think there is really need of better and more general restriction with regard to the ownership and care of dogs than at present. The disease is wholly preventable.

I would call to your attention especially the prevalence of diphtheria and scarlet fever throughout the state for the last two or three years, and I have with me several charts relative to the same which you can all examine at your leisure later on, and which have been prepared from the reports to the State Board of Health. It seems to me that in addition to the many causes which have been spoken of as means of communicating diseases, there should also be included that of railroads. Too little attention has been given to this point in the past, and much can be done in the way of railroad disinfection in the future. I have been especially interested in noting the high death-rate from diphtheria in many of the towns along the route of the Boston & Albany Railroad, and wondering how much of it was due to this cause.

I do not think that bad sanitary conditions are in themselves the sole cause of diphtheria, but I do believe that filth, bad drainage, etc., serve as mediums for the development of its germs.

MASSACHUSETTS ASSOCIATION OF BOARDS OF HEALTH

ORGANIZED 1890.

| Vol. I. | January, 1892. | No. 4. |

QUARTERLY MEETING

OF THE

MASSACHUSETTS ASSOCIATION OF BOARDS OF HEALTH.

Held in Boston, Friday, July 24, 1891.

THE sixth quarterly meeting of the Massachusetts Association of Boards of Health was held in Boston, July 24, the members being the guests of the Boston Board of Health. Sixty-five members of the Association assembled at Battery Wharf at one o'clock, where they went aboard the steamer "J. Putnam Bradlee" and proceeded down the harbor. The Moon Island outlet of the improved sewerage system was first visited, for the purpose of observing the discharge of the sewage into the bay.

The reservoirs contained about twenty-five million gallons of sewage, which was discharged in half an hour. No landing was made here at this time, but the cruise was continued down the harbor below Boston Light, where the Barney dumping scow was awaiting the arrival of the Association. As the "Bradlee" approached the dumper a signal flag was waved, and the boat was seen to divide lengthwise from the bottom, and discharge her cargo of refuse into the sea.

The steamer's prow was again headed onward, and another visit was made to Moon Island. This time a landing was made, the party went ashore, inspected the reservoirs for storing sewage, the methods of filling and emptying them were explained, and the system of flushing the reservoirs was shown. Boarding the "Bradlee" again the company proceeded to Galloup's and a landing was made there. In

the storehouse tables had been laid and a clambake was waiting
The menu consisted of fish chowder, baked clams, with corn, boiled
lobsters, cold tongue, watermelon, coffee and cigars, with rolls,
crackers, etc.

After justice had been done the spread, the meeting was called to
order by the vice-president, Dr. Durgin, chairman of the Boston Board
of Health, in the absence of the president, Dr. Walcott of Cambridge,
who was unable to be present

The records of the last meeting were read and approved.

VICE-PRESIDENT DURGIN — The first business before the meeting
will be action on the propositions for membership.

THE SECRETARY — I have the following list of applicants for membership who have been passed by the Executive Committee, and are
recommended to the Association for election : —

> E. EDWIN SPENCER, M.D., City Physician, Cambridge.
> B. F. THOMAS, Quincy.
> CHARLES D. BURRAGE, Gardner.
> JOHN W. COSDEN, Boston.
> JOSEPH E. CLARK. M.D., Medford.
> ALLEN GREENWOOD, M.D., Waltham.
> SAMUEL FRIEBE, Waltham.
> E. Irving SMITH, Waltham.
> F. HERBERT SNOW, City Engineer, Brockton.
> CHARLES SMITH, Fitchburg.

By vote of the Association all the foregoing parties were unanimously elected to membership.

Vice-President Durgin then introduced Mr. Frederic P. Stearns,
chief engineer of the State Board of Health, who read a paper
describing the present system of intercepting sewers in Boston.

At the close of the reading Mr. Stearns was greeted with hearty
applause.

Vice-President Durgin then introduced Mr. E. P. Fisk, clerk of
the Metropolitan Sewage Commission, who spoke in place of Engineer Carson, relative to the present condition of the work on the
Metropolitan systems of sewerage.

A vote of thanks was unanimously adopted to the Boston Board
of Health for its hospitality. The members then returned to Boston
on the steamer

[RECENT OUTBREAKS OF SMALLPOX IN MASSACHUSETTS

AND

PROTECTIVE INFLUENCE OF VACCINATION]

Massachusetts Association of Boards of Health.

Organized 1890.

[This Association as a body is not responsible for statements or opinions of any of its members.]

VOL. IV.   APRIL, 1894.   NO. 2.

QUARTERLY MEETING.

THE Massachusetts Association of Boards of Health held its regular meeting at the Parker House, Boston, on the afternoon of Thursday, April 26, 1894. The meeting was called to order by the President, Dr. Henry P. Walcott, who stated that the reading of the records of the last meeting would have to be dispensed with, owing to the absence of the Secretary.

On motion of Dr. S. H. Durgin, Dr. Farnham, of Cambridge, was appointed Secretary *pro tem.*

The PRESIDENT. The Executive Committee have to report to you the following names for membershlp in the Association: Dr. W. P. Bowers, of Clinton; Dr. J. A. Douglass, Dr. J. A. Fitz-Hugh and Mr. H. Cooper, of Amesbury; Dr. E. L. Warren, of Melrose; Mr. Edmund M. Parker and Charles Harris, of Cambridge.

The above named gentlemen were elected members of the Association.

The PRESIDENT. The Committee also recommend to the Association for action at this time, the following resolution:

" *Whereas,* an amendment is now before the General Court of Massachusetts exempting all children from vaccination upon presentation of a certificate of any reputable physician that they are not in condition to submit to it, therefore —

" *Be it resolved,* that the Massachusetts Association of Boards of Health considers that this amendment will largely nullify the objects of the bill, and will obstruct the efforts of boards of health in enforcing vaccination, and that it believes the amendment should not pass."

In explanation of that, it should be said, as many of you probably know, that an amendment to the vaccination law has been introduced, by which any person can present in behalf of a child, a statement from any physician whatever, stating that this child is not a proper subject for vaccination, and under that certificate the child at once enters the school, notwithstanding the present law that makes vaccination necessary. The Executive Committee feel that the influence of this Association should be thrown into the scale, if possible, to prevent this, and they therefore recommend this Association to adopt the resolution which I have read to you. Is there anything to be said about it?

Dr. DURGIN. This resolution is offered, I presume, for the reason that this subject is being discussed in the State Senate, and may be acted upon this afternoon, having been acted upon favorably in the House, and if the resolution meets the views of the Association, that expression ought to reach the Senate this afternoon. It seems to me that as a representative body we ought to speak upon this question, and it seems to me also that the Legislature would be glad to hear from this body upon this important subject, for the amendment undoubtedly breaks the whole force of the present excellent law on vaccination. I therefore move that this resolution be adopted.

The motion was seconded, and the resolution was adopted.

Dr. DURGIN. I would also move that a copy of this resolution be sent immediately to the chairman of the Committee on Public Health on the part of the Senate.

The motion was seconded and adopted.

The PRESIDENT. Is there any committee to report at this time? If not, the Association will proceed with its regular business for the afternoon, which is, first, a general discussion of the recent prevalence of smallpox in Massachusetts and the lessons taught by it. I will call upon Dr. McCollom to say something concerning the recent epidemic in Boston.

Dr. J. H. McCOLLOM. Mr. Chairman and Gentlemen: Smallpox in Boston has been a rare disease until within the last six or eight months. Perhaps it will be well at this time to look back to the earlier history of Boston previous to the discovery of vaccination. Previous to 1789 there were five distinct epidemics of smallpox in this city. These epidemics were so severe that in each of them nearly one-third of the inhabitants succumbed to the disease. It was during one of the later of these epidemics that inoculation came into use. In order to ensure the full benefits of inoculation, a hospital was established at Noddle's Island, one at Point Shirley, and one at Brookline, to which the people of Boston were allowed access. Inoculation diminished the number of deaths from smallpox, but it also served to keep alive the disease. It is interesting to notice that out of 5,075 inoculations at Point Shirley, there were only five deaths, showing that inoculation did diminish the severity of the disease.

In 1800, vaccination, the discovery of Jenner, came into use. I have here a paper published by the Board of Health of Boston in 1801, proving the protective power of vaccination, and in these days when so much is heard from the anti-vaccinationists that vaccination does not protect from smallpox, it is extremely interesting to notice that nineteen children were vaccinated in the first place, and passed through the disease of cow-pox in the natural way. Shortly after they were vaccinated, these nineteen children, together with two unvaccinated children, were inoculated with smallpox. The nineteen vaccinated children were exposed to smallpox for four or five weeks, and did not contract the disease, whereas the two who had not been vaccinated contracted it. The report of the Board of Health is as follows:

"REPORT OF THE BOARD OF HEALTH.

" The Board of Health for the town of *Boston*, are happy to have it in their power this day, to announce to their fellow-citizens the result of one of the most complete experiments which perhaps has ever been made, to prove the efficacy of the Cow-Pox, as a preventive against the Small-Pox; and while they take the liberty to congratulate the public on this important discovery, they do earnestly recommend its introduction generally, and are confident that it will be the means of preserving the lives and adding to the happiness of millions.

" The utmost care has been taken, during the experiments; and a detailed statement of facts are subjoined, for the gratification of every enquirer.

" In June, 1801, Dr. Jackson addressed a letter to the Board of Health, requesting their countenance in certain experiments which he contemplated making, to prove the efficacy of the Cow-Pox, as a preventive against the Small-Pox; to which application the avocations of the Board would not permit that attention which the plan proposed by Dr. Jackson required.

" In June, 1802, Dr. Waterhouse made a similar application, accompanied with a very minute history of that disorder, from himself, and also various documents in proof of its utility, from Societies in *New York* and elsewhere, who had associated for the purpose of making experiments similar to those proposed to be made by Dr. W., by which it appeared, that the public in those places, were deriving incalculable benefits by a pretty general inoculation. About this time the Small-Pox was raging in the family of Mr. Holden, *Fifth Street*, and three persons out of five, under the care of the Board of Health, had died. The Cow-pox had obtained much credit.

" The Board of Health, deeply affected with the fatal ravages of the Small-Pox, in the family before mentioned, and viewing their Institution as founded, under God, for the 'preservation of the health of their fellow-citizens; and believing, as they did, that this mild and safe disorder, " *the*

Cow-Pox," might be substituted for that fatal and distressing one, the Small-pox; so that if generally adopted, completely to annihilate and blot it from the catalogue of human woes; determined, under the influence of these considerations, to prove by experiments, to be made under their immediate observation, whether their faith in the efficacy of the Cow-pox was well founded or not.

"With this view, the plan of the experiments proposed were published in the newspapers, for the consideration of their fellow-citizens. The Secretary of the Board was also directed, in their name, to desire the assistance of Doctors Lloyd, Danforth, Rand, Jeffries, Warren, Jarvis and Waterhouse, who, agreeably to the invitation of the Board, met them at the Health-Office. Various impediments presented themselves in carrying into effect the plan as published. It was alleged, that the distance of *Rainsford's Island* from town, would prevent attendance of the gentlmen concerned, as often as would be requisite; and to make them in town, it would be necessary to have the permission of the town, in town-meeting, it being contrary to law to inoculate with the Small-pox without it. It was therefore determined to apply for this privilege; and the town being assembled for that purpose, it was objected to, on the grounds that it would alarm the country, and injure the trade of the town. After much debate, it was voted by the town — 'That the Board have power to make the experiments proposed, without the limits of the town; and to take up suitable buildings, etc. for that purpose.' It was with much difficulty a place could be obtained, comporting with the vote of the town. But started in the pursuit, the object, the happiness of mankind, the Board was determined that no difficulties which perseverance could surmount, should divert them from their purpose.

"At length Mr. Williams gave permission to erect a small building on *Noddle's Island*, and to make the proposed experiments there. Thus provided, on the 16th day of August, nineteen children, viz. :

DANIEL SCOTT, Chambers-Street.	THOMAS TRUMAN, Dogget's Alley.
ALMARIN CLARKE, Cornhill.	E. L. TRUMAN, Dogget's Alley.
JOHN SILSBY, Prince-Street.	JOHN WYER, Dogget's Alley.
OZIAS GOODWIN, Charter-Street.	SETH KING, Dogget's Alley.
GEORGE GOODWIN, Charter-Street.	GEORGE FORBES, Market-Square.
SAMUEL WATTS, Charter-Street.	WILLIAM AUSTIN, Market-Square.
SAMUEL RICHIE, Charter-Street.	JOHN HARRIS, Fifth-Street.
ROBERT WILLIAMS, Cole Lane.	THOMAS SPEAR, Friends-Street.
HENRY WILLIAMS, Cole Lane.	WM. GREENE, Hanover-Street.
REUBEN LORING, Willson's Lane.	

Were inoculated with the Cow-pox, at the Health-Office, in presence of the Board, and of a number of gentlemen invited. The physicians who attended were Drs. *Lloyd, Rand, Jeffries, Warren, Waterhouse, Wells, J. C. Howard,* and *T. Danforth ;* and the children went through the disorder to the satisfaction of the gentlemen, physicians and of this Board.

"Fresh Small-pox matter being obtained, through the politeness of Dr. Weeks, the proprietor of the Small-pox hospital at *Falmouth* — on the ninth of November, twelve of the children before named, together with *George Bartlett,* son of Dr. *Bartlett,* of *Charlestown,* who had the Cow-pox two years since, were inoculated at the hospital erected on *Noddle's Island,* with the Small-pox, from the matter obtained from Dr. *Weeks* — and at the same time two children of Mr. *Christopher Clark* of *Hinchman's Lane,* viz. *Thomas* and *John,* who had never had either the Cow-pox or Small-pox, were also inoculated with the latter ; and in the proper time the arms (of the two *Clarks*) become inflamed — the symptomatic fever, and usual appearances attending the Small-pox, appeared — and finally pustules to the amount of about 500 on one, and 150 on the other, put forth and matterated, as has been invariably the case in all instances ·of the small-pox within our knowledge. From these two children, thus effected with Small-pox, fresh matter was taken ; and the thirteen children before named, who were totally unaffected with the first inoculation with Small-pox, were again inoculated on the 21st day of November ; and the other seven children who had the Cow-pox as first mentioned, were also inoculated with fresh matter from the *Clarks ;* and the whole remained together in the same house, in the same room, and often in the same beds, without producing the least appearance of the Small-pox, either by uncommon soreness of the arm, headache, the least degree of fever or pustules — and this we certify to the public, having daily visited the Hospital ourselves, and made the most critical observations and inquiries, which are confirmed by the report of the physicians who attended the experiments (hereto annexed)and therefore are confident in affirming, that the Cow-pox is a complete preventive against all the effects of the Small-pox upon the human system."

"THE PHYSICIANS' REPORT.

"With a view of ascertaining the efficacy of the Cow-pox in preventing the Small-pox, and of diffusing through this country the knowledge of such facts as might be established by a course of experiments instituted for the purpose, and thereby removing any prejudices, which might possess the public mind on the subject, the Board of Health of the town of Boston, in the course of the last Summer, came to a determination to invite a number of Physicians to co-operate with them on this important design; and with a liberality becoming enlightened citizens, erected a Hospital on *Noddle's Island,* for carrying it into execution. Accordingly, on the sixteenth of August last, nineteen boys, whose names are subjoined, were inoculated for the Cow-pox at the office, and in presence of the above-mentioned Board, with fresh, transparent Cow-pox matter, taken from the arms of a number of patients then under this disease. These all received and passed through the disease to the complete satisfaction of every person present, conversant with the disease.

"On the ninth of November, twelve of the above children, together with one other, George Bartlett by name, who had passed through the Cow-Pox two years before, were inoculated for the Small-Pox on *Noddle's Island*, with matter taken from a Small-pox patient in the most infectious stage of that disease. The arms of these lads became inflamed at the incisions, in proportion to the various irritability of their habits, but not to a degree greater than what any other foreign, virulent matter would have produced. The Small-pox matter excited no general indisposition whatever, through the whole progress of the experiments, though the children took no medicines, but were indulged in their usual modes of living and exercise; and were all lodged promiscuously in one room.

"At the same time and place, in order to prove the activity of the Small-pox matter, which had been used, two lads, who had never had either the Small-pox or Cow-pox, were inoculated from the same matter. At the usual time, the arms of these two patients exhibited the true appearance of the Small-pox. A severe eruptive fever ensued, and produced a plenteous crop of Small-pox pustules, amounting by estimation, to more than five hundred in one and two hundred in the other.

"When these pustules were at the highest state of infection, the thirteen children before mentioned, were inoculated a second time, with recent matter, taken from the pustules, which said matter was likewise inserted into the arms of the seven other children, who were absent at the first inoculation. They were all exposed, most of them for twenty days, to infection, being in the same room with the two boys, who had the Small-pox, so that, if susceptible of this disease, they must inevitably have received it, if not by inoculation, in the natural way.

"Each of the children was examined by the Subscribers, who were individually convinced from the inspection of their arms, their perfect state of health, and exemption from every kind of eruption on their bodies, that the Cow-pox prevented their taking the Small-pox, and they do therefore consider the result of the experiment as satisfactory evidence, that the Cow-pox is a complete security against the Small-pox.

"JAMES LLOYD.	BENJAMIN WATERHOUSE.
ISAAC RAND.	JOSIAH BARTLETT.
SAMUEL DANFORTH.	JOHN FLEET, jun.
JOHN JEFFRIES.	JOHN C. HOWARD.
JOHN WARREN.	THOMAS DANFORTH."
THOMAS WELSH.	

(Then follows a certificate made by Dr. Bartlett.)

"CHARLESTOWN, Dec. 15, 1802.

"This may certify, that my son, George Bartlett, at the age of eight years, was inoculated for the Cow-pox," (of course, in these days we would say he was vaccinated, but that was the term in use at that time,) "on the eleventh day of November, 1800; that the appearance of his arm, and the symptoms, so fully corresponded with the plates and publications I had then seen, as to convince me, and others of my medical friends, that he had the disease.

"JOSIAH BARTLETT,
"*Fellow of the Mass. Medical Society.*
"To the President and Members of the Board of Health,
"Boston."

"BOSTON, December 8, 1802.

"We, Susanna Truman and Lucy Learned, nurses attending on the experiments corroborating the efficacy of the Cow-pox do certify that there was not the least sickness or appearance of Small-pox among any of the children who were subjects of the same, during their stay at *Noddle's Island*, excepting the two boys, Thomas and John Clarke, who had never had the Cow-pox, and were inoculated for the Small-pox, with a view to render the experiment more complete.

"SUSANNA TRUMAN.
"LUCY LEARNED."

"Health-Office, BOSTON, December 16, 1802.
"Published by order of the Board of Health.
"ISAIAH DOANE, President.
"R. GARDNER, Secretary."

It seems to me that this is an extremely valuable and very interesting document, and I will present it for your inspection.

On this chart you will see the deaths from smallpox in Boston for forty years — from 1852 to 1871, and from 1874 to 1893. The slight epidemic of 1872 and 1873 has been purposely omitted, as this was an exceptional time, and no reliable deductions could be drawn from it. During the twenty years commencing with 1852 and ending with 1871, when the average population was 187,969, there were 1,197 deaths from smallpox in this city. In 1852 there were 12 deaths; in 1853, 6; in 1854, 118; in 1855, 132; in 1856, 78; in 1857, 2; in 1858, 3; in 1859, 156; in 1860, 162; in 1861, 7; in 1862, 13; in 1863, 11; in 1864, 113; in 1865, 115; in 1866, 51; in 1867, 144; in 1868, 8; in

1869, 6; in 1870, 32; in 1871, 28. As I said before, the total is 1,197, with a population of 187,969.

You must also bear in mind that communication with foreign countries was not nearly so rapid as now, and that a person, during the years from 1852 to 1871, if he contracted the disease in Liverpool, would be very sure to be taken ill before the vessel arrived here. During the twenty years from 1874 to 1893, with an average population of 402,000, there were only 36 deaths. The number of deaths each year is as follows: In 1874 there were 2 deaths; in 1875, 1; in 1876, 2; in 1877, 4; in 1878, 0; in 1879, 0; in 1880, 1; in 1881, 6; in 1882, 8; in 1883, 1; in 1884, 1; in 1885, 2; in 1886, 0; in 1887, 0; in 1888, 2; in 1889, 2; in 1890, 0; in 1891, 0; in 1892, 0; in 1893, 4.

I would like to call your attention to this diagram that was taken from the report of a smallpox epidemic in Sheffield, England, from 1887 to 1888. You will see that there are six large squares, and that each of the large squares is divided into ten smaller squares. The squares divided by diagonal lines represent cases; the black squares represent deaths.

It will be seen from this diagram that of 4,493 vaccinated people exposed to smallpox under ten years of age, only 7.8 per cent. had the disease, and only one-tenth of one per cent. died; that of 13,423 vaccinated people of ten years of age and upwards, 28.1 per cent. contracted the disease, and 1.4 per cent. died; that of 18,220 vaccinated people of all ages 23 per cent. had the disease and 1.1 per cent. died. On the other hand, it will be seen that of 263 unvaccinated children under ten years of age exposed to the disease, 86.9 per cent. contracted it, and 38.1 per cent. died; that of 469 unvaccinated people ten years of age and upwards, 68.6 per cent. contracted the disease, and 37.1 per cent died; that of 736 unvaccinated persons of all ages exposed to smallpox 75 per cent. contracted the disease, and 37.2 per cent. died. The difference between a death-rate of one-tenth of one per cent. in vaccinated children under ten years of age, as compared with a death-rate of 38.1 per cent. in unvaccinated children under ten years of age, can only be explained by the protective power of vaccination; and a similar remark is true regarding the difference in death-rate between the vaccinated of ten years of age and upward, as compared with the death-rate of the unvaccinated of ten years and upwards.

In Boston during this present epidemic, or, I should hardly say epidemic, but during this outbreak of the disease, we have had ninety-five cases of smallpox, or, to speak accurately, we have had ninety-six cases, because there has been one case reported since I came to this meeting. There have been twenty-six deaths. No vaccinated person has died. I have seen the arm of every person who has been at the hospital. I have searched carefully for a scar in every instance, and in no instance where I have seen a scar that was satisfactory to me, or a scar on account of which

I should have given a certificate to allow a child to go to school, has a person been seriously ill.

Much has been said about the possibility of making a diagnosis before the appearance of the eruption. It is absolutely, morally and physically, impossible for anybody to make a diagnosis of smallpox before the eruption appears, and when I speak of the eruption I mean the eruption of smallpox. I do not mean the initial rash. Smallpox in a vaccinated person is very frequently so mild that it is almost impossible to make a diagnosis unless the physician is familiar with the disease. In regard to the isolation of persons who have been exposed to smallpox, it does not seem to me that this is important if other precautions are taken. It has been our custom in Boston, after a case of smallpox has been removed to the hospital, to have the patient's house visited every day or every other day by some physician. The moment that there is any appearance of illness in any member of the family, that person is placed under the most rigid supervision, and as soon as the eruption appears is removed to the hospital.

[At this point Dr. Walcott was obliged to retire from the meeting, and Dr. Durgin was called to the chair.]

The CHAIRMAN. Dr. Chapin, tell us something about smallpox up in Chicopee.

Dr. CHAPIN. Mr. President and Gentlemen: I do not know much about smallpox in Chicopee. I am not from Chicopee. I am from Springfield. Smallpox appeared in Holyoke some few weeks ago and later appeared in the city of Chicopee, about three miles north of Springfield. It appeared in a — there is nobody here from Chicopee, is there, Doctor?

The CHAIRMAN. No, sir; I think not.

Dr. CHAPIN. It appeared in a tenement house belonging to the Dwight Manufacturing Company of Chicopee. I think there were about twenty-eight people in the tenement house. The case that was discovered was some two weeks old. The whole population of the tenement house had been exposed, together with certain other people working in the mill. The Board of Health quarantined the tenement and the people in the building, and the disease has not extended much outside of the building in which it appeared,— I think not more than half a dozen cases. We are very closely connected in Springfield with Chicopee, but fortunately no cases have appeared among us. A few cases have sojourned with us, but those cases left the town the day before the eruption appeared. That is all I know about smallpox in Chicopee.

The CHAIRMAN. Dr. Field, of Lowell.

Dr. FIELD. Mr. Chairman: Dr. McCollom has said that we cannot make a diagnosis of smallpox before the eruption breaks out. The trouble has seemed to be with us in Lowell that we could not make the diagnosis after the eruption broke out, because some of our oldest physicians there, physicians whom the Board of Health employed, thinking they knew more about smallpox than we did, were unable to tell the disease when they saw it. The first thing I thought of this afternoon when that paper was passed around was, if the physicians of Boston ninety years ago were convinced that vaccination prevented smallpox, we ought to be ninety times as much convinced of it. As they were then, we ought to be cranks on the subject of vaccination just as much as some of these people are cranks on anti-vaccination. We ought always, in season and out of season, to urge vaccination upon the people. If we are members of a board of health, we ought to have our neighborhood and employees vaccinated, and keep them vaccinated all the time. As physicians, when school children come to us in the fall to be vaccinated before they go into school, we ought to advise their parents and older brothers and sisters to be revaccinated. Do not put off vaccination until the epidemic occurs, but keep the inhabitants of the city vaccinated all the time.

In Lowell we had a very severe epidemic of smallpox in 1881, one hundred and eight deaths occurring. Since then in two or three years there have been outbreaks of smallpox, with a few deaths. Last Christmas the present epidemic occurred. On the afternoon of that day we found a young bartender had been laid up for more than a week, and on the next day we found two girls who had been ill four or five weeks, so there were three cases which had been ill this length of time. This young bartender was attended by a physician who was dismissed just as the eruption began to break out. On the next day a young man who had never seen smallpox was called in and treated the case as a case of chicken-pox. The case was so much advanced that when I saw it, the day after Christmas, the pustular stage was already reached. At that time we had established a vaccination office in the barroom in which the young man was employed, but some members suggested that if we use such a very attractive place for a vaccination office the whole city of Lawrence would come up there, and so that idea was abandoned.

Our consulter, whom we called in on that case, for we had not seen more than four or five cases of smallpox, remarked that the first cases were the two girls whom he had seen three or four weeks ago. We found the house and found the two girls convalescing, but covered all over with scars, about two thousand, although they were not counted.

The history of the disease was that of a mild disease, but from these girls we traced it to this man, and afterwards to another person, tracing the contagion from one to the other. It seemed impossible that two girls had been suffering from smallpox for four or five weeks. and that persons had been in and out of the house during that time. Dr. Abbott, who came up afterwards to see the case, made a diagnosis, not from anything he could see on the patient, because you could see nothing but scars, but from the history of the contagion, spreading from these girls to this man and to others.

So we had three cases of smallpox at the start to which people had been exposed in great numbers. Afterwards we had other cases, nine in all, with three deaths. One case was a bad case, which we traced to this man, and which we sent to the hospital. The eruption came out when the vaccination sore on the patient's arm was at its height.

We had two other interesting cases. One was a milkman, who, when the eruptions were on his forehead, had been delivering milk about the city. Another was a nurse in a smallpox hospital who had had smallpox in her childhood, and we made the mistake of not vaccinating her, and after all the other patients had come down, she finally came down with the disease, and recovered.

Our treatment was to send every patient to the hospital. Following out the suggestion of Dr. McCollom, our hospital too was on the land, and I think almost every city, excepting those on the seaboard, would have to have a hospital on the land. We disinfected the premises as far as possible. I wish that we and all the cities in this State might have an apparatus for the disinfection of clothing by steam, the way they do in Boston. Our clothing we took to the cremator and burned up.

On vaccination I do not want to say anything. That subject comes up later. I simply want to speak of the large portion of the inhabitants of Lowell who were vaccinated. When we found that that milkman had been distributing milk throughout the city, we ordered a house-to-house vaccination in all parts of the city which he visited. About one-sixth of the city must have been vaccinated. In addition to that, some ten thousand were vaccinated at the City Hall and eight thousand at the hospital. 26,500 in all vaccinated out of 87,0000 inhabitants.

We believe in Lowell most thoroughly in quarantining a house, and we have an idea that if the houses had been quarantined in Boston, possibly we might not have had the smallpox in Lowell. We cannot prove that, but we know some of these patients who afterwards came down with smallpox would have gone off, and what town they would have gone to we do not know.

The CHAIRMAN. Mr. Bayles, of Lowell.

Mr. BAYLES. Mr. Chairman: I can only talk of smallpox from the point of view of the layman. I feel like taking some exceptions to Dr. McCollom's view of isolation. The cases of smallpox in Lowell occurred in a very compact community. The two girls who had been sick for five weeks were in a house adjoining the house which was first reported to us. The young man had been visiting back and forth. He was acquainted with the young women, and his sisters were in the habit of going back and forth; in fact, the space between the two houses was only about five feet. The morning after Christmas, when we found these two girls sick, the question arose as to what we should do. It was a very serious question with us, but we finally decided that the best thing to do was to quarantine both houses, so we put a guard there. We employed policemen, but I should advise any Board of Health of any town not to employ policemen, because they are very expensive luxuries. [Laughter.] We found we had to pay the policemen three days for one. Then we had to keep them pretty well supplied with stimulants, because they had the idea that if they had plenty of rum they would not have the smallpox. [Renewed laughter.] We subsequently employed our own men who had been appointed constables, and the results were more satisfactory. They were better satisfied with what they got, and satisfied with reasonable compensation. We quarantined those two houses.

When the next case broke out it was across the street, distant perhaps about fifty yards from the first two houses. In that case the young women had visited back and forth in the house where the young man had been sick and where the two girls had been sick. We quarantined that house, which was over the barroom in which the young man was employed.

The next case occurred around the corner, distant perhaps about twenty yards from the house in which the first patient was found, that is, the first patient that we were apprised of, and then we put that quarantine there. We had a very compact district, and there was no difficulty whatever in keeping people within bounds. They took to it very kindly. We had to provision them and give them everything they wanted, in fact, a good deal more than they wanted, for some of them were very shrewd, and they discovered that they wanted barrels of flour, and we found subsequently in one place where we had sent a barrel of flour that after quarantine was removed sixteen days later, the barrel of flour was still intact. We had six families in quarantine. The clothing and furniture in the rooms of two of the patients were destroyed. Had we suitable apparatus for disinfecting we would have been spared that expense, but we had no means of disinfecting other than sulphur, although I have not much faith in it. I think the policemen who went anywhere near the place went in and smoked themselves two or three times a day.

We directed a rigid quarantine and a very thorough vaccination, which tended to shorten the outbreak. I do not think that it would have been possible for us in Lowell to permit any of the people living in the house of the patient to go about at their work, because the popular sentiment there is very much opposed to anything of the kind. People have a great dread of the disease, and as we have so many factories there, everybody knows everybody else, and in a large mill it soon became known that Mary Flynn came from a house where they had smallpox, and we were obliged to establish a quarantine. As it was, we had numerous complaints from officious people who were always watching about for a policeman carrying cans to the people who were quarantined, and we had to shut off their beer. There was a great deal of complaint about that.

In regard to the moving of patients. We had a very antique and ancient vehicle, which in its palmy days had been used as an express wagon. It was impressed into the smallpox business about 1871, then carefully stored away in a shed, and reproduced again in 1893. We used it for an ambulance, and at night we used for a hearse. We learned from that that there was no reason why a person afflicted with smallpox should be treated with any such indignity, and it resulted in our purchasing an ambulance, which we have now, a very respectable vehicle, for conveying our patients to the hospital.

With regard to the hospital. In the old days it was considered anything was good enough for a small-pox patient. A person afflicted with the disease was treated much as a criminal would be,—hustle him out—

> " Rattle him over the stones,
> Only a pauper whom nobody owns."

And so, in 1871 the city of Lowell erected what they called a pest-house. I trust the members of the Board of Health will never use that term. It is a very ominous and very objectionable term. It has great effect on ignorant people, who regard a pest-house as something terrible, something without hope, whereas the term "hospital" has not the terror that the name "pest-house" has. We have been trying up there to get the new set of men, when they make their reports, to drop the term " pest-house." I think it should not be used, just because of the effect it has upon the minds of the people. We found it very difficult to remove people to the pest-house. They did not want to go there because they thought they would not be well treated. Perhaps they were not treated well in the old days when they went to the pest-house. We tried to give them the best treatment we could under the circumstances.

Our hospital is a large barn-like structure having seven rooms. It has no ventilation, no sewerage, no water, no gas, and no heating apparatus— only stoves—and in the winter when the temperature was low and the wind blew, it was a very difficult matter for us to keep all the patients comfortable.

There is no reason why a smallpox patient should be treated any differently than a patient suffering from typhoid fever or any other disease.

Common humanity should teach us to do the best we can for them, and one of the lessons we have learned from this epidemic is that the city of Lowell needs a new hospital, and is going to have one.

I do not know that I can say anything more about the matter. We have simply learned this: that we believe in quarantining all cases, and we believe that when a patient is submitted to our care or when we take charge of a patient, we are in duty bound, not only from a moral sense, but the sense of humanity, from every sense we are bound to give the patient the very best care we possibly can. [Applause.]

The CHAIRMAN. There are still a few minutes more which we can spare upon this subject before taking up the second one on the programme, and if there are other gentlemen who would like to say a few words on the lessons taught by the recent prevalence of smallpox, I should be glad to hear from them.

Dr. SWIFT, of New Bedford. Mr. President: You may be interested in a report of a few cases which we had in New Bedford summer before last, and I will read a short report of these cases.

On June 3, 1892, my attention as city physician was called to suspicious illness in the middle tenement of house numbered 944 South Water street.

The investigation showed a young man, John Andrews, in the pustular stage of smallpox; two children of George Rivers, at the beginning of the stages of desquamation; a young woman, Andrews, who had had a mild case of varioloid in the desquamative stage; and a baby of George Rivers two years old, in the pustular stage of smallpox.

Upstairs in the same house a French family lived; a man named York, with his wife and child, were visiting them. This child was in the pustular stage of smallpox.

The attending physician had considered these cases chicken-pox, and asked me to see them as interesting cases of that disease.

I asked him if he considered them suspicious, and he said he did not. I think the community is exposed to much danger by the ignorance of practitioners in regard to smallpox.

Exactly how physicians are to be trained in the diagnosis of this disease I do not pretend to say; but if there ever is a law passed regulating the practice of medicine in Massachusetts, I trust this Association will insist on at least a thorough theoretical knowledge of smallpox as one of the requirements.

The smallpox hospital had not been open for eleven years; but everything had been kept in readiness for cases, and the patients were all transferred to the hospital on the same day.

On the next day, another suspicious case was reported at 646 South Water street. It was found to be a case of smallpox in the beginning of the pustular stage, the patient being Charles Andrews, a brother of John Andrews. He was immediately transferred to the smallpox hospital. The other people living in both infected houses were transferred to the old poorhouse on French avenue, where a quarantine station was established for persons who, it was thought, had been in any way exposed to the disease.

The cases had been going on for at least two weeks, and it was impossible to say how far the contagion had gone.

On June 8, it was reported that William Andrews, a brother of the men who were already in the hospital, was ill. On investigation, he was found to have a mild case of varioloid. He lived at the east end of Coffin avenue. He was transferred to the hospital, and the other people in the house, to the quarantine station.

On June 9, a case was reported at 305 South Second street.

It proved to be a boy with a light case of varioloid. He was quarantined at home, and another family living upstairs in the house was transferred to the quarantine station.

On June 10, one of the children of the French family named Lemaux, who had lived upstairs at 944 South Water street, came down with smallpox at the quarantine station, and was at once transferred to the smallpox hospital. On June 14, the other Lemaux child also developed smallpox, and was transferred from the quarantine station to the hospital.

On June 15, Joseph Francis was found to be suffering from smallpox at 169 South Second street. He was employed by a grocer, and had taken provisions to the Rivers family. He was at once transferred to the hospital. He was seen at the beginning of the vesicular stage.

The day after he was transferred he had profuse hemorrhages from the nose, mouth, kidneys, and bowels. There were very few pustules, but ecchimotic spots appeared on his extremities, and on the calf of the left leg there was a slough about two inches across. He died the night of June 16, and was buried the next day in the burying-ground near the hospital.

The smallpox hospital, being a small building, was crowded, and it was thought best to construct a cheap building, to be used in case other patients had to be brought to the hospital.

A building was pnt up with eight rooms in it. It was not necessary to transfer any case to this building, but it was used for disinfecting purposes. One of the Rivers children, aged two years, had a severe confluent case of smallpox, and died from exhaustion. It was buried in the burying-ground near the hospital the next day.

On June 18, a case of smallpox was reported at 592 South First street. This was a French boy who worked in a cotton mill, and had no apparent connection with the other cases. He was at once transferred to the hospital. He lived in a large three-story tenement house, and it was impossible to take all the inmates to the quarantine station. Only the families living on the same floor where the case occurred were transferred. The others were advised to leave the house, and they did so.

After the discovery of this case, it seemed probable that the epidemic might be extensive, and a general vaccination was advised and ordered by the board. This was carried out in all the factories in the city, and in the schools. A house-to-house vaccination was also ordered in the vicinity of the infected houses. There were 14,456 vaccinations made.

The physicians were instructed to vaccinate all persons who had not been vaccinated within five years.

All the tenements where cases of smallpox had been found were thoroughly fumigated and cleaned. All the furniture, carpets, and clothing that had been exposed were destroyed. The tenements were washed with corrosive sublimate solution, and were entirely repainted and papered.

The patients were kept in the hospital until all signs of desquamation had cleared up. Meanwhile they were washed with corrosive sublimate solution and soap. When they were released, they were thoroughly washed with a corrosive sublimate solution and given an entire outfit of new clothing. They were allowed to take nothing away from the hospital.

After being thoroughly disinfected in this way, they were transferred to the quarantine house, and kept there several days before they were allowed to come to the city.

No expense or trouble was spared to do this work thoroughly, and the result was that no new cases developed, either from the infected tenements or from the patients themselves. In my opinion, the importance of the quarantine station in this epidemic cannot be overestimated.

It enables us to vacate the infected houses at once, and not to have them occupied again until they had been thororghly disinfected; it removed the persons living in these houses at once from a possible source of infection in the house, and it gave us the opportunity to watch the persons who had possibly been exposed to infection.

Establishing a quarantine station to which all persons who lived in the houses where cases of smallpox occurred were transferred, had much to do, I believe, with our success in stamping out this epidemic.

We had no power to compel them to go, but told them they must either go or be quarantined at home. If they remained at home they would not be allowed to work, but if they went to the quarantine station we would pay them their ordinary wages. Even on these terms we had much difficulty in persuading them to go.

We consulted our city solicitor in regard to this matter and he told us we had full power to quarantine people who had been exposed to smallpox in their houses, but no law gave us power to compel them to vacate their houses or to transfer them to a quarantine station.

I think the importance of vacating the infected houses cannot be over-estimated. In almost all tenement houses certain parts are used in common and people living in infected houses may be exposed to infection in this way. It is almost impossible to properly clean a house with people still living in it. It seems to me power should be given boards of health to vacate houses where cases of smallpox are found and transfer the people who may have been exposed to the disease to a quarantine station for observation.

Two cases of smallpox appearing in the quarantine station showed the wisdom of this precaution. There were thirteen cases in all; one a case of hemorrhagic smallpox, the patient dying before the pustular stage had developed; one case of confluent smallpox in a child of two years, the patient dying of exhaustion; two severe cases of smallpox in John and Charles Andrews; three confluent cases in the two Lemaux children and the York child; all these three children were very ill, but recovered; three cases were mild smallpox,— the two Rivers children and the French boy; and three cases of varioloid.

A point that came up during the epidemic may be instructive to the Association. The law of 1883 requires that when a case of smallpox occurs in a city or town, unless the local Board of Health notify the secretary of the State Board of Health within twenty-four hours of the occurrence of the case, the city or town loses its chance of reimbursment from the State, in case the patient proves to be a State pauper.

The clerk notified the secretary of the State Board of Health on the postal cards supplied to local Boards by the State Board for the weekly report. On this card one space is left for cases of smallpox. The cases were reported at once as one, two, or more, as they occurred.

This notice was not considered sufficient by the secretary of the State Board of Health and he failed to notify the Board of Lunacy and Charity, as he is required to do. Captain Shurtleff, secretary of the Board of Lunacy and Charity, held that he had received no notice and that we had forfeited our chance for any reimbursement. The matter was finally referred to the Attorney-General, and he decided that our notice was sufficient, as all that was required by law was a notice of the occurrence of a case of smallpox within twenty-four hours of the time it was reported to the local Board. Mr. Shurtleff, secretary of Board of Lunacy and Charity, however, held that for their department a special notice was required, as their general rule was to give no aid until after a report in full was made of a case. This view was not in accordance with that of the legal gentleman in the Attorney-General's office, but as the matter of the amount of money to be reimbursed is left by law entirely to the decision of the Board of Lunacy and Charity, we went no further to test the question. It seems to me that all these laws need thorough revision, and that this Association should take some action in regard to this matter.

Dr. W. G. McDonald, of Boston. Mr. Chairman: I did not intend to say anything on this matter, but since the discussion has started there are two or three points which have come to me. In the first place, in regard to Dr. Field's statement about quarantining in Boston. If Boston had been quarantined better, there would have been less smallpox. I can say this, that after a case was found in Boston, there was no question about keeping the patient in the house. The patient was removed to the hospital. The clothing, bedding, and such things were fumigated. Not only was that done, but the patient was questioned as to where he had been during the last few weeks. The patient's family were questioned, and every trace was followed up as far as possible. Every person who had come in contact with the patient was chased and followed for the next two weeks. It was stated that in Lowell one person knew the other. In large cities each one cannot know the other. Conditions have changed in large cities in the last twenty-five years. We have had a large tide of emigrants and a much different class of emigrants in the last twenty years. We have now one hundred thousand inhabitants more than in 1872, and a different kind of emigrants. At that time the most of the people who came here were from the British Empire or from Germany. They were people who came here to settle and become citizens of this country and become amenable to our laws and follow our habits. They are not so to-day. We have to-day Russian Jews; we have Italians, we have Portuguese and Chinese. We have a different class of people who come here to follow their own customs,— people whom it is very difficult to trace. We have in every instance tried to trace the case to its origin, and we have tried to follow it to its conclusion. In many cases we have failed in tracing it to its origin because of the difference in the people who are here to-day. That was one of the important lessons of this epidemic, different from any other epidemic that we have had.

Besides that, we have the question that has been raised already as to pest-houses. People dread a pest-house. We have, not a pest-house, but a hospital, with the most approved appliances, the most careful nursing and scientific treatment. That should be considered by the people, and the people must be educated in order to appreciate these things. There are cases where people have concealed themselves, and we found them only when the eruption broke out.

We have also the question of the education of physicians. That is a very hard thing, because smallpox is a rare disease, and being rare, a student may go through his course without ever coming in contact with a smallpox case; and if in his course a smallpox case arises, we cannot show it to him — we cannot show it to the entire class. The only education the students can get is a theoretical one, and that they are as apt to forget as they are the types of any other disease which we do not happen to have in this climate. But we can teach them in varicella. We have had here one such case where they followed an advanced case of varicella, and each student, I think, should be taught in that as well as vaccination.

Dr. FIELD. Mr. Chairman, I think the conditions in Lowell are very different from the conditions in Boston. Possibly if Dr. McCollom was in my place in Lowell he would quarantine his smallpox patients there, and probably if I were in his place in Boston, I would not quarantine my smallpox patients here. In Lowell the people largely know each other. I do not mean the patients, I mean the families, Doctor. The families in this locality were all related directly or indirectly through marriage, and they may have been visiting backward and forward, and we felt sure that after we had quarantined the houses we would have no walking cases of smallpox. Under the circumstances, we think it was the part of wisdom to quarantine.

Mr. BAYLES. Mr. Chairman: In Lowell our conditions are very different from those in Boston. Our people work in the factory. In the first instance, where we took that young man, our first case, there were eight persons living in that house. One of those persons was taken sick with the smallpox ten days after we had removed the case. That young woman worked in a factory employing about two thousand people. You can readily see the danger there would be in allowing that family to go to work in the mill among all these people. There were three of the quarantined people working in a factory employing two thousand, two in a mill employing three thousand, and two in a mill employing five hundred. The agents of those mills were extremely solicitous that we should allow no one from the infected houses to come to work, and they absolutely refused to admit them into the mill. They feared that the disease might be brought into the mill, and that they would be subjected to great expense and annoyance in disinfecting their goods before they could ship them to market.

I may also say in respect to the daily examination of the people living in infected houses, that Dr. Field went every day and made an examination of all the people who were quarantined.

Dr. McCOLLOM. Mr. Chairman: I would like to say that this person could not have communicated the disease until she was taken ill. That was just the point exactly. After having been exposed to smallpox, and after having the clothing thoroughly disinfected, the person could not communicate the disease.

Dr. FIELD. Don't you think she could carry the disease?

QUESTION. Don't you practically quarantine all other diseases, as, for instance, where children go to school where children have had scarlet fever?

Dr. McCollom. We do not have anything to do with that. I think it would be better for the children to be inspected in every case of scarlet fever and diphtheria. I think by inspection, although it will require a great deal of work, much more good will be accomplished for the community, and will stamp out the disease much more thoroughly than by quarantining. If we watch them and disinfect their clothing before they come down with the disease, it is impossible almost for them to communicate the disease.

Mr. Bayles. Sometimes they are too slippery to watch, Doctor.

Dr. ———. Mr. President: It seems to me this method of Dr. McCollom causes a good deal of trouble. Of course, it may be all right as far as the people are concerned, but the rest are put to considerable trouble. I think if the house had been quarantined in the first place, they would not have got to Lowell.

Dr. Swift. May I ask a question? When cases have been coming on in a house for some length of time, is it not a safer method to vacate that house? There are certain parts of tenement houses that are used in common; for instance, the basement usually, and possibly the water-closets; and is it not a safer way to vacate the house, if that is possible, at once, and to have it thoroughly cleaned: remove the people, if they have not already been exposed to the disease, and to permit them to come back when the house has been thoroughly cleaned and thoroughly disinfected, and in case of the patients being sent to the hospital, when the people are perfectly well return to the house? It seems to me that is the most thorough way of proceeding, if it is possible to do it. Of course, I do not mean to say it is always possible. In such a place as New Bedford the houses are small, and it is possible in most cases. The houses, as I have said, in this small outbreak were vacated and the people were not allowed to go back. We did not absolutely control them, but we persuaded them not to go back until everything was perfectly safe for them to go back. Meanwhile we supported them,— bribed them to stay away.

The Chairman. It is getting rather late, and in justice to our next subject I think we shall have to take it up now,—"Vaccination and Its Results." I will call on Dr. Abbott, Secretary of the State Board of Health.

Dr. S. W. Abbott. Mr. Chairman: The transition from smallpox to vaccination is so natural, that I may say a word about smallpox before referring to vaccination. There may be some here who have never seen a case. Here are some photographs taken at the smallpox hospital about ten years ago, which give an excellent idea of its appearance. I will pass them around so that you may see what the typical cases are. There are five or ten pustules to each square inch of body, not quite confluent, but very nearly so. The photographs show the stages from the very first day of the outbreak to the fifteenth day or thereabouts.

Another point is in regard to the time of incubation. Dr. L. Parkes has published a most excellent summary in regard to infectious diseases, in which he gives the least time of incubation at nine days and the longest time fifteen days. Not less, I should say, than fifteen days, would be a pretty good rule for quarantine purposes. Upon this question of vaccination the information to be obtained from the medical journals is slight. In fact, in America, almost throughout the whole country, statistics are entirely wanting on this subject. I have here a tabulation of all the cases that have been reported to us, which probably constitute about all in the State, at least nine-tenths, — from the first of January, 1893, and also a more complete summary for ten years. There have been since that time, that is, in about fifteen or sixteen months, some 188 cases reported to us in the State, all of which, excepting eleven, have been reported within the past seven months. Those eleven were in the early part of 1893. Then there were none for several months until the outbreak began in October, and increased. Then I have a tabulation of cases including the most of those back to 1885. The total number of cases reported to the State Board of Health was 267. There have been enough within the last few days to bring the number up to about 300 or 310. The percentage of deaths is 19 1-2. This is about the average fatality for smallpox. Generally the fatality of it is about 18 to 20 per cent., and that is just where the anti-vaccinationists at the State House always attempt an argument,— that the fatality in this century is no different from what it was in the last century, but they say nothing about the comparative fatality of the vaccinated and the unvaccinated.

I have carried this out as far as possible, and taken the fatality among the vaccinated and unvaccinated in Massachusetts. Of course, there are some cases that have to be thrown out altogether; the facts are unknown or indefinite, based entirely upon some hearsay statement of the patients themselves after the eruption has broken out, and you cannot tell whether they were vaccinated or not. Out of 104 persons who were vaccinated only 6 died, while of 122 persons unvaccinated the deaths were 35, or 28.7 per cent.— nearly five times as high a percentage. The doubtful cases were 41. Deaths among these were 11, a percentage of 26.8, nearly the same as the unvaccinated.

The proof of vaccination statistically is made in several ways. Some methods are more convincing than others. For instance, one proof is that the mortality from smallpox in this century is very much less than it was in the last century. For instance, there were 840 deaths in Boston in 1721, out of 12,000 people, which would mean about 25,000 deaths to-day in the population of Boston, which would be enormous; but it is nothing in this century to what it was in the last; it is nothing now to what it was twenty-five years ago. But that is not sufficient. It is not true that the State Board of Health, and even local Boards of Health, have accomplished all this. They have accomplished a great deal, but not all.

Another and much better proof is to take a vaccinated community, thoroughly vaccinated, and compare it with a partially vaccinated community. We have the fact that whereas Germany has forty or fifty millions of inhabitants, surrounded by other countries partially vaccinated, Germany has its law (which is not only a law, but it is an enforced and absolute law, for it is an imperial government), that a child shall be vaccinated practically before it is eighteen months old. Then every scholar must be revaccinated at the age of twelve years. Now about the only unvaccinated persons in that country are persons who have come there from Russia, where the law is very lax, or from Italy, or from France, or from Spain, or some other neighboring country; and when any of these die in Germany, of smallpox, of course the death is credited to their death-rate.

Now, the death-rate of Germany for the year 1891 from smallpox was almost nothing when compared with that of these neighboring countries.

Then another very convincing argument is the fact that in the last century smallpox was almost absolutely a disease of children,—a disease of children under ten years of age. The figures upon that subject are not very many or very great, but they relate to a few cities where old registers have been kept very carefully by the schoolmasters, town clerks and others in England, and also in the city of Geneva, Switzerland, and a few other places, where they show that smallpox was confined almost exclusively to children under ten years of age. For instance, out of a thousand persons in two or three English towns who died of smallpox, there were not more than ten or a dozen over ten years of age. We do not have that now. A very considerable percentage of the deaths from smallpox are among people who are over fifteen or twenty, simply because they have been protected by primary vaccination, and the disease is thrown forward to later ages; and as they have neglected revaccination, then we have mortality among the vaccinated, and that is where this adult mortality comes from. There are deaths among the vaccinated because they have neglected revaccination.

Now a word about those who claim to have been revaccinated, and yet have had the smallpox. If those persons had been examined carefully, we should have found that they had not been revaccinated, or that the vaccination was of a very limited character. Every person in Germany who is vaccinated is vaccinated three times on each arm, and it is very thoroughly done. I do not know that that is the law, but that is the custom, and I think in London also.

There is another point in regard to the London statistics which is shown in the law upon that subject. Every child who is vaccinated, at any rate every one who is vaccinated at the public expense, must by law, under a penalty, be brought back to the public vaccinator at the end of one week to be examined. That is a very useful law indeed, because a great many physicians might otherwise vaccinate children and let them go without further inspection. It is a very lax mode of procedure to allow the child to pass out of your sight without seeing it again at the end of a week.

Then in regard to methods of selling vaccine lymph. In many cases we know nothing about the mode of obtaining it. That may come up hereafter. I won't speak of that now, but there is one thing which affects this question, — the age and freshness of lymph. Dr. Corey's vaccinations in London are made with fresh lymph. The calf is vaccinated at his station, and the children are brought there when the lymph is to be taken fresh, and the fresh lymph is inserted into the child's arm.

I think that would be a very good addition to our law, but perhaps it could not be enforced except where children were vaccinated at the public expense.

The CHAIRMAN. I would like to ask Dr. Abbott if he can give us some brief data as to the difference in protection between one and many scars.

Dr. ABBOTT. Well, upon that point the principal authority is Dr. Marson, of England, who has made that one point a specialty, having examined a great many cases. It is true that a thorough vaccination is more protective than a limited one. Dr. Marson gives the ratio. I cannot state what the ratio exactly is. It is a diminished one, according to the number of scars. That is, the number of persons who took smallpox with one vaccination mark was greater relatively than those who had two, three or four, or five, or six, as the case might be. It is a fact that old lymph, that is, three, four, or five weeks old, might not produce so large scar, when it produces any at all, as that which is fresh from the calf. I have noticed that myself: that sometimes lymph that is just losing its efficiency will give you a little vesicle perhaps no larger than a small pea or the head of a pin. Perhaps you may have noticed that, Dr. McCollom.

Dr. McCOLLOM. Yes, I have noticed it, although I never use lymph that is more than two, or three, or four days old.

Dr. ABBOTT. If we could do away entirely with the selling of vaccine lymph, and have it issued directly from a station, as it is in many foreign countries, directly to the physician who uses it, coming from a source that he knows he can rely upon as to the date it is taken from the animal, and not simply the date that it is sold to him,—as I have known here in Boston,— then we should have something that would be of value to us.

Dr. GAGE, of Lowell. I have been asked to say a word or two upon the technique of vaccination, and I will speak of these points : First, what we do when we vaccinate, and how we do it, and the responsibility of boards of health in seeing it done right.

I am not going to give an argument. I am simply going to state my belief and leave to you the discussion of it.

What do we do when we vaccinate? I suppose we introduce into the body a living organism. Possibly the living organism is the cause of small-pox. That is what we do theoretically. Practically we have introduced something besides this bug into the body, a germ which causes the formation of pus in the body.

How do we do it? I will tell you now how I do it. The arm of the patient is first made clean with scrubbing with soap, and water, and brush. By "clean" I mean sterilized. Then a fresh point is scratched upon the arm; and third, the arm is kept clean by putting on a sterile dressing, which is sealed on, and remains until the vaccination has taken.

Now, as I say, sometimes we do more than this. We introduce besides this living germ which causes pus,—and I want to state as my belief here that the germ, if it be that, or what we introduce for vaccination, does not cause a formation of pus.

I do not believe that is produced by the germ introduced for vaccination. I believe that is caused by filth, and that we are reprehensible for those results.

Now I want to speak of another matter in which boards of health are interested, and it is based upon my observations. I am going to speak right out in meeting. There is a law which compels corporations to vaccinate their employees, and when a board of health notifies a corporation that they must do it, they are obliged to do it. That is, it is done by the order of the board of health directly, not as a matter of law. Now, the corporations at home vaccinate in this way: They make a contract with some doctor to come there and vaccinate the employees, and I happen to know as a matter of fact that a large number of corporations at home made a contract this year to have their employees vaccinated in their mills at four cents a head. In order to make anything out of that, the doctor must vaccinate a given number of people in a given time, and he has vaccinated from sixty to eighty people an hour, and one woman claimed she vaccinated one hundred and twenty. That means two persons vaccinated in a minute. I think such methods are reprehensible. The boards of health are established for the promotion of the health of the community, and they should see that their orders are carried out properly. I believe that they should insist upon these three points,—a clean arm, a clean operation and clean dressing. I believe it is incumbent on boards of health, when they issue these orders to the agents of corporations, to see that this is done in accordance with sound principles. That is all I have to say on this subject.

I would like to say a word about vaccination as a preventive of small-pox. Dr. McCollom spoke of the isolation of the patient in a smallpox hospital. I think, if I could have only one of the two, either isolation or vaccination, I would give up isolation and take vaccination. I believe vaccination is always cheaper than an epidemic.

I do not agree with Dr. McCollom. I think the time will come when it will be a reproach to any city to have any epidemic, and I believe that time will come when we establish a quarantine.

Dr. ABBOTT. I would like to say one word in reference to the supposed insusceptibility of certain children. I do not believe it exists. Dr. Corey has vaccinated fifty thousand children in succession, without a single break. Some of those had to be revaccinated in order to make it take, to be sure, but they all took. (See Dr. Corey's testimony in Report of British Parliamentary Commission of 1889.)

The CHAIRMAN. It seems to me that this subject is not exhausted so long as there is anything to be said concerning the repetition of vaccination, its thoroughness and the susceptibility found in different individuals. We have those here who have done a great deal of this work. I would state, as a matter of fact, we have seen one case here in Boston where vaccination had never been successful, and that person was a nurse in the smallpox hospital for nearly twenty years, and never contracted the disease. That would represent one of the extremes, and I presume there are other extremes where we might find that a person would show a susceptibility to vaccination about as often as it was applied. Has Dr. McCollom any data that he would like to give us on that point?

The CHAIRMAN. The case to which I referred, Doctor, was not a man; it happened to be a woman, in the person of Mrs. Powers.

Dr. McCOLLOM. I do not know that I saw Mrs. Powers all the time she was there.

The CHAIRMAN. I think in her case vaccination had never succeeded, and she had never taken smallpox, although she was a very old nurse in the hospital.

Dr. DAVENPORT. Mr. Chairman: During the epidemic of 1871, when I was vaccinating for the city, one case I vaccinated where there was a scar of smallpox, and the vaccination took. As far as I could see, it was a typical take.

Dr. McCOLLOM. We have had half a dozen cases of a second attack of smallpox. In one case a man had a third attack of smallpox and died.

Dr. DAVENPORT. And there was an infant less than one year of age who died of a second attack.

Dr. C. C. ABBOTT, of Andover. I will report one case where we had a patient who had had smallpox, and showed the characteristic pitting on the face markedly, and as all the inmates of the house were vaccinated, I vaccinated him, making two marks on the arm, and he had two typical, well-marked vesicles. They came out, the scabs came off, and no ulceration followed, but the typical scar is very marked in his case. He had smallpox two or three years ago in some foreign country, and came here as a sailor. He said they let him go on account of the scars on his face.

The CHAIRMAN. Is there anything further to be said on this subject? If not, a motion to adjourn will be in order.

Adjourned.

ANTI-TOXINE.

BY DR. HAROLD C. ERNST.

Mr. President and Gentlemen,— What I have to say this afternoon will be distinctly a talk, not a formal paper : and I hope that, if I do not explain everything that you would like to know, you will question me, and I will answer to the best of my ability. Dr. Durgin asked me some ten days ago if I would be willing to appear here; and, of course, I expressed my readiness to do so, and to explain as well as may be what this so-called anti-toxine of diphtheria is, and perhaps to give some sort of guess of the methods by which it works. But, in the first place, before I can attempt to tell what it is,— for very few of us know exactly that,— I think you should understand the difficulties which there are in the way of preparing it, and know something of what the process is, and the reasons for it.

In the first place, before one can produce anti-toxine, he must procure the toxine of diphtheria. The toxine of diphtheria is a fairly well-known substance that is produced in cultures of the bacillus of diphtheria in the laboratory, and not only there, but also in the living body during and after every attack of diphtheria. The toxine of diphtheria is the active factor in producing the worst later symptoms of the disease, leaving an especial action upon the nervous centres, and, as a result, producing the unfortunate sequelæ of diphtheria, the paralyses of the soft palate and of various regions of the body. This toxine, after a long series of experiments, was shown to be produced, as I have already said, by the cultures of the bacillus of diphtheria, as they are carried on in the laboratory. And the result of the work that has been done shows that this toxine is produced in varying degrees and amount of intensity by different cultures, or rather by cultures of bacilli of diphtheria coming from different sources. That is one of the peculiar effects that has to be recognized, and is one of the causes of the long time necessary to produce anti-toxine. In cultures of the bacilli of diphtheria coming from two cases that appear to be of equal degree of malignancy, or a culture coming from a case of extreme malignancy and one coming from a case of apparently mild type, the chemical manifestations may or may not have the same degree of virulence in each instance. There are some cultures of bacilli of diphtheria from different sources that have the peculiarity of being what are called good toxine producers : and this is the first step in producing anti-toxine,— to secure a good toxine producer,— because, before one succeeds in producing anti-toxine, one must have the toxine.

Now, the way in which one goes about it is to obtain, if possible, a culture of the diphtheria bacillus that upon inoculation into guinea pigs will kill those animals within a certain limited time, the extreme limit being forty-eight hours. And, if death can be produced in less time, so much better is the prospect of getting a good toxine producer; but this is not certain at all. Having secured this culture, the next step is to develop it in what is called nutrient bouillon, consisting of a watery extract of meat which has been boiled. the coagulable albuminous material removed after boiling, and certain proportions of salt and peptone added to it.

Then there are two ways of procedure. One is that of the French that has been devised by Roux and Yersin, which consists in the placing of the cultures of diphtheria bacillus in this nutrient bouillon. in an apparatus where they may be maintained at a temperature of 37.5° C., and so arranged that a constant current of air may be passed over them, so that there will be a constant supply of oxygen, and also a supply of moisture, in order that there shall not be undue evaporation. Now, the reason of taking so much trouble is because the toxine produced by the culture of diphtheria in this bouillon is formed more rapidly under these conditions, while under the ordinary conditions in the incubator the toxine is produced in ten or twelve weeks or more. This method of passing the air over the material reduces the time necessary to produce it to about three weeks. This is the method which has been adopted in the preparation of the toxine by me for the Boston Board of Health; and I have here a diagram of the incubator used for producing it which has been specially constructed, and which will show what is going on at the present moment in the laboratory. This diagram shows the outline of the incubator, which is kept at a proper temperature by a small burner underneath supplied by gas passing through the regulator,— that part is according to the ordinary method. In the interior are these flasks, each of which contains a small amount of nutrient bouillon and the culture of the bacillus of diphtheria. There are tubes and other flasks in which are growing cultures of various degrees of virulence. There is a recording thermometer, giving us the exact temperature night and day. The wall on one side is perforated by brass tubes which run into the body of the incubator, and each of which has a stop-cock on the outside. There are twelve of these, four upon each shelf of the incubator. They are all led into one tube finally, which passes overhead, and is connected with the water supply through a filter-pump which, by a very small stream of water, draws the air through these tubes. And we can see how fast the air is running through each of the flasks by means of flasks filled with sterilized water, which also furnish the moisture. Now, each of the brass tubes passing through the outside of the incubator is arranged to have connection with six flasks in the interior. Each series of flasks may be cut off from the outside, and each individual one can be cut off by a pinch-cock. The apparatus, of course, had to be got up rather hurriedly; but I have not seen anything that has worked more perfectly than this since it started: it seems to serve the purpose exactly. The door is of heavy plate-glass, and over it is placed a curtain; for cultures, as a rule, grow best in a dark chamber rather than in one exposed to varying degrees of light. The cultures are grown in flasks which have two tubes passing through the stoppers. One goes close to the bouillon, taking the air to the culture; and the shorter tube is simply the exit.

The cultures, having been started in the incubator, are cultivated for at least three weeks; and then it is not simply the process of taking them out and getting rid of the bacilli, and starting with the animals, whatever they may be, but one must get the toxine to a certain degree of virulence. It is of no great use to begin these experiments until one reaches that point where the material is spoken of as normal toxine, which means a toxine produced in this way, and of such a degree of strength that one-tenth of a cubic centimetre will kill a guinea pig weighing five hundred grams within thirty-six hours. One must reach that degree of strength of toxine. Having arrived at such a point with the culture that the toxine should be about ready, the next step must be to take these flasks,— such as I have shown you,— and pass the fluid, which is full of virulent and dead bacilli, through a filter of unglazed porcelain. We have a special filter for that. The toxine, having been passed through this unglazed porcelain filter, comes out as a perfectly clear fluid, amber-colored, and entirely free from any bacteria at all: the bacilli are left behind. Then it must be tested, to be sure that it reaches, or perhaps surpasses, this standard which I have given you, which is that one-tenth of a cubic centimetre will be sufficient to kill a guinea pig weighing five hundred grams within thirty-six hours.

Then only is the next step to be begun,— the preparation of the anti-toxine in the animal that has been selected. The horse has been chosen for the purpose of producing the anti-toxine for several reasons. The same results can be obtained with almost any animal: but the reasons for employing the horse are, in the first place, that he is less susceptible to the poisonous effects of toxine than other animals, which are apt to die when least expected, or to become dangerously ill while undergoing immunization, so that the work done upon them may be all thrown away. This is true to a less degree of the horse, and to so much less a degree that the horse was considered safer to use. In the second place, horses furnish a much larger proportion of serum, and can be bled oftener than the other animals: and so they are less expensive.

The operations through which this immunity and the anti-toxine are obtained are delicate and prolonged, and may fail at almost any stage. The shortest time in which complete immunity has been reached that I know of is eighty days. the longest, eight months: and one cannot tell what kind of a horse one has got, and how long it will take to immunize him until the experiment is completed.

The method of immunizing is by the use of toxine subcutaneously, beginning with small doses, gradually repeated, the dose increasing in size until by experiment it is found that the stage of immunity has been reached. The process is something like this: the initial dose is one-half a cubic centimetre injected subcutaneously; and even that small quantity, if of normal strength, must be guarded by a mixture of iodine and iodide of potash. The results of the first inoculation are watched with much care, because upon them must be based further procedure. The use of the mixture of the gram solution is found to have less dangerous effects than the plain toxine. The proportion is about one-third in bulk of this mixture of iodine and iodide of potash and about two-thirds of toxine. Of that mixture on the first day there may be injected half a cubic centimetre. The result is usually fever, some local œdema, and some general disturbance of the horse, which passes away in two or three hours. Two or three days after a second injection of the same mixture may be given. It may be of the same size or slightly increased, and it may be repeated at intervals of two, three, or four days, never as often as every other day; say two, at the outside three times a week; sometimes at intervals of eight or ten days. This procedure is carried on until it reaches into the thirtieth or thirty-fifth day, when the dose should have been increased to such a size that thirty-five to sixty cubic centimetres of toxine may be injected at once without any more reaction, and even less, following than was produced by the injection of half a centimetre at the first. Such injections may run up to quantities as large as two or three hundred centimetres, and yet produce no marked result, no fever, œdema, or special trouble of any kind. Then only can one feel that one may have reached the point of immunity; and then only can one feel that this anti-toxic serum may have been produced for which one has been working for so long a time.

Now, the anti-toxine is contained in the blood serum of the horse. Precisely what it is I do not think anybody can explain. It may be, as some claim, the result of the increased activity of the nuclei of the various forms of tissue cells in the body. It may be produced by retrograde metamorphosis,— exactly what it is not definitely known. As far as regards toxine, there is something known about that, as was first shown by Wassermann and Proskauer. It is a definite body, and has definite characteristics, which seem to indicate that it is one of the proteids.

Then the question is, What does anti-toxine do? It is not, apparently, as shown by the experiments of Roux, a direct chemical antidote to toxine. This is a natural suggestion, that when one introduces the serum obtained by this process from the animal, and diphtheria ceases, what has apparently been done is to introduce a direct chemical antidote to toxine; but that is not so, and the most recent explanation of what anti-toxine does in the cure of diphtheria,— because it is not open to reasonable doubt that it does act in that way,— the most recent explanation is the supposition that it produces an increased cellular activity, making the individual cells of the body more resistant to the toxine. That is a tentative explanation, but it furnishes a working theory.

Now, in regard to the dose. When the use of it first began, it was necessary to have some standard upon which to base the question of dosage. There have been half a dozen different standards given. The same man has started at least three different ones, so that the confusion which may arise is a very natural one in the minds of those who are reading the literature. I have tried to put down here very briefly, and I think clearly, what the most easily understood basis of dosage is and should be. In the first place, as I have said, the normal toxine is the toxine of which half a cubic centimetre will kill a guinea pig weighing five hundred grams in forty-eight hours. The standard anti-toxine is that mixture of one-tenth of a cubic centimetre of anti-toxic serum added to nine-tenths of a cubic centimetre of normal toxine, making one cubic centimetre in all, which may be injected into a guinea pig of five hundred grams weight without producing any effect,— in other words, the one part completely neutralizing the nine parts. If you multiply that out a little, you will see that one cubic centimetre of such anti-toxine will neutralize nine cubic centimetres of toxine in five thousand grams of guinea pig, or will immunize that weight of guinea pigs. There you get a basis for dosage of human beings. If one cubic centimetre will immunize five thousand grams of guinea pig or of human beings, it will immunize a baby weighing from six to seven pounds: and for a person weighing more you multiply the number of cubic centimetres in proportion, and, to leave a margin of safety, the dose is increased a little. But it must be remembered that in practice we are peculiarly dependent upon the absolute honesty and accuracy of the producer of the material.

As to the future, it seems to me exceedingly promising. In the first place, if the anti-toxic serum of diphtheria proves successful, the next step in advance will be the complete isolation of the anti-toxine; and we shall be able to use it in small doses, precisely as we use morphia and other substances to-day. If there are any questions to be asked, I shall be glad to answer them.

The Chairman.— Professor Ernst's remarks are before the Association; and it is to be hoped we shall have other remarks and questions submitted to Dr. Ernst, for the gratification of those who are interested in this subject.

A Member.— How is the serum produced? In what manner is it drawn from the horse?

Dr. Ernst.— That I meant to have spoken of. It is drawn from the jugular vein. It does not require any very severe precautions. The blood is drawn with an ordinary canula, which has been washed with alcohol and ether, and is received in flasks plugged with cotton wool, and previously sterilized. The blood is allowed to clot; and, where the serum is separated, it is drawn off into sterilized pipettes. The time it is safe to keep it is not settled; but it is considerable,— weeks, perhaps months. It must be placed in vessels completely filled, to which have been added one-half of one per cent. of camphor. The toxine and anti-toxine both lose their power after a considerable time, but very slowly. How long is not definitely determined. It is a matter of weeks and months rather than of days; and there is no practical danger of putrefaction, though the serum must be preserved very carefully, or there may be unfortunate results in the future, which will be sure to be attributed to the material itself rather than to the handling of it. The material appears to be giving all the results that have been claimed for it. I have this week received a letter from one of my former students, written from Berlin, in which he says that Kossel claims that they have not yet lost a case of diphtheria that has been treated in the first or second stage of the disease.

A Member.— What length of time is to be allowed between the different administrations of the remedy, if it needs to be repeated?

Dr. Ernst.— In human beings the average is two doses, with about twelve to fourteen hours' interval. If the case has been so far of a bad type, showing malignant symptoms, affecting the bronchii, the dose may be doubled. If the case be handled in the first or second stage, before very malignant general symptoms have appeared, two doses are usually sufficient. I believe the first case treated in this neighborhood was by Dr. Rogers in Dorchester, in October; and its history is a very striking one. It was a case where the membrane had formed over the soft palate, and involved the pharynx and larynx. Within three hours after the first dose the membrane was manifestly loosened at the edges; and after the repetition of the dose the next morning the membrane came off in twenty-four hours, and never re-formed. It was a case which, under ordinary conditions, might have been expected to result in death within twenty-four hours. The child is well to-day.

Dr. Gardner T. Swarts.— The subject as explained by Dr. Ernst has been put exceedingly well, and is one which is going to be of extreme interest to boards of health throughout the country, as evinced by many of the boards taking the control in the disposition of the material by placing it where it can be dispensed to physicians; and, as the control of it in that way brings it to the attention of health boards generally, it is therefore of more interest to this society than the therapeutic detail. This matter of the anti-toxine of diphtheria is, of course, similar in its relations to what we have had in connection with other toxines and anti-toxines in other diseases; and it is not necessary to refer here to the immediate application of those. The application of this material is not only theoretically, but scientifically, correct; and, practically, the result of the experiments made by those who have used the material shows that the material does bring about that which has been expected of it. A question to be decided at present is the amount of material required in given cases. There is the well-known division of cases into the first, second, and third stage,— a distinction difficult to make in an arbitrary way, but it can be made for practical purposes, and in those different conditions different doses will be required; and as to what those doses shall be should rest with those who dispense the material, with the health boards or those who have control of it. The experience in Rhode Island has been thus far fortunate in the way of the control of the material. That which has been used has been introduced from the Pasteur Institute of New York; and through the kindness of the firm having control, Lehn & Fink of New York, no material was supplied the local druggists unless recommended or approved by the City Board of Health of Providence or by the State Board of Health. In that way the history of the work accomplished by every bottle that came into the State could be known; and it could be known that no false material came into the State. The details of all cases could be obtained. The anti-toxine was dispensed to such physicians as supposed they had actual cases of diphtheria; and a complete history of each case has been kept and the results noted. If every Board of Health would follow out that same course, we should have a mass of material which would be of immense service to the practitioners who will doubtless use this material as their chief remedy.

There are two or three questions I should like to ask of Dr. Ernst. First, as to the value of different products now on the market. There are the Behring product, the French product, and others,— some available, and some not. The Pasteur Institute sends out its material, with the legend attached "immunizing power, 1 to 50,000," while the Behring solution is supplied in three strengths,— 1 to 600, 1 to 1,000, and 1 to 1,500: but as to the comparative values I am at a loss, and I should like to inquire, in order to obtain some information, as to which product is to be preferred, and how the dose of one compares with the dose of another.

DR. ERNST.— I am afraid I shall have to decline to answer that question. I do not think it is fair for me to be asked to express an opinion. I can say this: I believe the Boston Board of Health has taken the proper course; that is, to make it itself. We have a very large community, and should have this matter under our control. If the smaller communities cannot make it themselves, I think they should combine; and I hope the Boston Board of Health will agree that, in case we shall have so large a supply that we can afford to do it, we will supply the smaller communities, if necessary, at cost of production. As to guaranteeing anybody else's product, I should not think of it, particularly in this material. I would not consider it a moment. Neither would I recommend any special one. I would recommend the use of the anti-toxine for diphtheria, but I don't think I should be called upon to name any particular product.

DR. SWARTS.— Is there any way of interpreting the values of the different products?

DR. ERNST.— Those of New York are based upon the standard I mentioned, I believe. The Behring and others are based upon the German standard; and, as Behring has already had three standards of nomenclature, I do not know how many more he will have before he gets through. You must take the directions that come on each bottle.

PROFESSOR T. M. DROWN.— How much serum is obtained, and is the horse bled more than once?

DR. ERNST.— The horse may be bled indefinitely. Roux has been bleeding one for three years. They are bled about once a month, and furnish from one to three litres. That involves the question of maintaining the degree of immunity which the horse has attained, whether it is to be done by an injection, after the first bleeding, of a large quantity of toxine or whether the immunity is to be maintained by repeated doses of a smaller quantity. These differences of manipulation are shown by the differences which occur in different methods. The French never inject at one time more than 250 centimetres of toxine. The Germans have been seen to inject 4 litres in bulk; but, whether it is toxine pure or toxine mixture. I do not know.

A MEMBER.— What is the mixture?

DR. ERNST.— Nobody knows.

A MEMBER.— What is the mixture of the normal anti-toxine for injection? What is the vehicle?

DR. ERNST.— It is just itself.

A MEMBER.— In a case of malignant diphtheria would the doctor separate the other children or wait until they have an attack? Would he inoculate the other children with the anti-toxine?

DR. ERNST.— The routine thing is not only to treat the patients who have the disease, but the injection is made, as a matter of course, with all the persons who have been exposed before the symptoms appear. That reminds me of a curious fact. The immunizing of animals was secured four or five years ago by Fraenkel, Kitasato, and Brieger. The first paper upon the subject came out four years ago last fall, and that immunity was obtained by the continued use of toxine before the anti-toxine was known. Immunity is practically obtained now, but the two immunities are entirely different. Immunity after the use of toxine is slow in coming, difficult to obtain, and dangerous: but it is permanent. Immunity obtained by anti-toxine is easy to obtain, but is very fleeting, only lasting about two weeks. That is a very curious difference.

THE CHAIRMAN.— Professor Kinnicutt, have you a word to say?

PROFESSOR L. P. KINNICUTT, of Worcester.— I have been very much interested, but I know nothing absolutely about the subject. I have learned a great deal from the remarks of Dr. Ernst, and I express my personal thanks to him for his illustration of the matter.

DR. J. A. FITZHUGH, of Amesbury.— I represent a small community free from diphtheria, and I hope it will continue so: but I may have a case. I understand that the Boston Board of Health is not prepared to furnish us with anti-toxine, and that the available material is the French, or from Pasteur's Institute in New York. In a case of necessity what ought we to do at the present time?

DR. ERNST.— I should not suppose it would be possible to supply the entire demand for this article at the present time. If I were sick or had a case to treat, I should take the first supply I could reach, and trust to that.

DR. SWARTS.— Is there any one present who has used these different anti-toxines? and has the experiment shown a satisfactory result, as indicating whether the anti-toxine which is supplied by the Pasteur Institute, or that of Behring or Schering, is to be preferred?

THE CHAIRMAN.— I am told that Dr. French, of Clinton, has had some experience with anti-toxine; and we shall be glad to hear from him.

DR. C. L. FRENCH, of Clinton.— I have had a little experience in the use of anti-toxine. As soon as I knew it could be obtained in this country, I ordered a supply from the New York Institute. with instruments for using it: and within three days' time I had a case,— a child, five years old, who had a very suspicious membrane in his throat. I made a local application to the throat, and within twelve hours the membrane was almost entirely gone. The patient continued comfortable: but the membrane returned, and a second application removed it as before. Two or three days afterwards symptoms of croup developed, and those symptoms became very severe; and I considered that it was a case of membranous croup. The child was growing worse, suffering from difficulty of breathing. Then I decided to try the anti-toxine, which I had just been able to procure. First I took a culture from the throat, and sent it to Dr. Ernst. I injected at four o'clock in the afternoon fifteen cubic centimetres of anti-toxine, and from what I had known of it I didn't expect marked results under twenty-four hours. I expected to have to perform tracheotomy on the child; but at 7.30 that evening it was evident to me that the child was breathing easier. There was a little rattle there which I didn't get before: there was an elevation of temperature which I expected. The child grew no worse. He was not markedly improved, but it was evident he was getting no worse.

In twelve or fourteen hours after I injected ten cubic centimetres, making the whole number twenty-five. The child had a very hoarse cough, and I didn't feel entirely at ease about my patient. In forty-eight hours after the first injection he had grown no worse, and there was a little improvement. After that the improvement was more marked; and he made a perfect recovery, and is now well. When I took the culture, there was no membrane to be seen, and it seemed to me doubtful if I should get a report of " diphtheria "; but the report came from Dr. Ernst that it was a case of diphtheria. So, while I took from the throat material that showed no appearance of membrane, it seems he had the bacilli of diphtheria there; and it seems to me that no greater proof is needed that diphtheria may develop into membranous croup. Within a week or ten days I had a second case of croup, which, it seemed to me, was of a membranous character, though there was no membrane in the throat; and this was in a family where I had six weeks before performed tracheotomy for membranous croup on a child who afterwards recovered. The other children in the family were sent away at once to another house; and they afterwards developed sore throats, which had a look of diphtheritic character, but it was very mild, and they both recovered. But this second patient developed membranous croup, and the case was getting so bad I decided to treat him the same way. I took a culture which I sent to Dr. Ernst. My second patient had very much the same experience as the first. He was growing constantly worse, and I gave the injection of anti-toxine; and I gave a second injection in twelve or fourteen hours, as in the first case, and in two or three days the breathing was satisfactory, and he made a good recovery. But my report upon this second case to Dr. Ernst was that no bacilli were found. That is all I have to say about those cases.

I should like to ask Dr. Ernst what are the chances of our missing a correct diagnosis; whether on taking one culture from the throat, and on examination bacilli are not found, it is pretty positive proof that there are none there. I sent a culture yesterday from a case which, it seemed plain to me, was one of diphtheria: and I received a report to-day that it is not so.

Now, I suppose it is not; but I should like to ask that question. Perhaps I am not very expert in taking a culture, but I should like to know what the chances are in taking a culture of making a miss of it.

DR. ERNST.— In nine cases out of ten the method is more accurate than the clinical examination, but there are chances for error that it is almost impossible to guard against. Before I would advocate this method for general application, during my work with Dr. McCollom in my laboratory last year we carefully studied the whole subject, and asked for cases of sore throat where diphtheria was not suspected, and with the very purpose of determining how accurate this method of diagnosis might be made. As the result of that year's work, something like 800 cases were submitted to us for examination, and of them about 125, I think, were diphtheritic, and we learned a great deal; and the first thing was that, if this method is properly followed out, it is very accurate. I don't know whether the directions that are printed on the boxes that are sent out are definite and clear, and, if they are not, we should be only too thankful to get suggestions; but, if they are followed, it seems to me the results are very accurate. We have had cases sent to us where we have not found bacilli, and on the second examination we found them. A culture was sent within a fortnight that was negative, and the case died. Before the case died, the culture was said to have been made as accurately as it could be. It was made by a gentleman working in my laboratory; and, if he did it properly, I should not feel it was a case of diphtheria. The second point last year's work appeared to confirm was this: that there may be a formation of membrane or there may be none, the case following the exact clinical course of diphtheria, where it is *not* true diphtheria. If we take as the standard that disease which is produced by the bacillus of diphtheria,— and that is what we are working upon now,— that other bacteria may produce similar symptoms I think is true, but not common. As to treating those cases with anti-toxine, the practice in diphtheria hospitals in Berlin is not even to wait for the culture diagnosis; but every child that comes in is treated with anti-toxine. It does no harm; and. if it is a true case of diphtheria, no time is lost.

There is another little point which has created some criticism: and that is the method of making these cultures which we have adopted, by the use of the platinum wire, and not the cotton swab. We sought to determine the advantage of one over the other; and we came definitely to the conclusion that the platinum wire is the best thing, though somewhat more trouble to use, for the reason that with the cotton swabs we tried some of the cultures we got gave a negative result. The reason appears to be this: that the cotton swab may be several hours in being transported. and the material may get inside of the meshes, and it takes time to get it out again: and, in the second place, the wire takes a smaller quantity (at the same time all that is necessary), the culture is made at once at the bedside, and the growth begins then, if it begins at all. It begins then, and there is less chance for an obscure result. So it appears to me that the wire is the best thing to use.

A MEMBER.— We have only been using it for three weeks. I am the agent of the Board of Health, and what the physicians have told me is this: We have furnished in all some eleven bottles for cases that have occurred this year. Four were serious ones : the physicians told me they were in a very bad way. We have had no deaths whatever : the four bad cases entirely recovered. The hospital had three of them, and the clinical record there is very interesting. The only unfavorable result which has been noticed from the use of anti-toxine furnished by the New York institute has been a slight case of heart disturbance. That was the effect of its use on one of the nurses. A slight attack of heart trouble was experienced, but other than that nothing of the kind.

DR. ERNST.— One of the Newton physicians tried it on himself, and it had the same effect.

DR. S. W. ABBOTT.— I should like to answer a question that has been asked as to how this material may be procured in the future. The State Board has already initiated the proper procedure for producing anti-toxine. It has been at work for several weeks. We have five horses under treatment, and we hope to be able to issue the material to those Boards of Health that may require it. Just how it will be issued and how soon it may be ready I cannot state.

DR. J. E. CLARK, of Medford.— I will mention the case of a woman fifty-five years old, to whom anti-toxine was given. She had been suffering several days with a severe laryngeal diphtheria. At the time of the administration of the serum there was decided improvement as to the throat symptoms, the membranes having nearly disappeared : but the heart action was weak. Accordingly, 15 centimetres of the New York (Pasteur) preparation were used. The next morning, twelve hours after this treatment, the patient was visited, and found greatly improved in every way, a speedy, uneventful recovery following. As this person was very enthusiastic as to the efficacy of serum treatment, the question arose how much of the results manifested was due to anti-toxine and how much to " suggestion."

Several members of the family of this patient were immunized. No unpleasant effects followed.

As to the value of taking cultures : I had a case of diphtheria in the latter part of December. The diagnosis of the disease was made by the usual methods of inspection, etc. The patient, a lady. having a nursing child about six months old, was advised to send him away as a matter of precaution. Before returning, a culture was taken, although the patient was apparently well, and her throat had been perfectly clean about a week or ten days. The test revealed the presence of diphtheritic bacilli, and the parents advised against the return of the child till the cultures should prove negative. In a recent case of obstetrics one of the children in the family developed a sore throat of a very suspicious aspect. To absolutely determine its nature, a culture was taken, proving negative. By this measure much anxiety was quickly allayed.

From what I have stated the culture test is necessary in making absolutely certain diagnoses of the existence or not of diphtheria. My attention has been called to cases with simply running at the nose, but afterwards were found to be diphtheritic. In such the culture test is demanded.

I think physicians, particularly boards of health, should require cultures to be taken in all cases where the disease has existed previous to permitting school children of the infected premises to return to school, and the parties affected going about and mingling with the public.

Mr. Coffey.— I should like to instance a case which occurred at Worcester. It was that of a child three years of age, who had laryngeal croup. Two or three cultures were made, without finding Klebs-Loeffler bacilli. The child subsequently died, and an autopsy was performed, and cultures taken from various organs of the body: but the subsequent examination failed to show the diphtheria bacilli. Streptococci were found in large numbers, however; and, in the opinion of our bacteriologist, death was due to that cause.

Dr. Dike, of Melrose.— I should like to ask Dr. Ernst if other measures are advised in addition to the use of anti-toxine: the usual measures.

Dr. Ernst.— The routine is nothing but supporting treatment.

Dr. Dike.— You would not advise any other measures?

Dr. G. T. Swarts.— It has been stated in some of the foreign articles upon this subject that the use of carbolic acid or corrosive sublimate as a gargle or application to the throat was objectionable, inasmuch as it might neutralize the action of serum. I have had experience in injecting the serum in but fifteen cases. In ten of these the examination of the sections from the throat showed the presence of the Klebs-Loeffler bacillus. Four of these cases were of the severe type; that is, the membrane had extended into the larynx and nares, accompanied with extreme prostration and short and rapid breathing and that ashy, waxy look which appears in the severe cases. The results in these cases were most gratifying.

In the recommendation of Dr. Ernst that a platinum wire be used, and inserted under the membrane, it has seemed to me that by the previous heating of the wire for the purpose of sterilizing it, in the presence of the patient, especially in the case of a child, will make it difficult to convince the patient that the wire has cooled.

In the case of a struggling child, or where only a quick, hasty examination of the throat can be made, the physician will be more successful in obtaining the secretions from the back of the throat with the use of the cotton swab, which has been sterilized in a test tube before being delivered to the physician.

The use of the swab precludes the possibility of doing injury to the mucous membrane, and the physician will feel freer to search about in the pharynx than with a sharp wire. To the objection to the swab suggested by Dr. Ernst, that the organisms dry up in the meshes of the cotton, I would say that it is presupposed that the culture is made at once upon a serum tube sent with the swab in the same box. This is the method adopted by the Board of Rhode Island, and is copied from the practice of the Boards of Health in New York City, Brooklyn, and in the District of Columbia.

Our Board, as also that of the city of Providence, has thus far supplied the serum, free, to all cases where the patients were unable to pay for the same, and have also supplied or loaned the syringe, the first injection, wherever practicable, being applied by a member of the Board. In this way there has been no delay in applying the material either for supply or for want of instruments,— an essential feature in a disease which does not wait for the movements of the physician.

It was moved and seconded that Dr. Ernst receive the thanks of the Association for his able and interesting remarks, and the notion was unanimously carried.

The meeting was then adjourned.

MASSACHUSETTS ASSOCIATION OF BOARDS OF HEALTH.

Organized 1890.

[This Association as a body is not responsible for statements or opinions of any of its members.]

VOL. VI.   January, 1896.   NO. 1

JANUARY QUARTERLY MEETING

OF THE

Massachusetts Association of Boards of Health.

NOTE.— It will be observed that the present issue of the *Journal* contains several items of sanitary news in addition to the usual report of the Association. It is hoped in time to print each quarter a careful *résumé* of everything which occurs throughout the State of interest to sanitarians : and sanitary officers everywhere are cordially invited to send to the editor, in care of Maynard & Small, P.O. Box 2510, Boston, any material of general interest which may come to their notice. All such information will be gratefully acknowledged, and, if available, used in the *Journal*.

The January quarterly (or annual Boston) meeting of the Massachusetts Association of Boards of Health was held at the Parker House, Boston, on the afternoon of Thursday, Jan. 23, 1896. In the absence of the President, H P. Walcott. M.D., the Vice-President, S. H. Durgin. M.D., presided. The meeting was called to order shortly before three o'clock, and the Chairman called upon the Secretary to read the records of the last meeting. The records were then read, and declared approved, no corrections being offered.

THE CHAIRMAN.— The next business will be the report of the Executive Committee, which will be read by the Secretary.

THE SECRETARY.— The Executive Committee recommends for membership the following-named gentlemen : —

> A. D. HOLMES, M.D., Hyde Park.
> J. C. LINCOLN, M.D., Hyde Park.
> EDWIN C. FARWELL, Hyde Park.
> Prof. H. C. ERNST, M.D., Jamaica Plain.
> THEOBALD SMITH, M.D., Jamaica Plain.
> JOSEPH S. BIGELOW, Cohasset.

It was moved and seconded that the gentlemen whose names had been read should be elected members of the Association. The motion was carried.

THE CHAIRMAN.— The next business will be the reading of the Treasurer's report.

The Treasurer's report was then read and accepted. It is as follows : —

ANNUAL REPORT OF TREASURER FOR 1895.

Receipts.

Balance from 1894	$390.66
Received from annual assessments	336 00
	$726.66

Expenditures.

Stenographic report of meetings	$101.65
Postage	34.97
Printing	31.65
Typewriting and stationery	6.55
Extra dinner and cigars	5.70
Total expenses	$180.52
Balance to 1896	546.14
	$726.66

Respectfully submitted,

JAMES B. FIELD, *Treasurer.*

Examined and approved as correctly cast and properly vouched for.

JAMES C. COFFEY, *Auditor.*

JAN. 23, 1896.

THE CHAIRMAN.— The next business in order is the election of officers for the ensuing year. How shall this be done?

THE SECRETARY.— I move that a committee of three be appointed by the Chairman to present a ticket to the Association.

The motion was carried, and the chair appointed Messrs. Coffey, Pillsbury, and Newhall.

MR. GEORGE F. BABBITT.— Mr. Chairman, I do not know what this Association is going to do with the enormous surplus they have; and some of us have thought that a large surplus is a menace and danger to any organization. I know there was a motion presented at the last meeting, and I think adopted, that for the coming year the assessment be reduced to $2. I do not know why it should not be reduced to $1. I say this to bring it before the Association. I am not particularly anxious about it; but such an assessment would be ample to carry on the business of the Association, as I understand.

THE CHAIRMAN.— It would be in order to give notice that such an amendment to the by-laws would be presented at the next meeting. It has to go over to another meeting.

MR. BABBITT.— Well, then, I do that; but it is in order for discussion, I suppose, if anybody wants to discuss it.

THE CHAIRMAN.— No. I think it has to be discussed at the next meeting, but a written notice now would be in order for the next meeting.

The committee appointed to present a list of officers for the ensuing year then returned; and Mr. James C. Coffey, of Worcester, presented the report of the committee, as follows : —

MR. COFFEY.— The committee have attended to the business committed to them, and are ready to report. I must say that we are fortunate this year, as we always have been since the organization was founded, in not having any candidates for the offices. Consequently, the committee brought in the old list of officers just as they were last year, with the exception of Mr. Babbitt, who declines to serve on the Executive Committee; and we have substituted Mr. William H. Gove, of Salem, in his stead, so that the report of the committee is as follows : —

President.
HENRY P. WALCOTT, M.D.

Vice-Presidents.
S. H. DURGIN, M.D.   S. W. ABBOTT, M.D.

Secretary.
EDWIN FARNHAM, M.D.

Treasurer.
JAMES B. FIELD, M.D.

Executive Committee.
W. P. BOWERS, M.D.   G. L. TOBEY, M.D.   NATHANIEL HATHAWAY.
W. H. GOVE.   W. Y. FOX, M.D.

I move that that list be accepted and elected, and that the Secretary cast the ballot of the Association to that effect.

The motion was seconded and carried.

THE CHAIRMAN.— It is a pleasure to me to take it upon myself to thank the Association for the entire list. [Laughter.] The next business before the meeting is of a miscellaneous character. If any one has a motion to make, it is now in order.

DR. S. W. ABBOTT.—Mr. Chairman, I would like to say a word or two in regard to the publications of the Association. They have now completed the fifth year of these publications, and I understand they are becoming somewhat popular outside the State. There are some taken outside, and probably the number will increase. Their value is increasing as they grow older, and I think it is desirable to make these publications as good as they can be. I want to say there are in the series, if you wish to bind them, some five volumes now. There are two defects in the series. The first number of the second volume never was issued, and the third number of the third volume. So, if you desire to get those numbers, I think it is doubtful whether you can. I never have been able to find any. I do not think they could have been published. The old publishers have left the State, and it is impossible to obtain any knowledge of them; but otherwise the series would be complete. And, in order to make this publication still better, I thought I would make this motion, " That the Publication Committee of this Association be authorized to print from time to time in the quarterly transactions of the Association any items of information which said committee may deem useful to the local boards of health in Massachusetts, in addition to the regular business transacted at the meetings of the Association." I do this for the reason that sometimes during the three months between the meetings there are things that come up that might be somewhat useful. Here is a pamphlet, for instance, that was published only a few days ago, with some things in it which might be preserved in our records, and would be useful to certain boards of health. For instance, there are at least twenty-five public institutions in the State of Massachusetts. There are post-offices in every town. There are custom-houses and light-houses on our coast. And there is a question as to what authority local boards of health have over the government of such institutions. There was a question which came up in the town of Concord not long ago, where the board of health of the town of Concord submitted this question to the attorney-general, having reference to the State prison, whether the board of health of the town has authority over it. Now, this question is liable to come up anywhere,— for instance, in the new hospital to be erected in Rhode Island, or in insane asylums or the State prison, or a dozen other such places; and I think this pamphlet has some things in it which would be desirable to have published in our own *Journal.* I think anything of that sort that might come up during the year would be desirable for the Publication Committee to publish.

Mr. Edmund M. Parker.— Mr. Chairman, I wish to second the motion which Dr. Abbott has just made, and, in seconding it, to say the subject to which he has referred is one that has often come before us in the local board of Cambridge. We appreciate the value which has already been given the publications of this Association, and which may be given to future publications ; and, in saying that, I have no doubt I voice the sentiment of those present. We shall be very glad to see those publications take a wider range and have a still greater usefulness than they possess at present ; and perhaps in such publications may be found a remedy for the evils which have been already referred to of the enormous surplus, which I should be happy to see reduced by such a publication. I second the motion of Dr. Abbott.

The Chairman.— I would say that it will not cost the Association one dollar more for this extra publication, and that it will be a comfort to the printer to have this material brought for insertion in the report. It is moved and seconded that the Committee on Publication be authorized to print from time to time interesting matters which may affect the interests of the boards of health of the State in the quarterly *Journal*. Those in favor of the motion will say aye.

The motion was carried.

The Chairman.— I would give an invitation to any and all members of the Association to send such items to the Committee on Printing, and they will receive early notice. As I understand this vote, it is to be left in the discretion of the Committee on Publication as to whether any particular item shall be printed or not. Is that the intent of this motion? There should be some guard of this sort, otherwise the committee will be flooded with a great variety of things which it might or might not desire to insert in the *Journal*.

Mr. Parker.— Mr. Chairman, there is another matter to which I would like to refer, under the head of miscellaneous business, if the present one has received all the discussion desirable. I desire to make this motion, if it is proper for me, that the Legal Committee be requested to consider such amendments to the present law as may be desirable for increasing the power of the local boards of health in reference to quarantining and isolation of contagious cases, and disinfection. There are chances for improvement in this matter, and possibly there are more needed powers which we do not at present possess which might well be added. I refer to one instance in particular, and that is the question of our power over people who have been exposed to disease in houses from which a patient afflicted with disease has been removed. There may be, I think very probably there is, considerable question as to the exact extent of the power of a local board of health over people who have been so exposed and have not yet come down with the disease. I should like very much personally to see enacted in this State a law similar to that which obtains in our sister State of Maine, and the motion I make is that the committee be authorized to present such legislation as is needed to the present legislature for enactment.

The motion was seconded.

THE CHAIRMAN.— I do not know as I shall be able to follow the motion exactly; but. as I understand it, it is moved and seconded that the Committee on Legislation be authorized to consider the necessary amendments to the existing laws concerning contagious diseases and the powers of boards of health for quarantining the same, and appear before the proper legislative committee to favor such amendments. Is that near enough, Mr. Parker?

MR. PARKER.— Fully.

The motion was carried.

MR. J. C. BRIMBLECOM.— Mr. Chairman, I would move that the same committee, in considering the subject of quarantining and isolation and disinfection, also consider the subject of the present laws relating to the powers of boards of health to remove patients from their homes to a hospital. It seems to me that the present law is not adequate or is complicated in its method. and that the committee be requested to consider the advisability of simplifying and strengthening the law which will allow boards of health to remove persons to hospitals.

THE CHAIRMAN.— I should be inclined to think that that was embraced in the previous motion; but, if the Association feels differently, we will take that as a separate motion and act upon it.

MR. BRIMBLECOM.— If the motion already adopted includes that, I shall be glad to withdraw mine; but I thought the matter of quarantine and isolation did not cover removal.

THE CHAIRMAN.— Does any one second Mr. Brimblecom's motion?

The motion was seconded.

THE CHAIRMAN.— It is moved and seconded that the Legislative Committee be authorized to consider what amendments may be necessary to make the duties of boards of health clear as to quarantining, isolation, and removal of cases of contagious disease.

The motion was carried.

DR. EDWARD A. SAWYER.— Mr. Chairman, in connection with this same matter that has been brought up for consideration, I should like to ask for information for myself, and I find there are others who would like the same information, what authority or what power local boards of health have over parochial schools in this matter which we have just been considering.

THE CHAIRMAN.— I think there are legal gentlemen present who might make this clear. I would say as my own expression that it has seemed to the older boards that the health authority has the same jurisdiction over the parochial school that it has over any other school. It has not been clearly decided whether the local boards of health have a right to close those schools. In some places it has been found necessary for the board of health to order the school closed. I do not think that question has been tested. In most places, however, the advice of the board of health to the school committee has been sufficient to accomplish all that was desired. I should be very glad to have the legal gentleman answer such questions. I think Mr. Parker might say something.

MR. PARKER.— Mr. Chairman, I feel that the Association has already been very indulgent on account of the time I have taken up. I cannot say much in addition to what you have already said; but I will say that we have come to the conclusion in Cambridge, which you have already so clearly stated, that the power of the local board of health over the parochial school is the same as it is over any other school. I will amplify that a little by saying that, if the local board of health felt that the adoption of a certain regulation was necessary to prevent the spread of contagious diseases in a city or town, there was nothing in the law which exempted a parochial school from its operation. I think you told me once, Mr. Chairman, that the Board of Health of Boston had been advised in regard to the attendance of children in the public schools something to the effect that no scholar who had been affected with a contagious disease or who came from a household in which such disease existed should be permitted to return to the school without a certificate of the Board of Health; and the same rule can be applied to the parochial school, when it is necessary to prevent the spread of contagious diseases in the community. We know of no reason why the parochial school, by reason of being a parochial school, should be exempted from such a condition.

THE CHAIRMAN.— We have a statute law in reference to public schools, but the parochial school would not be regarded as within that provision. The parochial school is to all intents and purposes a private school, but with us in Boston there has been the most hearty co-operation with the Board of Health in every regulation and every step that we have taken affecting the schools; and the parochial school management has very generously acquiesced in all the requirements, so that the question of right has never arisen here.   Is there any other miscellaneous business?

THE SECRETARY.— I hereby cast a ballot for the officers of the Association for the ensuing year, which has been read by copy.

THE CHAIRMAN.— My thanks were a little premature, but I repeat them.   [Laughter.]   Is there any other miscellaneous business?

MR. BRIMBLECOM.— I would like to move "that the committee on legislation be requested to appear at the hearing before the Legislative Committee on Health upon a bill, which is an annual bill, which has been before the committee for seven or eight years, prohibiting the feeding of city garbage to food animals."   I was very much astonished last year when I came before that committee, and a bill was before them, to find there was no one representing this Association present in favor of the bill.   It was unanimously opposed by the Market Gardeners' Association, and was amended so that it was of no practical value to the boards of health as to the care of garbage.   Dr. Osgood told us at our Brookline meeting that 99 per cent. of the cases of trichinosis reported to the Cattle Association was traced to the feeding of garbage to swine, and it seems to me that anything so vitally affecting the health of animals which are intended for consumption should cause this Association to urge upon the legislature the passage of the bill which is now before it.   I move you, sir, that the committee be requested to appear in favor of that bill.

The motion was seconded and carried.

MR. COFFEY.— Mr. Chairman, I want to move that the Legislative Committee be increased by two.   It now consists of but three members, and there are times, of course, when it might be impossible for one or more of them to be present; and, if the committee were increased, of course we could rely upon it that perhaps two or more might be able to attend whatever hearings might be held, and I would move that the chair be empowered to increase the committee by the addition of two members at some future time.   I do not intend he shall do it immediately.   I want to give him an opportunity to look the field over and select two men at some future time, and he can notify them of their selection.   I make that motion, that the Legislative Committee be increased to five.

The motion was seconded and carried.

THE CHAIRMAN.— I am reminded of an omission to ask the vote on increasing the publication of the *Journal*.   You heard the motion which has been seconded concerning the admission of items to the *Journal*.   Those in favor of this motion will say aye.

The motion was carried.

DR. SAWYER.—Mr. Chairman, I suppose under the head of miscellaneous business it will be proper to take some action in regard to our next meeting; and I will be just as brief as possible in stating what I have to say. That matter is one of some considerable importance, as there seems to be a growing feeling among the members of this organization that we are not spreading out as much as we ought to; that we are somewhat exclusive, not because we wish to be so, but in the natural course of events; and some members have suggested that, as we had no standing invitation to any of the western towns or cities, we vote ourselves to hold our next meeting at some one of the western towns or cities. Wherever the organization is known and its objects understood, a great deal of interest is taken in this body. Its publications are of great value, not only to the local boards of health, but, I think, to all who are interested in health matters; and it seems to me that, if there is any way by which we can extend our influence and our helpfulness, we should do so. On the other hand, we have a very cordial invitation from the city of Salem to hold our next meeting there; and, in order that the sense of this meeting may be taken, I desire to ask the Chairman if he will put the matter to vote whether we shall hold our next meeting in Salem or whether we shall vote to hold it at some western town or city.

THE CHAIRMAN.— I would say one word to the effect that we might suit one side of the question in April and the other in October. It will be necessary for some motion to be made as to this question. If some one will make a motion, the chair is ready to hear it.

MR. GOVE.— Mr. Chairman, as Chairman of the Board of Health of Salem, I desire to extend the invitation which has been referred to. I make a motion that the next meeting be held in Salem, and we will try to entertain the Association suitably if it chooses to come there.

The motion was seconded and carried.

THE CHAIRMAN.— Is there any other miscellaneous business?

DR. CLARENCE W. SPRING.— Mr. Chairman, we have about 55 cows on our list of inspection in our town. We have a quarantine station. The towns of Sterling and Lunenburg are sending milk into our town without being inspected, and we have done everything we can to stop it. I should like to ask for information if there is any way we can stop Sterling, Fitchburg, and Lunenburg sending their milk into our town without its being inspected.

THE CHAIRMAN.— That would be hardly germane to this part of the meeting.

DR. SPRING.— All right.

THE CHAIRMAN.— Is there any other miscellaneous business? If not we will proceed at once to the discussion of Dr. Abbott's report on Death Certificates, printed in the last *Journal*. I will call on Dr. Farnham to start the discussion.

DR. FARNHAM.— Dr. Abbott's Report on Death Certificates is one of which the Association may well be proud, and its thanks are due to him for the clear and able manner in which the subject has been treated. So well has the work been done that little remains to be said save in the way of approval. The time is past when it was necessary to contend that our death certificates needed some alteration; for all who have given the subject attention know that upon the correctness of these certificates depend, among other things, the value of the statistics dealing with the death-rates of the various diseases, and of the liability of certain ages and of the sexes to be affected by particular diseases. As some members of the Association are not obliged to read death certificates, and so remain in ignorance of the vexations of those who have to bring some order out of the chaos at times prevailing among them, I will give briefly a few facts gathered from the returns made in Cambridge during one year. The subject has already been treated by Dr. W. Y. Fox, in a paper read at a meeting of the Association held at Cambridge in October, 1894, and published in the *Journal*.

Among the causes of deaths classed as ill-defined, those of most frequent occurrence during the year 1894 were convulsions, marasmus, inanition, debility, natural causes.

Debility must be an accompaniment of most causes of death, if we except sudden deaths from violence.

Natural causes is presumably intended to convey the impression that there is no suspicion of foul play. Neither debility nor natural causes conveys any idea as to what the disease was of which the person died.

Inanition is defined to be " starvation, due to deficiency or mal-assimilation of food " (Century Dictionary). If deficiency of food is meant, it had better be called starvation. If the term means mal-assimilation of food, that is the result of some morbid condition, either unknown or not stated.

Marasmus is defined to be " a wasting of the flesh. The term is usually restricted to cases in which the cause of the wasting is obscure " (Century Dictionary). It is thus the result of a condition unknown or not stated. A convulsion is defined to be " involuntary contraction of voluntary muscles " (National Medical Dictionary). This is obviously a phenomenon that may be due to various morbid conditions seated in different parts of the animal economy.

In the year 1894, under these five terms were grouped 122 cases, about 8 per cent. of all deaths recorded that year.

There were 22 other deaths certified as due to the following causes : —

Abdominal disease, 1; asphyxia, 3; atrophy, 1 ; dentition, 1; dropsy, 2; exhaustion, 2; heart failure, 9; malarial consumption, 1; neurasthenia, 1; stomach trouble, 1.

There were some other cases, which, though obscure to me, may have had a meaning for the certifying physician; and I have therefore passed them over, giving the certifier the benefit of the doubt.

After physicians have been educated to make out proper death certificates, there will still remain a number of obscure cases in which fuller information is necessary to render the certificate satisfactory; and for the investigation of these cases a body of experts will be needed. It has been shown by our esteemed Vice-President, Dr. Durgin, that there is already in existence a body of officials eminently fitted to discharge this duty, the Medical Examiners. If we can secure the adoption of Dr. Abbott's form for certificates, and the passage of an act requiring examination of and report upon deaths resulting from obscure causes, by the Medical Examiners, then a great step in advance will have been made.

The Chairman.— Dr. Macdonald.

Dr. W. G. Macdonald.— Mr. Chairman, I have been very much interested in the matter as presented by the committee. I had a number of death certificates from five or six cities of the country, but they have disappeared from my pocket during the dinner. I do not know what has become of them. However, I do say that at the time of the report I sent to Chicago, New York, Brooklyn, Philadelphia, Baltimore, and New Orleans, in order to get copies of their death reports, which I ought to have here, and which I will let the gentlemen see at some other time. As the result of a comparison of them, I found that our own returns seemed to me to answer the purpose better than anything else. In the first place, in our own reports we have a return which is the right size for binding or the right size for folding as a legal document; second, we have a return that gives the date of death, name, occupation, etc., and it is to be signed by a responsible man, according to his knowledge and belief. We have not yet a list of the diseases that is furnished in Dr. Abbott's report. I believe that in some cities — New York, for instance — there was a book sent around to each one of the physicians, which had a stub like that of a check-book, and the return can be torn off after the physician has filled it in. That return is passed to the board of health. The law obliges the physician also to fill in the stub, so that, if in any way the original report is lost, he will be able to furnish a duplicate. We have not got that, and I do not know that we need it. In some papers I found this at the top, " The physician or undertaker"— whichever might be the responsible individual, in a particular city — "shall return this record within twenty-four" or "forty-eight hours," some within thirty-six, "to the board of health." That, I believe, ought to be incorporated in our return, for this reason. There are many times when an undertaker makes out a return that is imperfect; and, when it gets to the board of health, it is found to be imperfect, and cannot be taken. The undertaker keeps that return two or three days, and then brings it in within a very short time of the funeral. We are then obliged either to accept an unsatisfactory record or to seriously inconvenience the family of the deceased by compelling a postponement of the funeral. Therefore, I believe in our return we should have at the top, "This return must be presented at the board of health office within twenty-four or thirty-six hours from the time of death." Then at the bottom of the return, on its face, I think we should have the general statute relating to the furnishing of death returns by the physicians. This is already printed on the return blank in some of our cities. I believe, instead of putting that on the back, we ought to put it right on the face of the certificate, where it can be easily seen. This statute says, " A physician who has attended a person during his last illness shall, when requested, forthwith furnish for registration a certificate stating, to the best of his knowledge and belief, the name of the deceased, his age, the disease of which he died, the duration of his last illness, and the date of his decease ; and a physician who has attended at the birth of a child dying immediately thereafter, or at the birth of a still-born child, shall, when requested, forthwith furnish for registration a certificate stating, to the best of his knowledge and belief, that such a child died after birth or was born dead." That is very important on account of succession of property, for instance. In many cities — Brooklyn, for instance — they have three different death certificates, pink, yellow, and blue. One color gives the ordinary return, the second one gives the return in case of still-born, and the third gives the coroner's return. In one of the other cities — Baltimore, I think — they have a still-born return besides the regular one. It is a different color and size, so that in every city of importance this "still-born" is seen. We have not so carefully followed that out in Massachusetts. In the Boston Board of Health we have been in the habit of acting in this way. If a return came in and no age was placed against it, we compelled the undertaker to take that back to the physician, and the physician added the words "still-born" to it, if it were a still-born child, or else put the time that the child lived. The rest of the statute says, "If a physician neglects or refuses to make a certificate as aforesaid or makes a false statement therein, he shall be subject to a fine not exceeding fifty dollars." That is also important. Most physicians do not understand there is any penalty attached to their not certifying the facts on the death return. I have known of cases where the physician who had been in attendance had refused to sign the certificate because the people had not paid him his fee. If that notice of penalty is placed at the bottom of the return, the undertaker can then compel the physician's signature or report him to the board of health.

Another statute which would be desirable to insert is that "a physician attending a soldier or sailor who served in the War of the Rebellion shall give both the primary and the secondary or immediate cause of death, as nearly as he can state the same. If the physician refuses, he shall forfeit the sum of ten dollars, to be placed to the credit of the town in which he lives." The reason for this is because on the question of pension this record must stand. If the soldier or sailor dies, and the family applies for a pension, the primary and secondary causes of death are known : and there is no chance for confusion, as the primary here means clearly antecedent. The idea is, evidently, to mention those diseases which he might have contracted during service.

Then as to the list of diseases. The list furnished by the committee, I think, is an excellent one. I haven't it about me, but I looked it over. I think in some cases, however, they have not included as many synonymes as they might have done. For instance, I found the word "anasarca," but not "ascitas." A careful consideration of this point is necessary, because, if you leave a loophole at all for the physicians, they will leave out a word that they ought not to or they will put in a word they ought not to. Therefore, every time we need a synonyme we should put in that synonyme. Then I think a great necessity in this connection would be the idea of looking out for deaths from diphtheria. We receive constantly records of deaths from acute laryngitis, laryngeal spasm, cynanche trachealis, etc. It is probable that most of these deaths are from diphtheria, and yet it is hard to act on that assumption without causing some dissatisfaction in each individual case.

So that I think that at the bottom of the list of diseases there should be placed something like this. "It will be assumed in all cases of death," for instance, "from acute throat troubles, that the patient had diphtheria, unless the physician absolutely states to the contrary."

Then I think it might be well to place pyæmia and septicæmia in that list, which I think are not there, because they are always secondary to something else. It is necessary in some cases to know what that something else is. Then, gentlemen, it seems to me that, with the return which we have at present, the addition of these extracts from the statutes in their places, the return presented within twenty-four or thirty-six hours, whichever we wish to make it, and a list on the back giving the list of diseases already presented with the additions, we shall have almost an ideal certificate.

The Chairman.— I will call upon Dr. Chapin, of Providence.

Dr. William H. Chapin.— Mr. President, I do not know that I have anything to add to the discussion of the very excellent paper by Dr. Abbott. One of the greatest difficulties or troubles that we have to contend with is the ignorance of the community. They do not know the cause of death. In very many cases they do not know anything about it whatever. They do not know anything about the names which Dr. Abbott has set out, showing what is the cause of death. I would say, however, that there is one matter which I have used in Providence. I had our certificate printed with quite a large space for the cause of death, and I have encouraged the physician in questionable cases to write out as much as he could about the case. A great many of the physicians have taken to doing that, so that I get a much clearer idea of the cause of death in doubtful cases or in complicated cases than I could if they put the name of one or two or three diseases upon the death certificate without any explanation of the relation between them.

The Chairman.— The question is now open for general discussion. We have a few minutes more we might devote to this.

Mr. J. A. Burgess.— Mr. Chairman, in my experience as chairman of the Board of Health in my town, I have some queer opinions from doctors. I find they are a very curious class of people. There were born in my town some time ago twins, which were very small. One is alive to-day the other lived a few days. The doctor made the return of the one that died that it died of premature birth, and I suppose the other lived from premature birth.

The Chairman.— He did not say which one was born first?

Mr. Burgess.— He did not.

The Chairman.— Are there any further remarks to be made upon this paper?

Dr. Gardner T. Swarts.— Mr. Chairman, I wish to say that in Rhode Island we have some conditions which make our duties extremely irksome. I find a great deal of difficulty in separating the condition where insanity is involved: and I have had reports involving, for instance, the question of tuberculosis and dementia, and I would like very much to receive the assistance of this committee in connection with this list here, to ascertain what would be preferable in these cases, as to whether dementia was caused by tuberculosis or not, because I am told by the attendants at the State institutions that it is a difficult matter at times to determine in these cases of dementia as to whether they are brought on by conditions previously existing or whether there was some brain disease preceding the tuberculosis.

In the disease known as anthrax, I would like to ask the question whether the diagnosis should be accepted as correct when the physician reports anthrax, unless the actual condition of anthrax is present; that is, unless the bacillus is present, and found in the secretions of the abscess. I think that in all cases that should be learned by inquiry from the physician whether he has had a bacteriological examination made. If we do so, the interest of the physician will be encouraged to make more common use of this aid in diagnosis; and it will be of benefit to the profession at large.

On the question of heart failure the committee states that these terms should not be accepted if any more definite term can be given. And it seems to me a more definite term *can* be given in every case where death is caused by heart failure, except in a case where it may be from shock, a sudden cessation of action of the heart, in which case it should be entered as shock, if no previous history is ascertainable. In these cases I think it is as much an unknown cause as it is usually when it is signed in that way. And I personally should much prefer that the physician should sign his cause of death as unknown, owning up honestly that he does not claim that it should be put in a category, than give the indefinite term "heart failure," which is somewhat of a half confession. However, usually, by correspondence with the physician, the symptoms of some previous disease may be obtained; and the physician will in this way give information which he would not otherwise have done, and more accuracy in diagnosis will be the result.

One cause which is frequently sent into our office which is not mentioned in this list is peritonitis, which I do not let go by without learning, if possible, what the cause of the peritonitis was. If not ascertainable, I place it as peritonitis under "causes unknown": but for the peritonitis there must have been some cause. Sometimes it is a strain from lifting or a fall; but something must have been the cause of the peritonitis, and frequently by ferreting it out this can be ascertained.

I should like to ask in connection with this report, which is made here, whether it is the intention of our committee to go farther, and make a new nomenclature of diseases and classification. I hope that it will be possible for that committee to formulate something which all New England, and possibly other States, may follow, which will permit us to abandon the obsolete terms which at this day have no meaning.

THE CHAIRMAN.—If there are no other speakers on this question, I will call on Dr. Abbott to close the discussion. The time has come when we shall soon have to take up the next subject.

Dr. S. W. Abbott.— The committee, Mr. Chairman, have hardly considered the question of giving an entirely new nomenclature yet. It is one of those things that I suppose must come. Our old one is getting very fast out of date for reasons that are stated in this paper, but that has not been formulated. I do not know but it may be possible before long to bring some such list before you. Certainly, in regard to tuberculosis there is one very good point which is changing itself; and we know that it does not belong away down in the list under what used to be called constitutional diseases, but it is decidedly an infectious disease, and placed in the same list which used to be called zymotic, but the word "zymotic" is fast going out of date, like a good many others. The whole subject is a progressive one. We have to bear that in mind, and that no list that can ever be made will last forever. Just like all things in natural history and natural science, it is progressive, very much like the whole subject of the practice of medicine; and we cannot make any cast-iron list. Still, I think we shall be able before long to bring forward a list that will be up to the present day.

There is only one other matter I should like to mention; and that is to call your attention to the fact that there was last winter before the legislature, and I think it has been referred to this General Court, an entirely new bill upon the registration of births, marriages, and deaths, which includes some very good amendments, and more, I think, which are quite as objectionable, which did not emanate from any sanitary authority. If it did, I think it would be quite different from what it is. I should like to call attention to one passage on the 90th page, which states that "the records of all public institutions whatever throughout the State shall be required to make a separate report of deaths." I think that is a very important thing. You all know in your own towns and cities that your death-rate is increased by the number in the institution; that you may have in an institution a higher death-rate than the town itself, unless it be one for young people, vigorous boys, like the Lyman School up at the other extreme of the State. The State almshouse at Tewksbury has an enormous rate, twenty times that of the town of Tewksbury; and in some towns in their reports those are included. The Somerville Asylum, for instance, is always included in the reports of Somerville. At Westboro the deaths in the two institutions there go into the report of the town of Westboro, but they do not belong there. They are people from outside, and should be classed outside. Of course, they are part of the State death-rate; but they should be classed by themselves always in making up a general report. It is always so in every foreign country that has any amount of progressiveness about it. I do not know that there is anything further that I would say, Mr. Chairman.

PROF. H. C. ERNST.—Mr. Chairman, in conversation to-day and in the speaking I have noticed the same condition that apparently exists generally in regard to these diseases in the use of the terms "infectious" and "contagious." It appears to me that it is a pretty important matter to settle that definition. I should therefore like to move that this committee be requested to settle that definition, and adopt one term or the other for general employment in the designation of this class of diseases.

The motion was seconded.

THE CHAIRMAN.—It is moved and seconded that the Committee on Vital Statistics be asked to consider in their work the definition of "infectious" and "contagious"; that they adopt one or the other, the preference being given to "infectious."

The motion was carried.

MR. E. L. PILLSBURY.—Mr. Chairman, in order that more light may be cast upon the subject under discussion, I would move that the Committee on Vital Statistics be requested and authorized to give further consideration to the subject.

The motion was seconded.

THE CHAIRMAN.—It is moved and seconded that the Committee on Vital Statistics continue their good work in the consideration of death returns and nomenclature of diseases.

The motion was carried.

THE CHAIRMAN.—The next business in order is the discussion of Culture Diagnosis in Diphtheria, by Professor Ernst.

CULTURE DIAGNOSIS OF DIPHTHERIA.

BY PROFESSOR H. C. ERNST.

Mr. Chairman and Gentlemen,—In speaking of this question, which appears to be of importance, and of constantly growing importance, as I think I shall be able to show you by some figures that I shall give you, and in describing the methods employed, I shall give as accurately as may be those which we ourselves use in this city, which, we think, are the best, of course, —because, if we thought there were any better, we should have adopted them.

In the first place, the whole value of the culture diagnosis of cases of suspected sore throat depends upon the fact that the bacillus of diphtheria develops more rapidly than other bacteria that usually grow in the mouth, upon a special nutrient medium and at a special temperature; and these conditions must be fulfilled as nearly as possible, and, if any of them fail, by so much the accuracy of the diagnosis is diminished. In fulfilling these conditions, it is necessary to take into consideration the applicability of the methods adopted to a very large field; and these are the points that we have attempted to work out in our line of investigation in this direction.

The basis, of course, of the whole test is the proper preparation of the nutrient medium. We have seen no reason at any time to adopt any change from the original so-called Loeffler's sugar serum, which is a mixture of blood serum and bouillon, with a definite amount of grape sugar added. These are mixed in the proportion of two parts of serum and one of bouillon, and then sterilized. We have made a slight modification in the method of sterilization that is quite commonly used now, and consists of the addition of an average of one-half of one per cent. of caustic potash to the blood serum. This takes advantage of the fact that has been known for a long time to physiologists: that, if a certain proportion of a strong alkali, like caustic potash or caustic soda,—varying in percentage with the different forms of albumen,—be added to the albuminous material, this mixture of fluid·albumen and caustic potash may be coagulated by a high degree of heat without losing its transparency. This, of course, is a very great advantage in the preparation of albuminous nutrient media upon the large scale that is necessary in such a work as ours, because it shortens the length of time necessary at least one-half. After having added this proportion of caustic potash (0.5 per cent.), which is the alkali which we use, the mixture is at once placed in the sterilizer, the ordinary serum inspissator which is known in all bacteriological laboratories, and subjected to a temperature of a little less than that of steam, of about 98 degrees Centigrade, for an hour or two. That serves the double purpose of sterilizing and solidifying the nutrient medium, so that further sterilization may be completed in the same apparatus, and the tubes be all ready for use on the third day instead of on the seventh or eighth day. Just at present I am expecting daily a new form of sterilizer that I have had constructed in New York, consisting of a steam jacket somewhat similar to those that are used in some hospitals, but with changes which will enable this sterilization to be carried on under pressure and completed in the course of ten or fifteen minutes. This will again shorten the time necessary for the sterilization of the serum.

The second point in regard to the nutrient medium is the necessity for a free supply of blood serum. That we obtain — not without some difficulty, because we need a great deal of it — at the Brighton abattoir, where it is collected under the supervision of the veterinarian of the board, Dr. Burt. The serum is sent for from the laboratory at least twice, not infrequently three times a week, and is put through the method of preparation of which I have spoken. The tubes are the ordinary size used in the laboratory, 6 inches by $\frac{1}{2}$ inch. This is a matter of necessity, because it would be almost impossible to keep the different styles of tubes separate because of the constant call for the cases, and the confusion that would occur in the laboratory if one branch of the work were carried on with one size, and another with another. Still, I should not change the size of the tube now if it were possible, because of a point which I shall speak of a little later.

In making cultures, it is a wise plan to have plenty of the nutrient medium, because, by having a proper surface for the growth to develop upon, it enables a much more accurate diagnosis to be made; and, as will be seen with these (exhibiting tubes), after sterilization a small amount of water condenses. That collects at the base, and assists in keeping the nutrient medium for a greater length of time by keeping it moist. The drying is further prevented by covering the tubes with these rubber caps, which I at last succeeded in having made in this country at somewhere near the same price at which they could be imported. In fact, as it is now, I can secure them at exactly the same price as the cost of imported caps; and their importance lies, in the first place, in preventing the evaporation of moisture, because it is hardly necessary to repeat the fact that the cotton in the end of the tube acts not as a cork, but simply as a filter. It is not a plug to absolutely prevent the entrance of air, but simply a filter to filter the air, and filter out bacteria. In the second place, the cap acts to prevent the forming of moulds upon the surface of the cotton plug, and their gradual growth through the interstices of the cotton, which is one of the main causes of contamination in case the tubes of nutrient media are kept for a long time.

The next especial point of the method that is used in the diagnosis of diphtheria in this city is the use of these copper cases, which are the result of an evolution that has been going on for three or four years in the laboratory. We began when the call for tubes of nutrient media first occurred, by having prepared a rather expensive box with the old-fashioned velvet lining, and a good deal of elaborateness about it. That was altogether too expensive for any such demand as this culture diagnosis seemed likely to create; and we have had various forms of boxes, as our ideas have changed, until, finally, we have settled upon this, and we have now had them in use for a year. The supply has been increased as fast as we could have them made, and so far I know of nothing that compares with them for the purpose for which they are employed.

As you see, the box consists of the box proper and of the case, which has no bottom. The box is made of a single piece which is moulded, and contains a place for two tubes, and hollow for the wire, with a ring to assist in pulling it out. That is really unnecessary, because it can be pushed up from the bottom in that way (illustrating).

When these outfits are returned to the laboratory, the tubes are removed, the box is sterilized, and can be used over and over again with perfect safety.

The object, of course, of the stamp upon it, is to show where the box belongs. The object of the number is in order to keep some sort of control of them. When the boxes go from the laboratory, the person who takes them is charged with the number, and once a month or once in six weeks, as the case may be, the record is gone over; and, if we find that the boxes have been kept out for six weeks or more, we send notice, and request their return for inspection. The reason for this would make itself easily apparent if any one has to do with this sort of thing, because, in the first place, many physicians get them, and forget all about them. In the second place, as a rule, the life of the tubes without contamination is about six weeks. If the sterilization is very complete, and if the cap is put on before the moulds are enclosed beneath it, and above the cotton, the life is indefinite. But we cannot depend upon that, so we like to change the tubes once in six weeks ; and that is the object of the practice of sending out for them.

The wires are of the form devised by Dr. McCollom, consisting of platinum wire, which is swaged into a heavy brass wire, which again fits into a handle, making the outfit as nearly complete as possible.

Of course, the main difference between the method that is used here and that that is usually employed is the difference between using this platinum wire for the purpose of securing material for cultivation and the use of a cotton swab, a small piece of cotton wound around the end of a probe or piece of wire. The advantages of the cotton swab are that it is easier to use, that it is not common to injure the struggling child, and that with it you can take up a very much larger amount of material.

Now, in the first place, if this platinum wire be properly used, it bends very easily; and it would require a good deal of lack of skill to injure a throat with it, particularly as the point is bent over. If any of them go out of the laboratory where that is not the case, it is an oversight. As a rule, they will be bent over. In the second place, the wire takes up a very small amount of material, which is a great advantage rather than a disadvantage. It is necessary to have an extremely small portion of the material to be examined, in order to detect any bacteria that may be present. And, lastly, the method of inoculation furnished by the wire has a very great advantage that we see exemplified every day in our examinations. According to the directions that are sent out, the wire is to be touched to the throat, and then is to be drawn along the surface of the nutrient medium in three parallel lines one after the other without reloading. The object of this, of course, is to distribute the major portion of the material collected on the wire on the first stroke, and a smaller portion on the second, and, practically, all that remains on the third. In this way the bacteria are more or less separated from each other, and the culture, if properly done, practically amounts to a plate culture: and in innumerable cases we have it occur that there will be one fine dot representing a single colony of the bacilli of diphtheria that has been singled out by this method of isolation on the surface of the nutrient medium. I can only say now, as I have stated before, that the results seem to us to justify most emphatically the use of the wire for obtaining material for cultivation rather than the swab for the general purposes of a diagnosis, and the results are more accurate. It is a little more trouble to the physician; but, because the results are more accurate, it seems to me as though there were no question as to what should be used.

The culture having been made, the method of transportation to the laboratory is the next point. In the first place there are a number of stations scattered throughout the city, under the Board of Health, at which these cases may be obtained by those living in the neighborhood. A definite time is set at or before which each case must be returned to that station, in order to secure transportation that day to the laboratory. That hour has heretofore been twelve o'clock; but I believe that in the coming year the chairman of the board has in mind to make the hour still later in the afternoon, and to have a special agent of the Board of Health collect the cases and bring them to the laboratory rather than depend upon persons at the stations to send them. If the cases are not returned to the stations by twelve o'clock, as is the practice to-day, the physician himself must see to their transportation to us before six o'clock; and, if that be done, the tubes are at once placed in the incubator, and the resulting examination is made upon the following day, a point — that it does take over night at least to get the results — which the general practitioner frequently does not seem to realize. That is a length of time which seems to many practitioners to require shortening, but it is not possible to shorten it. The necessity of the test forbids the result being reached until the next day. But there are differences in the way in which those results may be sent out. The method that we have adopted is that the cultures are all examined together, the examinations beginning at about eight o'clock in the morning, the staining being started at that time. A single report cannot be sent out any earlier than all the rest: they must all go together, in order to secure the best average speed. But the microscopic examination never depends upon one man alone. That, it seems to me, is also a great point. Cover-glasses are prepared by two assistants, who may be spoken of as the two junior assistants. A probable diagnosis is written down by each one of them : and each record is gone over by what may be spoken of as the senior assistant, and the final diagnosis is settled. If there is any question in regard to any particular case or any difference of opinion, the matter is referred to me.

Then the reports are sent out upon blanks in accordance with these three. There is the first one. " The culture submitted by you yesterday from " . . . " shows the presence of the bacilli of diphtheria." That card is sent by mail. If there is any special reason for haste, there is a telegram sent as well; and frequently there is a special delivery stamp as between the two.

I have declined from the beginning to send any reports by telephone; and I am extremely glad I did so, because in either of these means, a communication by telegram, of which a copy is kept, by a letter or a card, of which a record is kept, we have some way of answering complaints, if they are made. A telephone is not only a great servitor, but it may be a great nuisance. If there is any mistake in the name or anything of that kind, in sending a message over the telephone, one has no record and no protection. So, as I say, from the very beginning I have declined to send reports by telephone.

The second of the blanks that we send out is, " The culture submitted by you yesterday from . . . does not show the presence of diphtheria." Which should be altered so as to read "does not show the presence of the bacilli of diphtheria."

The third blank is one which has been already modified. It reads now, " The culture submitted by you yesterday from . . . shows no growth. The test therefore is of no value. Will you be good enough to send us a second culture ? " and so far I have heard no complaint about this wording. As it was at first, after saying that " it shows no growth," the words used were, " There must therefore have been some error in technique," which was the most innocent expression on our part that could be imagined, but apparently it aroused the wrath of about every one who received the card. It simply meant what this card means, that for some reason there was no growth. It did not mean any criticism upon the individual at all.

These are the three blanks, then, that are sent by mail; and, as a rule, within the city limits the reports are received in the afternoon. We have made special arrangements with the postal authorities by which our mail is received after the closing of the regular mail; and the reports are all sent by the 1.30 post, or at the latest by the one following. And this does not mean only week-days. It means every day in the year, Sundays and holidays as well, which is one of the great points, that the work is never stopped; and I think the profession in Boston are appreciating that more and more every day. Last year we used to have a very large drop in the number of cases that were sent in upon Sunday. This year and with each succeeding week the number of cases is increasing upon Sunday, because the medical profession begin to know there is no stop to the work on that day. Cases are just as ill with diphtheria on that day as any other, and we have discovered that examinations can be made upon that day as well as any other day of the week.

One word more in regard to the cases. Three blanks are sent out with each case. The first contains directions for making cultures; and, with the exception of altering the hours, I have seen no reason for changing the wording at all since we began. The change of the hours will probably be made as the board perfects its further arrangements. There have been cards, one for each tube, sent out ever since the beginning, containing spaces for the patient's name and address, the physician's name and address, the date of the first, second, and third culture, and so on. Upon the back was simply printed the word "Remarks." As a rule, that blank did not bring us any clinical information; but it brought us many complaints [laughter], so that quite recently we have filled up that space, and, if complaints are to be made, they must be sent upon a special note from these new data, which we hope the profession will take pains to fill out, and I think they will. We expect to get some extremely valuable information. We request the questions to be answered as to the purpose of the culture, the age of the patient, duration of the illness, whether membrane is present or not, as to the presence of nasal and laryngeal symptoms, and a statement of the clinical diagnosis. Then there is a very small space at the bottom for any general remarks that one desires to make. I think that any one will see that, if these blanks are generally filled out, in connection with the work of the board with the anti-toxin of diphtheria, at the end of the year we shall have some extremely valuable information, not only as regards this method of diagnosis as compared with the clinical diagnosis, but also as compared with the use of anti-toxin in the various cases.

These blanks are sent back to us. Each case goes out with fresh ones; and, if the second culture is returned, the date and result are posted upon the original blank sent in the first place by the physician, all of which are filed according to the name of the patient, so that we have the records complete from the beginning. And if any question is raised in regard to what became of such and such a culture, and in regard to such a patient, when he was ill and so on, or when he received the culture, we have that information filed in the original handwriting. It would be extremely interesting, I think, to know how many cases come in, in which the physician takes neither the pains to fill in the name of the patient nor his own. We have an average, I should think, of ten cases a week where we have absolutely no data upon which to return a report; and then in the course of a week or so after that the shower begins. [Laughter.] "This does not amount to anything. You did not manage that right." And we show them the blank card, which we keep in a special box. It is very common to have incomplete data, and especially a number of physicians are accustomed to sigr. only their last name without any address, so that a number of reports have gone wrong; but, taking into consideration the amount of work we have done, it seems to me it has been done with absolutely as little friction as could be expected.

Now, in regard to this question of "No Growth." I have told you that on one of the blanks we send out the fact that no growth occurred; and it seems often, no doubt, to disturb the physician more than anything else, more than our saying he has a case of diphtheria when he thinks he has not or that he has not a case when he thinks he has. The fact that he did not get any growth at all seems to be particularly embarrassing to him. I think the reason for these no growths occurring is very largely because the physicians do not pay sufficient attention to the directions for making a culture; and I think this is certainly carried out by the fact that the proportion of "No Growth" cultures being sent to us is diminishing, and diminishing quite rapidly. As an illustration, in the last week there were three hundred cases sent in for examination. Out of those three hundred there were only two cases of "No Growth." The reports are sent not only to the physician, but, of course, upon request they are sent to the patient as well; and, as a matter of routine, every day a full list of the reports of the cultures, the name of the patient and the address, the name of the physician and the address, and the result of the examination, with dates in each case, are sent to the Board of Health Office, and in that way they have, as well as we, a complete record of every case that is examined and all the work that we do. In addition to that we have recently adopted the plan of reporting on the cases sent in for release directly and immediately to the board, and I believe that within the limited time that the plan has been adopted it has saved at least twenty-four hours in each case for the releasing of the patient and disinfection of the premises. Is not that true, Dr. Durgin?

THE CHAIRMAN.— Yes, twenty-four hours to three days.

PROF. ERNST.— Twenty-four hours to three days. So it seems as though that method were going to make the results available as promptly as can possibly be expected.

Now, in regard to the amount of work that has been carried on by the board during the last year, or rather during the last fourteen months. It began upon the first of November, 1894; and I have here a chart showing, by weeks, the number of cultures that were sent in, the number of new cases, and the number of positive cases during each week from that time until the first of January, 1896, which gives a total of 8,644 examinations made for physicians of this city during the fourteen months preceding this. And it is exceedingly interesting to see the variations in the curves. In the first of the time the rise is extremely rapid, because, in the month of November, 1894, the profession was becoming aware of the fact that these examinations could be made. Then the number sent in holds about the same until the time of the closing of the schools at the Christmas recess; and during the period from Dec. 23 to Jan. 6, 1894 and 1895, there is a very marked drop in the number of suspected cases, accompanied by a fall of the actual number of cases of diphtheria, as is shown upon the curves, as you can see when the chart is passed around. Then there is a marked fall in the number of cases sent in through the summer months, reaching its minimum in the last week in August. From the time the schools begin, as you can see, the rise has been very sharp until again we reach the time of the Christmas recess, when it falls. I think it is a very remarkable fact that is shown by this chart that the idea in regard to schools being extremely influential in the spread of this disease is a well-founded one. All the percentages for the various months are worked out at the foot of the chart.

The next question is a very practical one, and of general interest in regard to the relative value of this method of diagnosis as compared with the clinical diagnosis of diphtheria. That is, it appears to me, an extremely important point; and it also appears to me (and I mean no self-laudation at all in making this statement, because the result could not have been reached without the most active and generous support of the Board of Health, and without the active assistance of the gentlemen assisting me) that we have raised the percentage of accuracy of this method of diagnosis to a very high degree. And, as to individual opinions that this is so, we have had an extremely complimentary and voluntary tribute to the work in a recent number of the New York *Medical Record*, which was called to my attention yesterday; and also it happened yesterday that two physicians in the city, who have sent us as large a number of cases of this kind as any other two, I think, in the city, in the course of conversation said that, in every instance during the past year where their clinical diagnosis had crossed our cultural diagnosis, we had been shown to be right by subsequent events. I do not suppose that this holds in every case. It would be absurd to suppose so, to think it for a moment; but it does give evidence that the percentage of accuracy in this method may be raised to a very high degree, and that it is certainly an extremely important addition to the methods of diagnosis is, it seems to me, wholly unquestionable at the present stage of our experience.

This brings up another question of practical interest; and that is as to when the physician should report the case as one of diphtheria, whether upon his clinical impression or wait for the result of an examination. Of course, these cultural examinations depend entirely upon the honesty of the physician. As one gentleman said to me in the laboratory three or four weeks ago, "What would you do if I wanted you to decide, and I made a negative culture, having taken the culture from the patient's hand?" Well, of course there is nothing to be said. We depend in the first place upon the honesty, the conscientiousness, of the medical profession. It seems to me as if that was all we needed as evidence. As to whether a person should report a case as one of diphtheria before or after receiving a report from us, if it be true that the percentage of accuracy with these cultural diagnoses is very high, it would appear to me as if it would be well to wait until he received a report from us, having made the culture under proper conditions. The reason for this is illustrated by one of these physicians that I spoke of, who told me yesterday of a case in which he had been assured that there was diphtheria. There were all the clinical symptoms of it, according to his mind; and he went so far as to notify the Board of Health to put up the card, and on the following day he received a negative culture from us. He sent in two cultures after that, and received three negative reports. The patient had recovered practically, was practically well in three days.

It does not require very much extra isolation, if a patient has a bad sore throat. He should be kept quiet any way, and he can easily be isolated for the length of time that it takes to make this examination. Equally, of course, in such a case, if there was reason for expediting the report, that can be done if it is stated upon the card when it is sent in.

Then, again. as to how many negative cultures are necessary for release. That also is a point that can hardly be settled to everybody's satisfaction. It would appear to me that, if a patient clinically is well, one negative report is all that is necessary. I do not see any reason for keeping him in quarantine after the clinical symptoms have disappeared, if the report is negative. We had also an extremely interesting instance of that sort yesterday in a gentleman who has been ill with diphtheria, was ill last week. He has been one of my assistants, and entered the laboratory on Monday, and had a culture taken, which was negative. He came in again on Tuesday. A culture was taken in the laboratory, and he came in yesterday morning to see the result. The result was positive. He had diphtheria bacilli present; but he himself was apparently perfectly well, and at the time the health officials were fumigating his house. A third culture was taken at once, and again it was negative. Now, the point about that is that the bacilli were present; but they were not producing any symptoms in him. What we found in that second culture, a positive culture, was a minute focus where there were a few bacilli present; but to say that that person was affected with diphtheria would have been absurd, because he was really immune. He had just recovered from an attack, and it would not have been worth while to quarantine him further. ,

Another serious question is that of cases of delayed release; that is, in which the bacilli persist for apparently a long time. A point is raised as to whether these bacilli are or are not virulent, and that is left to us to decide. As to deciding it in individual cases, it is extremely difficult, for the reason that in every case in which we have attempted the decision the length of time necessary for securing a pure culture and the results of inoculation has been longer than until a negative culture from the patient himself was secured; and, therefore, it seems as if in delayed cases it was safer to depend upon successive cultures than to depend upon the inoculation experiment.

The last point of which I have to speak is as to how long these culture tubes will remain good, one that I have already touched upon. The length of time on the average is six weeks. Of course, a thoroughly sterilized tube, which has been plugged and kept under aseptic and antiseptic conditions, will keep an indefinitely long time; but, where from one to two hundred tubes a day must be prepared, haste is necessary, and moulds might get in between the cap and the rubber stopper, as is the case not infrequently, so that contamination may become manifest in the course of six weeks. We have had boxes brought back to us which were perfectly good at the end of six months, but it would not be safe to depend upon that length of time. They should be changed, as I have said, about once in six weeks, certainly examined as often as that.

Dr. Durgin suggests a statement in regard to the time after the culture is made before it should go into the incubator; and that should be, of course, as soon as it can reasonably be done. If a culture be made and sent to us, it should be got to us within a few hours after. If it be kept cool, it is a matter of practical indifference when it gets to us. That is to say, if the growth of bacteria be hindered by a low temperature, it may come to us at almost any time, and then be placed in the incubator, as is done as a regular thing in the late afternoon.

That is all I have to say, unless some gentlemen present desire to ask me questions.

MR. PILLSBURY.— In regard to the case that the doctor stated of the gentleman who had had no diphtheria bacilli present at one time, and then bacilli were present at another, and as to not having virulent diphtheria bacilli, and therefore not having diphtheria himself, I would like to ask whether there was any danger to the rest of the community from his being out, and as to whether he should not be still quarantined on that ground.

PROF. ERNST.—Yes, quarantined on that ground; but my point was that, as I believe has been shown by this second culture, and as I believe will be shown by any number of cultures taken on successive days, they will go on being negative, and the patient himself was free from danger.

QUESTION.— Would that be called a case of diphtheria?

PROF. ERNST.— I suppose, if it occurred originally, it would be reported as a case of diphtheria; but it had been already reported. He had been sick and gone through the symptoms and had recovered, so it could be hardly necessary to report it again.

THE CHAIRMAN.— I will announce the addition to the Legislative Committee as being Mr. Parker, from Cambridge, and Mr. Pillsbury, from Boston. I will now call upon Dr. Swarts.

DR. GARDNER T. SWARTS.— Mr. Chairman, I have a great deal of diffidence in attempting to approach the discussion of the remarks made by one who was my instructor. I hope that I may be excused if I should differ somewhat in the conclusions reached by the presentation of the subject. Another thing which leads me to speak rather closely and rather mildly is the fact that the number of cases naturally coming from the small State of Rhode Island does not begin to compare with the number in this city, and consequently must have less weight when compared with the numbers presented by Dr. Ernst. Therefore, I will merely give my experience as being an addendum, and bearing upon the results in Rhode Island.

One of the first difficulties which was met with by our board is that physicians do not fully understand the method of making the culture; and under that condition it results that the tubes, as has been stated by Dr. Ernst, are liable to be lost or liable to disappear. Out of four hundred tubes sent out during the first six months of the last year, two hundred have entirely disappeared. They were seized upon by the physician, and placed upon the shelf as souvenirs of the advance in medicine. The board, therefore, are now having a large number of dry tubes sent in; and that is the point which brings up the question of the method of taking the culture. The method which is adopted by us in taking cultures is the same as has been stated by Dr. Ernst, except that we use the swab. The culture is intended to be the same, the preparation of the culture may be the same, and the evaporation of the tubes is the same. The reason for using this form of distribution and transportation was simply the result of having copied from the city of New York, and are the same methods which are now being used in Brooklyn, Denver, Washington, and other large cities. The method, as some of you may be aware, is in the use of a smaller, shorter. These are one containing the nutrient serum and the other the swab, in a small box,—just an ordinary school pencil box; and, the tubes to be examined having been sent from the manufacturers in the first place in a rather heavy form, that condition has been retained, for the reason that, if the tube is dropped upon the floor, it is not so liable to break as a lighter tube, thus avoiding loss of the culture in transit and contaminating from the breakage.

In the use of the swab the additional advantages claimed by those who make use of it are that, in the first place, you approach the patient with less fear of doing injury to the mucous membrane of the throat. If you have a child in front of you, the mouth wide open, and several persons holding that mouth open, the opportunity of getting at the back of the throat is very small; and, if a wire only is used, it would be a difficult matter for the physician to reach the membrane that he was looking for, especially if he did not see that point. Assuming we desire to get at the membrane, and the physician is clinically able to distinguish a diphtheria membrane from one formed by the accumulation of micrococci, streptococci, or starch, and can see and touch that membrane, we may be able to get the culture that we are looking for.

But I claim that, if the mouth is entirely open and the swab can be swept over the arch of the fauces with a twisting motion, so that the swab will cover all parts of the arch and pharynx, we shall run a better chance of obtaining a better average of what there is in the throat than if we take it from one spot only.

If, as a laboratory expert, one could get the particular amount that we wanted, and could place it as a "streak culture" on the serum, it might be easier to isolate the given colonies.

The disadvantage of two cultures with a made wire probe is that it necessitates a second struggle with the patient, which, in many instances, increases the action of the heart, which is already sufficiently depressed by the action of the toxins present.

In this form of culture kit we have a wire which is just the ordinary coppered wire, wound with absorbent cotton; and the swab and wire are thrown away after being sterilized.

The use of the box is of no special advantage that I can see, except that it is small, and is somewhat more readily carried in the pocket of the physician. One advantage which Dr. Ernst has told us of is the rubber cap, which prevents the evaporation of moisture in the tube, and is a most important point. We endeavor to overcome that by wrapping the whole box in a piece of ordinary waxed paper; and in that condition, to a certain extent, it prevents evaporation, and also serves the purpose of preventing the chance of carrying the material from place to place.

In regard to the growth of organisms Dr. Ernst has laid great stress — and rightfully, I think — upon the length of time necessary. My experience has been, of course, limited; but it is that it requires at least fourteen to sixteen hours' growth before one would be willing to make a diagnosis or express an opinion upon the growth which has appeared upon the serum. Another advantage in the use of the swab is this, as has been frequently shown recently: The swab is used by the ignorant practitioner on dried serum, and it is sent to the laboratory with no moisture on the serum, but with the swab still infected. In these cases we have the swab, and it has been of great service in making a fresh culture at the laboratory. A great difficulty is found with us, as in this city, in the non-observance of directions by physicians. Frequently left in on top of the serum, which is one against the swab; but that is of course caused from the ignorance of the practitioner and a lack of attention to the instructions.

The question of making a positive diagnosis upon the first examination is one which I think will come up in the future. A culture is sent in, and the result is reported as negative: there are no bacilli present. Examination has shown in one or two instances, where the physician was doubtful about the bacteriological report, and sent in a second culture, and the second culture was positive, it may have been due to a lack of technique with the bacteriologist or on the part of the physician.

As to reports by telephone, it is a disadvantage especially to the ones who have to telephone; but it is an advantage where the message is received properly, and our practice has been that we will not give it unless there is some one who can receive it properly. By this means we cause a more rapid dissemination of knowledge, which is necessary to the physician. Our collections are up to five o'clock in the afternoon; but, if they come after that time, they are sent to my residence, and placed in an incubator there, for the purpose of carrying them over to the next day. All that are received by five o'clock can be usually reported on by half-past nine the next morning, frequently before the physician starts on his rounds. He has, therefore, the advantage of a little time there. Sometimes, if you are a little later with the report, the physician says, " It is not now necessary, as my patient is dead."

As to the method of raising the quarantine, I think Dr. Ernst intended to make it clear — I am not sure whether he did or not — as to the necessity of two negatives, as is to be the practice with us. Our experience has been that two negatives are necessary. The rule has not been fully adopted as yet, but it will be.

As to there being no growth, the physician may mistake the purport of the report. When he has the report sent to him that there is no growth, he may consider that there is no disease there whatever, since he thinks that he has made no mistake in his technique. The fact is that there is always something to be obtained from every throat.

A matter which I would like to have Dr. Ernst consider in his summing up is the question of the possibility, which has been proposed by some bacteriologists, of getting an immediate "snap diagnosis" from the swab, assuming the swab is used of course. It has been done with a certain amount of success by the authorities in Denver, by making a cover-glass preparation from the contents of the swab. In a discussion which occurred on this subject at Denver recently, Dr. Kenyoun, of the Marine Hospital Service in Washington, said that twenty per cent. could be obtained in that way. It is not a method to be depended upon; but, when one is in a great hurry, it might be of great service if the Klebs-Loeffler bacilli were found to be present, but could not be relied upon if the examination was negative.

As to the virility of the organisms in the throat, the necessity of quarantine has already been brought up; and I will not refer to that.

The blank which is sent out by our department asks for the name of the maker of the culture, which gives the information whether it was made by a physician or by some one else, or was left to the patient, as is sometimes the case, but should never be. It leads us to make a judgment as to whether the culture was properly made or not, the date, time, and occupation, the attending physician, the duration of the disease, in order to make a study of the character of the organism to a certain extent, and as to the location of the membrane; what, if any, applications have been made to the throat; if so, how long before taking the culture. I do not know that anything will ever come from that; but it might be that some local application may have had an effect to inhibit the growth of the culture, and might serve to tell us what we should use for a remedy. Of course, at the present day we know of nothing. Then the question as to the first or second culture follows after that in the questions to be answered.

The question of the examination of throats found to be suspicious is a question that comes up for consideration with us, so much so that Dr. Chapin, superintendent of the local Board of Health of Providence, has issued notice to all physicians, stating that all cases of sore throat must be examined or, if they are not examined, and a case comes to the notice of the health board, the health board will take the liberty of examining the throat, if possible, or placing a placard on the house, as may seem desirable. This, of course, seems to be an arbitrary measure to the physician; but it is grounded upon these points,— that, if there is a sore throat which is sufficiently bad that a physician should be called, he maintains that that physician is not upon his clinical examination alone able to make a correct diagnosis, and the diagnosis should be made negative or positive.

As to reporting cases to the health department. The physicians are requested to report all their cases of suspected diphtheria to the department; and, in case it is found to be a negative, a card is not put on the door, but, if deemed necessary, a card is put on and does not come down, nor can the child attend school without a negative result being shown twice.

THE CHAIRMAN.— Dr. Smith.

DR. THEOBALD SMITH.— Mr. Chairman, I have scarcely anything to add to the description which has been given by Professor Ernst and the remarks that have been made by Dr. Swarts. There is one point, however, which it seems to me should be emphasized; and that is that all diagnoses of diphtheria are tentative and liable to be erroneous. Any one who has ever given any attention to bacterial diseases of the mucous membranes knows how exceedingly difficult it is to isolate those bacteria. Diphtheria seems to be one of the fortunate exceptions to that rule, and it is something the medical profession should be thankful for that a diagnosis may be made from the mucous membrane. There are, however, for the reason given, limitations of the method; and it seems to me that any bacteriological examination of a diseased throat that reports negative results must be taken with a certain amount of reserve, and that any examination which reports the absence of diphtheria bacilli in the throat ten days, fifteen days, or twenty days after convalescence, must always be taken with a certain allowance. Recovered persons should not, within a number of months, kiss any small children or in any way make it possible for certain germs from his or her mouth to be transmitted to others. I think the organism of diphtheria, and I believe we all think so now, is conveyed almost directly from person to person. It is not very long ago when sewer gas was regarded as a fruitful source of infection. It is only a year or two ago when one of the prominent members of some State board of health spoke to me about the sewer-gas theory as one to be reckoned with. I, at that time, told him that the trend of bacteriology was in an entirely different direction, and that direct infection from person to person was far more probable. To return then to the first thought of my remarks, I would state that in all cases of negative diagnosis, or in all cases where diphtheria bacilli are supposed to have disappeared, or where the clinical and the bacteriological diagnoses fail to agree, the attending physician should not consider the diagnosis clean cut. He should at least inform his patients that caution is necessary. It seems to me that the direction which bacteriology is taking is away from very definite diagnoses. We know that in Germany during the past two years many persons have been found who carry cholera germs in their body during the prevalence of this disease. They have received the name of " cholera carriers " because the living germs have been found in their fœces. They are, as a rule, perfectly well. The same is true of diphtheria. We know that pneumonia germs exist in the throat, and it is probable that other disease germs are carried about by healthy persons. It is these facts of the possible unsuspected presence of disease germs which are going to give sanitarians most trouble in the future. The question has been asked whether diphtheria bacilli in the mouths of very mild cases or of healthy persons are virulent. To answer this question, I may state that there are two factors in the production of infectious disease. One is the person, the other is the germ. The person may be in such a condition that a virulent germ has no effect upon him. We know from experiment that in certain species of animals certain bacteria produce no effect, while toward other species they may prove very virulent. We can change experimentally a rapidly fatal septicæmia by immunizing the animal until either no effect at all is produced or else a mild or chronic affection only. So it may be with diphtheria. The presence of diphtheria bacilli, which do not produce disease, is no proof that they are not virulent. They may be highly virulent: they may even start a general epidemic. I simply speak of these as things for the physician to bear in mind in case difficulties arise which he may not have anticipated or provided for.

It seems to me that there is one point which has not been insisted upon by the gentlemen who have spoken, that is, that the returns should indicate absolutely the stage or duration of the disease when the culture was made. The rapid substitution of the specific germs of disease for other germs, such as streptococci, staphylococci, and putrefactive species on the mucous membrane, is something surprising, and accounts for the difficulty of finding bacteria in late stages of the disease. Hence, in those cases from which cultures are obtained comparatively late in the disease, a negative result is not to be relied upon as proving the absence of diphtheria bacilli. In regard to technique, we all know that every method has its advantages and its drawbacks. I think perhaps, on the whole, that the swab might cause the fewest negative results in the culture-tube, because more of the membrane or exudate would be taken with it and transferred to the tube.

The Chairman.— We should be sorry to leave this subject without the practical side being presented, and I will call upon Dr. Shea.

Dr. T. B. Shea.— Mr. Chairman and gentlemen, since the diagnosis of diphtheria has been referred to the bacteriologist, conditions have arisen which to us charged with the care of these cases occasion not a little worry and anxiety. I refer especially to those mild cases of diphtheria presenting in themselves no clinical evidences of the disease, and no history of exposure. These are the cases that try the health officers. For example, a report reaches the office that a child has broken through quarantine, and probably would be found in the street playing with other children. A visit is immediately made, and the parent or guardian is asked by what right he has violated the regulations. We are immediately met by the statement that the child is not sick, has not been sick; and sometimes, I am sorry to say, their statement is verified by that of the family physician, that he has examined the child and could find no evidences of the disease. What are we to do in this case? Examination is made. If any membrane is found, we make short work of that case by reporting the facts to the board; and probably an order issues for its removal to the hospital. But, if on examination we find the case is probably two weeks old, and no clinical evidences of the disease, a culture is taken and referred to the bacteriologist. The report is anxiously waited for, and it comes that the child has diphtheria. What, then? I am free to confess that in the majority of these cases after talking with a parent or guardian, showing them the danger to themselves and their family if the child is not isolated, they cooperate with us; and, if it cannot be properly isolated at home, they acquiesce in the removal to the hospital. But sometimes unfortunately we meet with people who have opinions of their own and are willing to defend them. What, then? If a child will not be isolated by the parent or proper guardian, what are we to do? That is a question for the bacteriologist. Can the bacteriologist tell us, "Is that child in his present condition dangerous?" — is that child a source of danger to the community? If he is, then we will remove the case to the hospital. But, when the culture is sent to the bacteriologist, and we learn that the child has bacilli of diphtheria in its throat, we want him to add that those bacilli are virulent and can do damage. If he can, our way is clear, and we can proceed.

I can tell some of the gentlemen here who have asked about the removal of cases that we have been at that work this winter. Cases where we have never been in doubt we have removed to the hospital; but, as I said before, we do meet with some cases and we do meet with some people that cause us anxiety how to proceed. There was a case that occurred in Dorchester where a child had been sick for over a month with nasal diphtheria; and, as usual, a report reached the office that the child was out playing in the street. I was sent to investigate the case. I saw the mother, and asked her why the rules and regulations provided for this class of cases had been violated. She told me she had a physician, and that she thought the interest of her child demanded sunlight and fresh air, and that we were doing wrong to qnarantine that child any further.

Now, that was a case where I thought the bacteriologist's place was to assure us at that time as to the virulence of that diphtheria. If it was virulent, then we would quarantine the child. If not, I think we should be doing an injustice toward the child as well as an injustice to the community and to the family.

THE CHAIRMAN.— Dr. Rogers.

Dr. O. F. Rogers.— Mr. Chairman, I thoroughly appreciate the privilege of being present and listening to this exceedingly interesting and instructive discussion of the subject.   I approach it as a general practitioner, and not as a bacteriologist.   The result of such cultures as I have been able to make in the last fourteen or fifteen months has been to establish in my mind the value and the accuracy of cultural diagnoses.   At the same time it has confirmed in my mind very strongly the belief that the diagnosis of most men, the clinical diagnosis, is in most instances accurate. The percentage of error is rather small.   My errors have been of two sorts. I have mistaken mild diphtheria, in a few instances, for tonsilitis, but the percentage is exceedingly small; but it is sufficient to warrant me in coming to the conclusion that it is the duty to-day of every man to make a culture in every case where he sees a deposit of any sort or kind in the throat.   I am aware that it throws a large amount of labor upon physicians to report the facts to the board of health: but it can be done without any expense to themselves, and I believe the best interests of the public demand that this should be done.   I confess that I am not always in the habit of doing it, but I certainly shall endeavor to do so in the future.   I am quite sure that no man, no matter how accurate he is, can always say whether a given case is diphtheria; and the errors that he will make will be in the way of overlooking and calling diphtheria something else.   Everybody has seen instances of that sort.   There is another error of diagnosis which is on the side of safety: that is. mistaking the streptococcus throat for diphtheria.   I do not know of anybody that knows whether or not a streptococcus throat is infectious, or, if so, to what extent it is infectious.   I, certainly, for one. would not want the streptococcus grafted on to my tonsil or placed in my mouth on the chance that there might be an abrasion, in which case I am quite sure I should be in very great danger of having streptococcus throat.   It has happened to me several times to make a diagnosis of diphtheria, because I found a membrane which had travelled off the tonsil toward the roof of the mouth to the anterior pillar, and on to the posterior wall of the pharynx, which seemed to warrant me in declaring the case to be one of diphtheria; and I think in three cases, perhaps more, I have reported them without waiting for the cultural diagnosis.   You can imagine my surprise when the word came back that the bacilli of diphtheria were not found.   Now. in such a case. I shall stand to my diagnosis.   Not that I doubt for a moment the truth of the statement of the bacteriologist.   I have the highest respect for that. but as a measure of self-protection. also as a measure of protection for other members of the family, I shall insist upon that card staying there : and as long as the board of health does not take it upon itself to say it is not a case of diphtheria because it has received a report from its bacteriologist that the case is not diphtheria, and takes down the card, it won't come down until I see fit to have it, which will be when the membrane has absolutely disappeared, and I have made some more culture, and the culture has shown no Klebs-Loeffler or streptococci present. These cases all got well, and yet three of them were very severe cases. When we look at them, and consider that they have considerable constitutional disturbance, perhaps the membrane extends clear to the end of the tongue, the corners of the mouth, the nose, the lip, the conjunctiva, and grows on every abraded spot into which it is rubbed, one asks, "Why should not that child be quarantined?" He ought to be. And yet the bacteriologist says it is not diphtheria. If the board of health saw fit to interfere, it would put the doctor in a bad place; but they do not do it, fortunately. It would be very desirable if some authoritative statement could be made in regard to whether or not such cases are infectious, and to what degree they are infectious, whether or not the card is rightly up in such an instance.

Then as to the differences between the clinical diagnosis and the bacteriologist's diagnosis. Occasionally it has happened that I have used anti-toxin (in fact, I now always use it that way, if I use it at all) before I get my report from the culture. Now, if I do use anti-toxin, and it turns out I have not diphtheria, then I am in a double hole. I have used anti-toxin, and I have got a card on the house; and the bacteriologist says there is no diphtheria. Well, the only way to do is to stand to your guns, and declare that under the circumstances you are perfectly justified in doing it, as I believe every man is; and I believe also, if he has diphtheria, he is not justified in any event in not using anti-toxin in every instance. And, strangely enough, in cases where I have used anti-toxin, and there has been a streptococcus growth in the culture, the results have seemed to be beneficial. I know that, in saying this, I am perhaps going contrary to the wise men of the world; but what a man sees he sees.

In regard to negative cultures, when they first began to make them, some men in Dorchester were a good deal cut up because the report came back, "No growth." I suggested that they spit in the tube to see if that would not do something. [Laughter.] I do not know whether they followed the advice or not, but I know they do not come back as they used to. But it won't do to say. If a man touches the wire to the throat, something will always grow. I made sure of that in one case. I managed to pick off a piece of the membrane and applied it in the tube, and then got nothing. But the negative culture settles itself very easily. As men learn to make cultures, I am quite sure there will be less and less trouble.

THE CHAIRMAN.— I should like to ask Dr. Rogers how he dealt with the family when he got the card up, and found a negative culture.

DR. ROGERS.—I told them that they had not the Klebs-Loeffler diphtheria, but a streptococcus diphtheria. [Prolonged laughter.] Up to date it has always floored them.

THE CHAIRMAN.— There is time to continue the discussion briefly.

DR. PIERCE.— Mr. Chairman, it seems to me that the bacteriological examination and clinical appearances should be brought much nearer together than they are at the present day. I speak of that because it has been admitted that we do find diphtheria bacilli in perfectly healthy throats. If that is admitted, it brings me down to a question which I would like to ask, as in case of a child whose throat contains diphtheria bacilli upon bacteriological examination, and that child has no clinical appearances, is perfectly well and about the streets,— whether the board of health is justified in isolating that child, though he is perfectly well himself; whether, because he is able to communicate to others, he should be isolated. Is the board of health under such conditions justified in removing that child to the hospital, forcibly removing him?

THE CHAIRMAN.— I am sorry the lawyer has gone, because we need more legal advice on this question. We want the lawyer to tell us when the responsibility of the attending physician begins and when it ceases. The statute law says that, when a physician knows of a case of contagious disease, he shall immediately report it to the board of health. I certainly hope that physicians will not be led to give up the evidence which clinical observation gives them, however valuable we think the evidence from the bacteriologist is ; and we all allow it the highest place. I hope the physician will continue to respect the clinical evidences and his responsibility under the law to report cases as soon as clinical observation will warrant.

The hour being late, I will call on Dr. Ernst to close the discussion.

PROF. H. C. ERNST.— Mr. Chairman and gentlemen, I have, as well as I am able, written down the points that seem to me to require reply as they have been brought up. Dr. Swarts has begun by expressing a very strong feeling in preference of the swab over the wire for obtaining cultures. Of course, that was true when the method began. The swab is much easier to use, and I recognized that fact when we began to use the wire. I also recognized the fact that the swab had been used very much more than the wire ; but, before we decided upon using the wire, we had been carrying on experiments for a year in regard to the comparative accuracy of results as obtained with the swab and with the wire, and I know of no place where those experiments have ever been carried on excepting by us, and we found unquestionably that the results were very much more accurate, as far as the discovery of the existence of the bacilli of diphtheria is concerned, if the wire were used than with the swab. It did require a little more learning on the part of the physician ; but it seems to me, on the whole, the general profession in this community are using the wire with quite as much ease as the swab. Our outfits have been carried to Germany in two instances this summer with a view of introducing precisely the same methods there, both in Hanover and in Hamburg. All the testimony that I have been able to get is this : that this outfit for the general purposes is as complete as has been suggested. I meant to have asked Dr. Swarts also how many cases a day came to his office for diagnosis.

In regard to the use of the telephone, as can easily be seen, if we should undertake to telephone our results (and we usually average 35 or 40 a day), it would require a special telephone and special service, besides giving a chance for its inaccuracies.

He asked a question also as to the possibility of a snap diagnosis from a swab as rubbed over the throat, and then a microscopic preparation made. In answer to that, I must say I should be absolutely sceptical of the results. That method of diagnosis has been wholly abandoned in Paris, and I have never seen any reason to rely upon it at all in this country. In fact, I think Dr. Williams at the City Hospital showed that it was unreliable.

I meant to have spoken in the first place in regard to our methods of staining. We use, of course, Lœffler's Alkaline Methylene Blue ; but we have also found that " Hunt's " stain is extremely effective in doubtful cases.

The question of the virulence of the bacilli in the throats of healthy persons has not been very accurately and extensively worked out. As far as the evidence goes, the virulence of bacilli in the throats of healthy persons, persons who have had no symptoms at all, is probably small. The investigation, however, is being carried on ; and some time during the coming year we hope to have very effective results from the work that is going on at the Children's Hospital.

With reference to what Dr. Smith said, it is perfectly true that any negative results are to be taken with a certain grain of doubt under ordinary conditions : but given the conditions of this method of diagnosis, given the thousands and thousands and thousands of examinations that have been made, it seems to me that experience shows very clearly that we can place much more reliance upon cultures made with proper precautions than would be the case without this experience. So that personally I have grown to put a great deal more confidence in a negative result I have obtained than I should have had two years ago. It seems to me that all the evidence tends to show that this method of diagnosis is more accurate as regards the results obtained than is the case with the microscopic examination for the bacilli of tuberculosis, or is the case with testing for albumen

in the urine.   If we are to rely upon these, we certainly are justified in re-
lying upon this cultural diagnosis.

The length of time of the disease is emphasized on this new blank, so
that that point is covered.

Then Dr. Smith also thought we should obtain less negative results by
using the swab.   I have the impression that he means less negative results
as regards no growth at all, not less negative results as to the presence or
absence of diphtheria from the swab; and that, of course, is perfectly true.
But the whole point of the observation in regard to the use of wires is as to
accuracy of obtaining the bacilli and the distribution along the surface of
the nutrient media, so that, when the bacilli of diphtheria are present, they
will have an opportunity to grow, and not be overwhelmed by the masses of
other bacteria that are likely to be taken up by the swab.

In reply to Dr. Shea as to the virulence or non-virulence of the bacilli
persisting in cases that have recovered, the evidence tends to show that
they are non-virulent.   I mean in cases where the diphtheria symptoms
have disappeared, and bacilli are still persistent in the throat.   Of course,
no positive statement can be made in regard to it; but the evidence shows
that or tends to show that.

I do not know why Dr. Rogers should have any hesitation in feeling that
the streptococcus in the throat is an extremely infectious one.   It is unquestionably so; and, if anything has been determined in this method of examination, it is that these cases of streptococcus in the throat are just as
infectious as cases of ordinary diphtheria.   The point of emphasis is that
it may not be far in the future before the board of health has a new form of
card, using the expression "a streptococcus throat," or some similar thing,
where the culture diagnosis shows the absence of diphtheria bacilli.   The
difference so far as the clinical evidence shows — that has been gathered
not only in our City Hospital, but elsewhere — is that streptococcus infection does not, as a rule, produce the severe symptoms, and it is not as a rule
as malignant in the percentages of mortality; but, of course, the separation
of this disease from true diphtheria is not exact, and we have not a great
deal to go upon.   In an article which I wrote upon diphtheria some years
ago I made the distinction between true diphtheria and other affections
that resembled it clinically.

Of course, every person who asks the question of me receives the advice
to use anti-toxin without waiting for the bacteriological result.   There is
no question about that at all, and the board in its forthcoming report shows
the wisdom of that absolutely.   In general practice there is no death reported where the serum was used reasonably early.   Anti-toxin does no
harm.   It has been shown that it can be used without producing any ill
effect whatever; and, even if it is not a case of true diphtheria, the clinical

symptoms are a guide as to whether one should wait for the result of a culture or give the patient the benefit of the doubt — and the anti-toxin.

I know, as every bacteriologist knows, that the mere touching of the throat with the wire is not invariably followed by a growth. It may occur to any one. as happened to me only the other day, where I undertook to make a culture with the wire, that no growth followed the passing of the wire over the nutrient medium. And I think Dr. Rogers has had that brought to his attention before, that, when the cultural diagnosis first began, it was apt to be found that scme antiseptic had been used in the throat, and that was the reason there was no growth.

As to the virulence of the bacilli occurring in the throats of healthy persons where there are no symptoms at all, I think Dr. McCollom's experiments show very perfectly that, unless a patient has been exposed to diphtheria and had a chance of carrying around the bacilli, that bacilli are not found. Dr. McCollom made a long series of investigations of the throats of healthy persons who had not been near, so far as he knew, a case of diphtheria. and never once found anything resembling bacilli of diphtheria. If bacilli are found, therefore, it seems to me the evidence shows that that particular person should be quarantined, at any rate for a time.

Now, the last point raised by Dr. Durgin, as to how much notice should be taken by the board of the positive results from the laboratory,— of course this question must be answered before a great while. I think Dr. Norton could give some information in regard to that of the case that occurred in Everett in the spring. A positive result was returned from the laboratory, and the physician refused to report the case as one of diphtheria. I do not know what the result was, but the Everett Board of Health took the matter in hand. It seems to me as if that was one question that must be settled.

These are all new points that are raised by this method of investigation : and, if there is any value in it, they must be carefully studied. It seems to me as if the evidence certainly is in favor of the value of the method.

THE CHAIRMAN.— We must bring this interesting discussion to a close, because I notice the authorities of the house are peeping through the small cracks to know when we are going to get through.

The meeting was then adjourned.

THE BROOKLINE PUBLIC BATH.

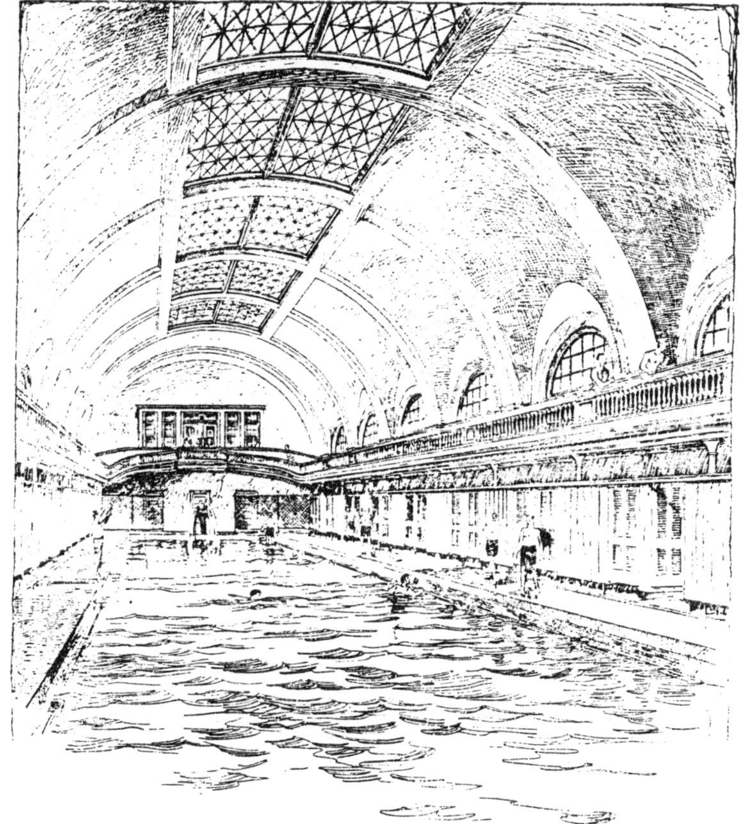

A MODEL PUBLIC BATHING ESTABLISHMENT.

Chairman Horace James, of the Brookline Board of Health, in his address of welcome to the Massachusetts Association of Boards of Health when it met October last in Brookline, stated that the town would consider in a day or two the question of providing improved public bathing facilities, and further expressed the conviction that the town would vote to have them. The town voted, as Chairman James predicted it would, to build according to the plans of the committee appointed in April, 1895, and appropriated $40,000 for the purpose.

The location is the centre of population of the town, and adjoins the principal playground and the new High School. Certainly, the location is the best possible and the surroundings most congenial. The handsome brick building will contain a number of improved shower baths (the so-called "rain baths" of the German army) and a swimming tank 80 feet by 26 feet, lined on the bottom and sides with white glazed brick. There will also be a few bath-tubs, a plunge bath 22 feet by 10 feet, meeting-rooms, and other interesting features. The architect is Mr. F. Joseph Untersee, a resident of Brookline. We hope after the opening, expected in August, to give our readers a further account of this model American public bath. The importance of frequent bathing as a sanitary measure and the value to a community like Brookline, which has no water front, of a place where her school children will all be taught the healthful and life-saving art of swimming, cannot be overestimated. We heartily congratulate the progressive town of Brookline.

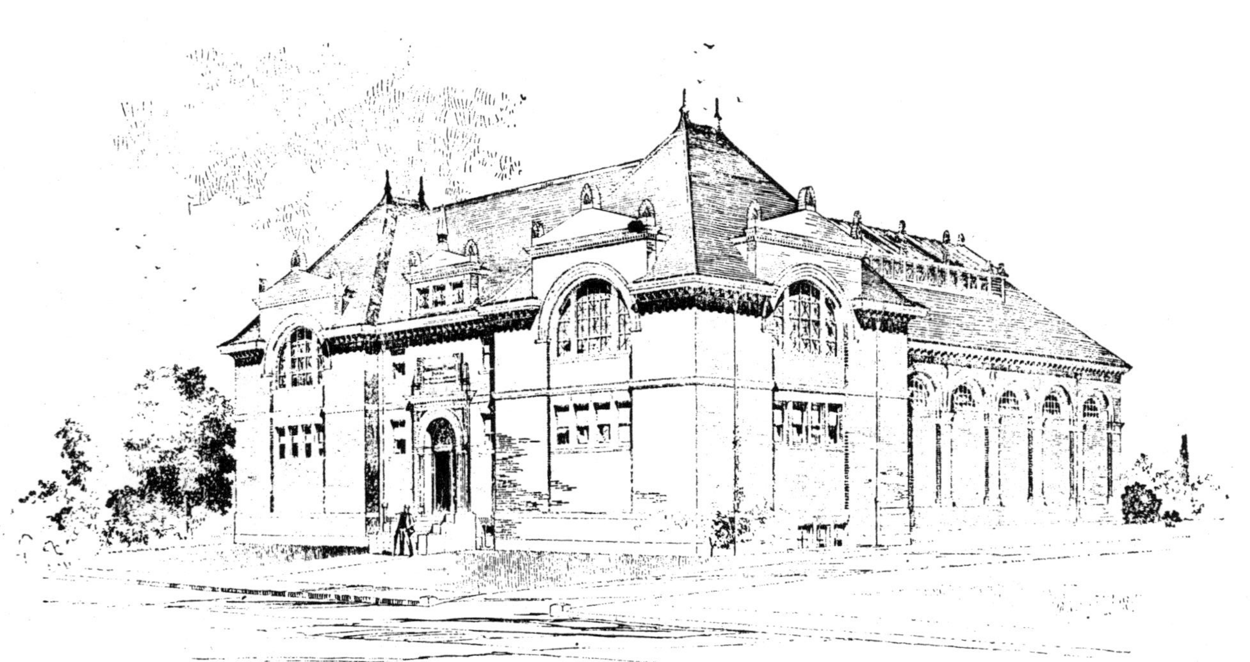

THE BROOKLINE PUBLIC BATH.

(From architect's drawing.)

THE AUTHORITY OF LOCAL BOARDS OF HEALTH OVER PUBLIC INSTITUTIONS.

The following extract from a pamphlet published at the Massachusetts Reformatory in Concord contains information which may prove useful to the boards of health of such cities and towns as contain public institutions or establishments within their respective limits.

A comparatively new question has recently arisen which will appear interesting to all local boards of health, since it relates to the authority which such boards may have over State or national institutions situated within the limits of the cities and towns. The Board of Health of the town of Concord recently submitted the following questions to the Attorney-General : —

(1) Has the Board of Health of the town of Concord authority to inspect the plumbing and drainage of that part of the Massachusetts Reformatory within the walls, or order changes therein?

(2) Has the said Board authority to inspect the houses occupied by the superintendent and deputy superintendent upon the front of the said prison building, or to order changes therein?

(3) Has the said Board authority to inspect the unattached tenements belonging to the said Reformatory and upon the land of the Commonwealth, and occupied by its officers, or to order changes therein?

(4) Has the Board of Health authority to make regulations concerning the keeping of swine by the Massachusetts Reformatory, and, if so, do we come under the regulation prohibiting piggeries to be within six hundred feet of the highway?

(5) Has the said Board of Health authority to order the discontinuance of the transportation of swill from the State Prison at Charlestown to the Reformatory piggeries?

(6) Has the town of Concord authority to demand that the dogs belonging to the Massachusetts Reformatory shall be licensed?

In replying to these questions the Attorney-General considered the subject at length, quoting decisions which had been made in other States on such matters, and summed up the questions as follows : —

The fountain of the police power of the Commonwealth is the legislature acting under the authority of the constitution. The legislature has seen fit to delegate a portion of this police power to local boards of health. Although this delegation is absolute in terms, it is not to be construed as exclusive of the authority of the Commonwealth or as against its public policy. It would certainly be against public policy to hold that a local and transient board should have greater authority over the property of the Commonwealth, cared for and controlled by the officers of the Commonwealth, acting under direct authority of the legislature, than those officers themselves. It is much more consistent to assume that in the delegation of police power to boards of health there is an implied reservation as to the property of the Commonwealth which is specifically and fully provided for by legislation, and the care and control of which is committed to boards and officers established for that purpose and acting under the direction and authority of the legislature. Any other position is inconsistent with the sovereignty of the Commonwealth. It follows, therefore, that, although the delegation of authority to local boards of health is general in its terms, and purports to embrace all persons and property within the limits of the town, there is an implied exception of such property as is cared for and controlled by the Commonwealth itself, and under its special and peculiar jurisdiction.

I am of opinion, therefore, that your first three questions relating to the authority of the Board of Health of the town of Concord to inspect and order changes in the plumbing and drainage (1) of that part of the Reformatory within the walls, (2) of the superintendent's house, (3) of the unattached tenements belonging to the Reformatory and on the land of the Commonwealth and occupied by its officers, must be answered in the negative.

The same considerations, in my opinion, apply to the keeping of swine within the limits of the property of the Commonwealth occupied by it for the purposes of the Reformatory. It is unnecessary to decide whether the penal statutes of the Commonwealth, or even such provisions of the common law as have the force of penal statutes, are in all cases applicable to the officers of the Commonwealth. Many of them, obviously, are so applicable. An officer of the Commonwealth, even under the direction of the superintendent of the Commissioners of Prisons, may not commit felony or any other grave crime or misdemeanor. On the other hand, statutes relating to hours of labor and to fire escapes, and even the ordinary rules of law relating to assault, are inapplicable to the conduct of the Reformatory. It may be a question whether, if the officers of the Reformatory permitted a preventable nuisance to exist upon the land of the Commonwealth, such, for example, as a decaying heap of vegetable matter, a filthy and offensive piggery, or other source of pollution of the health of the neighborhood, they could not be indicted and punished for maintaining a nuisance. It is not to be presumed that the officers of the Commonwealth will direct or authorize acts which are in violation of the rights of the community; and, if such acts occur, it may well be that the court would hold them to be unauthorized, or, if authorized, that the persons in charge exceeded their own authority. So, if the keeping of swine should become, in fact, a nuisance to the extent that people residing in the neighborhood were endangered in their health, it may be that the persons in charge or responsible for such keeping would be liable to be indicted therefor as for a nuisance.

But this is a very different question from that which involves the right of the local board of health to prescribe an arbitrary distance from the highway within the limits of which swine shall not be kept. That is a local police regulation in which a limit is fixed for convenience, and under which the question of the actual nuisance does not arise. An offensive and unhealthy pig-sty more than six hundred feet from the highway could not be complained of under such a rule, while, on the other hand, one that was clean, and in fact inoffensive, would still be unlawful within that limit. Even if the officers are liable for maintaining what is in fact a nuisance, it by no means follows that they are subject to the regulations of the Board of Health, with respect to the place where swine shall be kept, or that, in order to keep them, they shall be required to obtain a license from the Board. I assume that the keeping of swine is an incident of the business of carrying on the Reformatory, an institution which involves manufacturing, farming, and other industries, carried on under the exclusive jurisdiction of the State. For the reasons above stated with reference to the plumbing, I am of opinion that the rule of the Board of Health which prohibits the keeping of swine within six hundred feet of the highway does not apply to the land of the Commonwealth which comprises the Reformatory.

Question 5, relating to the right of transfer of swill through the public streets, stands upon a different principle. There is no exclusive authority over the streets of Concord conferred upon the prison officers. When they leave the property set apart for the uses of the Commonwealth and travel upon the public streets, they should be, and in my opinion are, subject to all reasonable regulations and laws, whether of the Commonwealth or of the town, or its officers, in regard to the use of such streets. And, if swill is carried by the officers of the Commonwealth through the streets of Concord in violation of the regulations of the Board of Health, I think the persons so offending may be persecuted and convicted; and that they cannot plead in justification any authority or direction of the officers of the institution.

The statutes of the Commonwealth (Pub. Sts., ch. 102) provide for the registration, numbering, describing, and licensing of dogs. This is a police regulation, made for the protection of the community. The license fee is not a tax. It is not authorized or designed for a revenue, general or local, but is in the nature of a license under a special police regulation, and is an exercise of the police power rather than the power to levy excises. (Desty on Taxation, 1404; Blair *v.* Forehand, 100 Mass. 139, 142, 143.) The object of the law may be said to be the identification and regulation of dogs running at large. There is, it is true, no exemption in the statutes of dogs which are not allowed to run at large; and it may be well that the legislature contemplated the possibility that dogs, which, although not beasts *feræ naturæ*, are yet less under subjection than neat cattle and other like domestic animals, would run at large. I see no reason why dogs kept by the officers of the Commonwealth, even though they be the property of the Commonwealth, should not be registered, described, and licensed; and, inasmuch as the fee is not in the nature of a tax, but for the registration and license, it should be paid as well in the case of dogs kept by officers of the Commonwealth or owned by the Commonwealth as in the case of other dogs. It would destroy the purpose of the law if any dogs were allowed to go at large unlicensed, and without the provision for identification prescribed in the statutes relating to the licensing of dogs. The Commonwealth, of course, may not be prosecuted for the keeping of an unlicensed dog; but whoever, whether a State officer or other person, keeps a dog, in my opinion, must have him licensed and pay the fee therefor, and is subject to the penalties of the statutes for failure so to do.

ON THE PROTECTION OF PUBLIC MILK SUPPLIES FROM POLLUTION.

BY PROFESSOR W. T. SEDGWICK,

MASSACHUSETTS INSTITUTE OF TECHNOLOGY.

ON THE PROTECTION OF PUBLIC MILK SUPPLIES
FROM POLLUTION.

BY PROFESSOR W. T. SEDGWICK,

MASSACHUSETTS INSTITUTE OF TECHNOLOGY.

The milk-supply question is to-day perhaps the most pressing problem in American sanitation. The public has become tolerably well informed in regard to the dangers of impure water. City officials, engineers, and members of boards of health, physicians, sanitarians,— almost everybody,— now know that with water, as with many other things in this world, appearances are often deceitful, and that in the innocent-looking, sparkling glass of cold water, once the symbol of purity and the emblem of charity, may lurk the germs of disease, the messengers of death. In many States much still remains to be done, to be sure, in educating the people and in providing them with pure water; but in our own fair State, thanks to a wise and able State Board of Health supported by an enlightened and generous public opinion, this great work of education and provision is well advanced. And this is the more fortunate as it bids fair to enable us as sanitarians and guardians of the public health to begin to turn our attention to another aspect of preventive medicine, which urgently demands our most serious attention.

Next in magnitude and in importance to the question of water supply is that of milk supply. There can be no question of this. The only question is whether it stands next before or next after in urgency and importance. Like water, milk is a liquid, and hence favorable as a vehicle for micro-organisms. It is less used than water, but far better soil for bacteria to thrive upon. It is more costly than water, but still cheap and deservedly of high repute as food. It wears a heavy veil of white,— everywhere the emblem of purity and innocence; but there is only too much reason to fear that milk is often nevertheless wolfish, though arrayed in sheep's clothing. Water is, in essence, inorganic and not subject to decay: milk is a direct product of living animal tissues and, being richly organic, is therefore highly putrescible. Water is usually served in towns and cities from tightly-closed pipes or vessels buried in the earth, so that it arrives in much the same condition as when it left its source. Milk is extensively manipulated by human agencies, transported in various vessels by wagon or by rail, and reaches the consumer in a totally different state from that in which it left its source,— the cow. The germs of most diseases die out in pure water. The germs of many diseases probably thrive in pure milk. In fine, milk, by virtue of its high reputation as a food, its veil of white, its richness in organic matters, its fluid consistency, and its cheapness, is an ideal vehicle for the distribution of disease germs, if these once find entrance into it. That disease germs do often find entrance into milk supplies is now a truism.

I have long dwelt publicly upon these facts, and from time to time, in epidemiological investigations for the State Board of Health, have had fresh and striking proof of their importance.

The great epidemic of typhoid fever in Springfield in 1892 taught Dr. Chapin and myself lessons in regard to milk and its dangers which we shall never forget. An epidemic of typhoid fever in Somerville in the same year led me to consider the part played in milk epidemiology by the *system of supply*, and similar epidemics during July, August, and September last in Cambridge, compelled me to return to the question. I had long suspected that the system of supply, or the handling, of the milk in Boston and vicinity was peculiar, and in some ways very objectionable from a sanitary point of view; and I was curious to know how it compared with the systems in vogue in other American cities and towns. On behalf of the State Board of Health I have, accordingly, recently visited the principal cities as far south as Washington, and made inquiries in cities as far westward as Chicago, in order to be able to compare the Boston system of supply with theirs. But, before describing the systems of supply in other cities, I ought, perhaps, to say something about the system in the Greater Boston, because, I dare say, there are members of this Association who are not familiar with the details of that system. In the matter of milk supply, as well as in other problems, it is necessary to go into details if one would fully understand the situation.

THE BOSTON SYSTEM OF MILK SUPPLY.

In Boston the milk is very largely railroad milk; that is, it comes from more or less remote towns as far west as the Hoosac Tunnel, and northward and southward nearly as far, and is brought in on trains in small cans,— small, I mean, as compared with those in use in other cities. As a result of what I have seen in other cities I am led to believe that in Boston the system is more differentiated, more highly developed, more admirably managed from an economic point of view than in any other city. It is controlled, according to a recent statement of Mr. Whitaker of the Dairy Bureau, largely by three men,— this railroad milk supply; and those men are known as "contractors." The trains, carrying the milk in eight-and-a-half-quart cans, come into the city, arriving, as a rule, about ten o'clock in the morning. The cans are then taken from the train by the local dealers, whom we may call local milkmen or pedlers, if we please, or dealers. They are not milkmen in the strict sense; at least, they are not cowmen, because they do not deal with the cows at all. They are local milkmen,— local dealers we may call them for convenience. The milk is taken by them to their headquarters or houses, which contain milk-rooms. These are too often closely connected with stables in which the horses are kept. It would not be fair to say exactly that the milk is handled in the stables; but the stables are generally only a few feet away, and the association of the horses with the milk is decidedly too close to satisfy good sanitary conditions. The milk-room is provided with ice-chests and the like and, what is of the highest importance, with one great "cooler," as it is called, or "mixer," a large tank holding the contents of a number of the cans,— perhaps ten, or even more in some cases. Over the top of this mixer is stretched, for a strainer, a cloth. At the bottom is a spigot.

All the cans, as soon as possible after they are brought into the milk-house, are "tasted." This is done often at the tail of the wagon, the can being simply tipped up on the tail-board and the plug knocked out; the man in charge "tasting" the milk to see if it is fresh. This is done as a protection to the dealer; for, if a can is sour, that can will be returned to the farmer from whom it came, and

of course the milkman does not pay for it. Now I cannot say that
this is the first objectionable operation in the handling. One should
begin, of course, with the conditions on the farm, in the stable, and
all that; but I will pass that by. The time spent on the train is another element. I ought to have said that the milk brought in at 10
A.M. is generally that morning's milk and the milk of the night before. Arriving at ten or eleven o'clock, it is tasted and handled
before noon. After the men have done their morning delivery in the
early hours of the day, they go to the trains and get the cans for the
next day's delivery, bringing them to the milk-house and tasting
them soon after their arrival, in the way that I have described.
Any sanitarian, I think, must stop right here, and say that this
"tasting" system is most objectionable, because, even if we do not
put the worst face upon it,— and I am very anxious not to do that
because this is an important industry and concerns the welfare not
only of dozens of farmers, but of dozens of other men whose living
depends upon their successful handling of the milk,— I say even if
they do not do the worst things that are suggested and said sometimes to be done (namely, take the milk into their mouths, taste it,
and then return it to the can in order to lose no milk), yet the mere
tasting and spitting of the milk out upon the floor is not a cleanly
operation, as I have often seen it conducted; and, if the man who
does it or the boy who does it happens to be suffering with an infectious disease, an early stage of diphtheria perhaps, it is not a pleasant thought that he has brought his lips in contact with a can the
milk from which may find its way to your table or to mine. The
tasting operation is, perhaps, almost essential, under our system, to
protect the milk dealer. But we are not now considering chiefly
what is essential or advantageous. We are considering what are the
facts, as a basis for proper sanitary interpretation of the conditions.
And at once we must set down the tasting operation, it seems to me,
as highly objectionable from every point of view. I may say I found
the same custom in most of the cities I visited,— Washington, Baltimore, etc.,— but not in New York. There is every reason to believe
that the custom grew up before any one realized the dangers of it.
All our ideas about infectious diseases are new. The germ theory
did not get established until about fifteen years ago in any reason-

able fashion; and the germs of the principal infectious diseases were not worked out until a little later than that. So that it is not strange that this custom, pertaining really to a primitive period, should have grown up as it has and remained as it has.

The milk having been thus "tasted," the cans are emptied, one after another, in Boston,—this is all about Boston thus far; and I wish to emphasize some of these points, because they are peculiar to us, different from what we find in any other city; and I wish, moreover, to draw the conclusion which I believe to be perfectly just, that the system, while admirable from an economic point of view, from the point of view of convenience and all that, is, from' a sanitary point of view, perhaps more objectionable than that of any other city that I have seen,—the cans, I repeat, are emptied through the cloth strainer into the "mixer," and their contents are thus mingled, the dealer often mixing milk that has come from several different farms, different dairies. I am thinking of one man who used about eighty cans a day. He derived them from as many, I should say, as eight or ten different dairies, some of course furnishing only one or two cans, others many more than that. And, as these are handled in the car and handled in the wagon, it is as likely as not that a can from dairy A may stand next to one from dairy B, and one from dairy B may stand next to one from dairy C; and then, one after another, their contents may go together into the mixer. Now, this is highly objectionable, because, if there is disease in the milk from any one farm, you have here a diluted mixture of the whole; and when the little cans are filled from the spigot below, as will shortly be described, an even dose, though perhaps a slight dose, is drawn off into each one of them. This "mixing" of various milks is also, not entirely but largely, peculiar to Boston, and objectionable from a sanitary point of view, as any sanitarian can see.

The next step is the filling of the little cans. And Boston is the only city that I have discovered in which the milkman furnishes such little cans, furnishes the receptacle for the consumer. In New York, Philadelphia, Washington, Baltimore, Albany, New Haven, Buffalo, Cleveland, and all other large cities that I know about, the consumer, except in the "bottle" trade, furnishes the receptacle.

The milkman deals out the milk from some receptacle of his own, which he uses over and over again. But once the milk has gone from his can, or whatever it may be, on the wagon, his connection with it has ceased; and, no matter whether there is typhoid fever or Asiatic cholera in the house which he serves, there is never any ready means of communication from the house back to his wagon. But see how it is in Boston. The milkman furnishes numerous quart or pint tin cans, which he fills at the spigot attached to the cooler. These small cans are then stowed in refrigerators and iced. If bottles are used, they are filled in the same way, essentially; and I shall have to say more about that in a moment. The small cans or bottles are filled from the spigot, with the hands of the operator passing over or near the mouth of the can. And if any one of those cans has received a germ or a number of germs from any source, although the ice reduces the temperature to a point at which growth is probably slight, yet there is possibility, especially if the ice happens to run a little short, of the germs growing in the little cans. These cans are kept on the ice until the next morning, thus of course adding to the age of the milk and giving further opportunity for germ growth. And this particular mixing and handling does not occur in any other city, because they do not put the milk in little cans at all. The milk stays in big (usually ten gallon) cans, the product of each dairy separate from that of every other.

Very early the next morning the dealer loads his wagon with the little cans and some eight-quart cans for the bakery and grocery and other "wholesale" trade. And the Boston wagon, I find, is also peculiar and not seen in any other city. It is very ingenious. One horse draws a good deal more milk here than anywhere else. We have arrived at a fine differentiation of the system, admirably arranged as it is from a business point of view. And those cans are left on the doorstep at an hour of the morning suggestive of freshness, although the milk they contain is really at least twenty-four, and often thirty-six, or even more, hours old. Now if the can which is left on my doorstep to-day was yesterday in a place where there was scarlet fever or diphtheria, or stood on a kitchen table in a tenement perhaps, there is a chance that it may have got contaminated, and then having gone back to the milk-house, and perhaps not having been thoroughly washed, it may bring to me the next morning the germs of disease. I say no other city, as far as I know, anywhere, has our peculiar system. It is very convenient for the consumer. We do not have to provide any receptacle for the milk we buy. The servant-girl does not have to look out and have a bowl ready or a quart-cup. The milkman does it all. But from a sanitary point of view this must be regarded as an objectionable feature, because this system furnishes a possible bond of connection and the transfer of disease from house to house.

To return for a moment to the spigot and the filling of the little pint and quart cans, and also to the emptying of the big cans. If one of the men in the milk-house is in an early stage of typhoid fever; and if, as generally happens, there is a privy near by to which this man retires, with a mild diarrhœa perhaps; and if, further, as too often happens, he does not thoroughly clean his fingers on returning from the privy, but proceeds to empty the big cans into the cooler or to fill the little cans from the spigot,— it is not difficult to see that we have here an opportunity for contamination. In the principal Cambridge epidemic of 1896 I had every reason to believe that it was in some such way that the infection took place. The milk-farms from which the milk came were all right, as far as any one could discover,— they were even unusually good. We believed that the milk when it arrived in the city was in good condition, and also when it arrived in the milk-house. It was the milk-house of a careful, honest, and intelligent dealer. But it so happened that he had three helpers there who were, successively, in what we believe to have been an early stage of typhoid fever, basing our opinion upon expert medical evidence. We know that these people worked over the milk; and we know that there were eighty-six cases of typhoid fever more or less clearly due to that milk. There was nothing out of the way on the farms; but there were these people in an early stage of the disease in the milk-house, and they were working over the cans in this way. We know that they retired frequently to the privy, because they admitted it. They had bowel complaint, as they called it. And the privy was conveniently near, and not of a high grade. It was very easy to imagine, though not to prove — for there was no proof, it was strong circumstantial evidence only — that the trouble might have come in that way.

Such, then, is the Boston system: railroad milk in large quantities and, at the sources, not differing much from the milk in any other city, brought on trains which arrive at ten o'clock in the morning,— a convenient hour for the milkman, but resulting in an age of the milk which is undesirable; taken to the milk-house and mixed in an unfortunate fashion; first tasted in a very unfortunate fashion, then mixed, drawn off into little cans through a spigot, by hand. And, if any one has watched that operation and knows how the "striker" operates, he knows how he throws the little cans in under the spigot one after another, his hands very often coming into the stream of milk, the connection between fingers and milk-can being of the most intimate sort, food and fingers getting mixed up in a very unpleasant way. And, finally, we have the system of little cans furnished by the dealer, and not by the consumer. It is necessary, it seems to me, to go minutely into these details, if we would inquire further into the methods of protection. We must know where the trouble comes from before we undertake to remedy it.

SYSTEMS OF MILK SUPPLY IN WASHINGTON AND BALTIMORE.

How is it in other cities? In Washington I find that quite a lot of railroad milk arrives in much the same way; but it comes, to begin with, not in eight-quart cans, but in forty-quart cans, big and heavy. These are taken from the station directly to the dairies, as they are called there, which correspond to our milk-houses. But there is no stable near, and no mixer. The cans are set right in big tubs of ice-cold water or ice, and the milk is kept *in the same cans* in which it arrives. The trains arrive at the same time as in Boston; and the next morning these cans are put into wagons, open in the middle, such as you have all seen in New York, but with a "churn," as it is called, beside the driver, in which the milk of one or two cans is mixed. It holds a good amount of milk, two or three cans, these being forty-quart cans: two, perhaps, are dumped into it, and then the milk is drawn out and sold. When that is drawn out, more milk is put in. But in both Washington and Baltimore, such mixing as there is is done only just before delivery; and in both cities the milkman sits in the wagon. In Baltimore he rings a bell, which is a nuisance to any one trying to sleep in the morning, the ringing of bells all through the city being enough to drive any one distracted, if he is not a good sleeper. On the ringing of the bell, a servant is supposed to come out of the house with a quart-cup, or some receptacle, and get the milk. The day that I was there it was very cold, and the milkmen I happened to see did sometimes carry the milk into the house in their measure. But they poured it into something in the house, and brought nothing out of the house except what they had carried in for the moment only.

In Washington they are doing a good deal of bottle trade. In Baltimore and Philadelphia that is also being done a good deal, and in New York. But in all these places the health authorities regard it as objectionable, because it is an approach to the Boston system of furnishing the receptacle for the milk, and thus making a bond of connection which may wind in and out from the houses of the patrons to the milk establishment. They might also object to it for another reason, which they have not yet become familiar with; namely, that in the process of filling these bottles the milk from different dairies is necessarily mixed. In Washington I saw an ingenious bottling establishment where a big reservoir runs on a track,—a big wooden tub it really is, a square tub which runs on a track. In the bottom of the reservoir is a series of holes, with plugs. The bottles are put between the wheels on the track, and this receptacle is rolled along over the bottles. As it arrives over each row, the plugs are pulled out, the milk runs in, and the plugs are then put back. In order to accomplish this rapidly, the milk has to be mixed. In New York the Board of Health has very strict rules about the bottling of milk; but, in general, I may say that it is objected to by officials more on account of the bottles, which go from house to house, than on account of the mixing.

We are plainly dealing with a system which has slowly grown up, and it is very interesting to see how it has been evolved. We start with one family having one cow. Then come one hundred families and one hundred cows and a middleman must come in: if we have a thousand families and a thousand cows, we must have more middlemen. And when we reach a hundred thousand families and a hundred thousand cows, we have to draw from all the neighboring States. The matter has become an immense *system*. It is evidently an evolution made necessary by the development of the community from village life up to urban life.

The Baltimore system is a good deal like the Washington system. I should have said that they have two deliveries a day in Washington. The reason for this is because it is a warmer climate. In Baltimore the reform administration has established some very good laboratories; and the chemical, and even, indeed, the bacteriological, examination of milk is undertaken to some extent. And yet their laws or rules are defective; the courts do not support them very well, and the principal remedy which they seem to have is what they call "spilling." They spill the milk at the borders or frontiers of the city, at the railway stations, if they find it bad. And while that does away with the milk, it does not of course really meet the case as well as the system of inspection and penalties that we have here. There is some mixing there, and there is some bottle trade; but most of the milk is delivered from the single can just as it comes from the farm, without having been mixed with the milk from any other dairy. Dr. Stokes, the bacteriologist of the health department, an excellent pathologist, has lately reported a form of diseased milk which was new to me. I should like to touch on it for a moment, because it seems to me a remarkable and interesting case. The milk inspectors in Baltimore noticed that one of the samples of milk seemed to be very rich and creamy, but at the same time somehow did not look right. On studying into it with a centrifugal machine and a microscope, they found that it was filled with pus. I quote from the original paper by Dr. Stokes and Dr. Clement, State veterinarian:* —

Dr. Clement "was called upon professionally in August to attend a herd of cattle which, as the owners said, were 'milking pus.' I found a herd of about seventy cows all affected to a greater or less extent. They were all nearly dry, and what milk could be obtained was of a thick, yellowish nature. The cows stood in a double row of stanchions. The history obtained, after careful inquiry, was that the disease first appeared in one cow; that the owner's attention was

* *Maryland Medical Journal*, Jan. 9, 1897.

called to the condition of the milk by the retailers who bought it. The infection spread to the rest of the herd with great rapidity, so that in the course of two or three weeks the whole herd had become affected.

"These cattle were at the time on pasture, fed twice a day on mill feed, and, according to the foreman's statement, milked regularly. Further inquiry brought forth the information that a strange man had hired out on the farm, who was an experienced milker, but who sought professional advice from the physician attending the family for a sore upon his finger, which he said he got from milking cows on a large dairy farm in York, Pa. This man left the place in about a week; and a few days after his departure the disease appeared in the first cow, soon followed by its appearance in the rest of the herd. Cleanliness and irrigation with warm water gradually caused the animals to become dry, in which condition they have remained up to the present time. A complete autopsy was made upon one of the cows, but nothing abnormal was made out, with the exception of a purulent inflammation of the somewhat dilated milk ducts. Cultures from the blood of the beast and the internal viscera remained sterile."

THE SYSTEM OF MILK SUPPLY IN PHILADELPHIA.

In Philadelphia the amount of milk which is used is of course great. A very large amount of it (seven-eighths) comes on the railway. It is taken from the trains in the original forty-quart cans directly to tubs of ice-water, and kept and cooled until the next morning. The trains arrive, as here, in the morning; and there is not very much to be learned from the Philadelphia system that I have not already mentioned for other cities, excepting with regard to a few points. In the first place, they have pretty strict rules about tuberculosis, regarding which the following Resolutions with Preamble attached were adopted by the Board of Health of Philadelphia on Oct. 16, 1894: —

Whereas it has been decided by competent authority that physical examination alone is an uncertain and therefore unreliable means of determining the freedom of cattle from tuberculosis; and

Whereas the tuberculin test is the only means of detecting many occult cases of this disease, and is therefore indispensable in arriving at the knowledge that a herd of cattle is free from tuberculosis,— therefore

Resolved, that the Chief Inspector of Milk be and is hereby instructed to indorse as *untrustworthy* all certificates of the freedom of herds of milch cows from tuberculosis that are not based upon the use of the tuberculin test by trained veterinarians.

Resolved, That the Chief Inspector of Milk keep a book in which shall be registered all herds of milch cows that supply the city of Philadelphia that have been certified as free from tuberculosis by the method approved by the Board of Health, also of such as have not been thus reliably certified, and which are therefore "suspicious," which records shall be open to the inspection of the public. Said records shall contain the names of the dealers supplied by such herds.

Resolved, That all producers of milk supplying the city of Philadelphia who fail after sixty days' notice to furnish a certificate or clean bill of health of their cattle, based on the method of examination demanded by experts and approved by the Board of Health, shall be reported to the board, and be liable to have their milk rejected as being "*suspicious*."

In this connection I may remark that in several cities grocers and small dealers in milk are obliged to keep posted in plain sight a placard stating the sources of the milk which they are selling, so that, in case an epidemic occurs, or anything of that sort, an inspector could see at a glance where that milk came from. I think that this would be a great help anywhere. One of the chief things an epidemiologist has to do in a milk epidemic is to hunt about and find out where the milk comes from, and this often takes a great deal of time and trouble.

One of the interesting things in Philadelphia is its attitude toward skimmed milk and what they call "creamery slop" or "creamery refuse." They make a special point of this. They say that skimmed milk is one thing; hand-skimmed contains 1.75 per cent. to 3 per cent. butter fat, dependent on the method of setting; while creamery refuse contains from 0.1 to 0.3 of 1 per cent. of butter fat. That is, one is 1.75 to 3, and the other is from 0.1 to 0.3 of 1 per cent. Inspector Burns is very earnest upon this subject: he has, as the phrase is, "no use" at all for the material left by the separator, the milk which we should commonly call separator-skimmed milk; and the Board of Health of Philadelphia does not allow it to come into the city at all, but designates it by such names as "milk refuse," and "separator slop." If any one is interested in it, there is a long legal discussion in the Report for 1895 in regard to these matters, with a charge from Judge Hare covering several pages, which of course I cannot go into now. I may add that in New York no skimmed, or otherwise robbed, milk — that is, no milk except whole milk — is allowed to be sold or admitted to the city *in any form*.

The New York Board of Health takes the ground that if they once admit such a thing as skimmed milk into the city, it will surely get mixed with the whole milk, even although it is printed on it that it is skimmed, in letters of Gothic, etc.: it is a great deal better, they hold, to keep it out altogether, and they take that stand very strongly and in spite of the possible food value of such milk. In Philadelphia they admit the ordinary skimmed milk, but refuse skimmed milk derived from the separator.

THE SYSTEM OF MILK SUPPLY IN NEW YORK.

New York is, on the whole, it seems to me, by far the most interesting and instructive of our neighboring cities in every respect as regards its milk supply, because, in the first place, although it draws milk from as far away as Pittsfield, Mass., and Hornellsville in the western part of the State of New York, it has a very useful set of maps and a card catalogue showing exactly the districts from which the milk supply is derived. Then they have no contractor system in New York. There are one or two rather large wholesalers, but not very large. And the milk which comes on the trains for New York and Brooklyn — for it very largely comes through New York to Brooklyn, Long Island not supplying milk enough — arrives and is delivered to the consumer from these great distances as fresh in point of time as the milk that reaches Boston from a town like Acton, a point relatively near to Boston. In other words, it is so arranged that the trains arrive in the city from 9 P.M. to 7 A.M. They do not come in, as they do with us, at 10 in the morning: they arrive in the evening and the night. And the dealers, who are in communication with the farms from which the milk comes, — they are not buying through great contractors for the most part, — go to the train, take the cans, which are forty-quart or twenty-quart cans mostly, upon the wagons which are familiar to all visitors to New York, — those wagons having an opening in the middle, the man sitting with some cans in front of him and some cans behind him. They do not take the cans to milk-houses and taste them there. They do not mix their contents at all. They do not put the milk in little cans. The consumer furnishes the receptacle. So that it actually turns out that the milk delivered in New York is first, as fresh as the milk delivered in Boston; and it is delivered in the " original packages," so to speak, which is, I hold, a very important sanitary matter, because, even if there is infection in one forty-quart can, it is limited to that can, it is not mixed up with a lot of others and sent about in numerous little cans.

And the care of the milk and the rules for the registration of the dealers are remarkably good. Here, for instance, is a blank. I should say, right here, that a great deal of the milk that comes to New York comes from creameries, the creamery not being always what we understand as a creamery in the first instance, but really a milk-house in the country, a sort of clearing-house in a country town. A great deal of the milk also is condensed milk,— not what we buy as condensed milk, but more like what the New England Kitchen sells as evaporated milk. And the New York Board of Health obliges each owner of a creamery or condensary to fill out a blank such as I have here. This bears the name of the owner of the creamery, shipping station (county and State and railroad), states at what time the milk is shipped, how many hours in transit on the train, the nature of the water supply in the creameries, the number of cans per day, the number of quarts in bottles. A good many bottles are shipped, but the Board has a very strict rule about bottles. Then below you have the name of the farmer, number of cows, breed of cows, system of water supply for washing cans, etc. The rules which govern these things are very strict. I won't go through all of them. With regard to their skimmed milk, the rule is this, the first rule of the sanitary code governing milk : —

SECTION 186. No milk which has been watered, adulterated, reduced or changed in any respect by the addition of water, or other substance, or by the removal of cream, shall be brought into, held, kept, or offered for sale at any place in the city of New York, nor shall any one keep, have, or offer for sale in the said city any such milk.

With regard to bottling in the city : —

Milk must not be transferred from cans to bottles or other vessels on streets, or on ferries, or at depots, except when transferred to vessel of purchaser at time of delivery.

And further with regard to the bottle business : —

Milk shall not be sold in bottles except under the following rules : —
Bottles must be washed clean with a hot-water solution of soap, or soda, or some other alkali, and then with hot water before filling with milk.
Bottles must not be filled except at the dairy or creamery, and in the city only in rooms so situated as to prevent the contamination of the milk by dust from the streets or other impurities.
Bottles must not be washed or filled with milk in any room used for sleeping or domestic purposes or opening into the same.

Regarding store licenses : —

Store permits must be posted in stores so that they can be easily seen at all times.

Of course, as everybody knows, all rules and laws depend for their value upon the way in which they are carried out. But I was given to understand that in New York these rules are carried out with marked success. Dr. Martin, to whom I am especially indebted, seemed to me to have an admirably equipped department admirably administered.

My time, I see, is gone ; and I ought to stop here. But I want to make just one remark upon the recent report of Mr. Whitaker, of the Milk Producers' Union. Mr. Whitaker, after saying that the year has been an excellent one for production, says that there has been, if anything, an overproduction, and yet not quite that. Here are his own words, "One cause of the surplus in Boston is under-consumption." Mr. Whitaker goes on to say that the public does not realize the food value of milk. I should doubt that. It seems to me the public has been brought up to believe that milk is the one thing we can rely on, that it is remarkably cheap and digestible ; that if we want a convenient, cheap, and digestible food, milk meets those requirements. But Mr. Whitaker says: "The public does not appreciate and realize the food value of milk. When hard times come on and economies are necessary, milk is regarded as a luxury to be curtailed." I doubt that very much. "Truer economy would insist on using more milk and less meat. The consumption of milk has been decreased by the increasing use of condensed milk, which comes from greater distance, and by the increasing use of cream," etc.

Now I think one great reason for the diminished use of milk —
for Mr. Whitaker shows there is actually less of it used *per capita*
than before — is that the public is beginning to get waked up on this
matter. The public is beginning to feel anxious about the sanitary
condition of milk. I confess I have done a good deal to stimulate
that uneasiness, and I intend to continue doing it; for I believe that
the milk-supply problem is one of the very serious things of the day,
from a sanitary point of view. And instead of claiming that the
public does not understand the value of milk, I think it would be
a great deal better for persons interested to try to take pains to
assure the public that the milk is in the best possible sanitary condition. I think there is grave danger that the public shall lose confidence in milk. At a meeting which I attended a few evenings ago
some one suggested that the only safe attitude in regard to milk is
total abstinence. That, certainly, if it became common, would
diminish the use of milk still further than it has been diminished
thus far.

There are many other interesting points in this subject which
I should like to touch upon, with regard to the standard, for example.
It seems to me that Mr. Whitaker is very wise there. He does
not believe in any reduction of the standard, because that would
let in more milk, and milk of lower grade.

The conclusion of this whole matter, as far as I am concerned,
is that, in my opinion, the detailed administration of the milk business leaves much to be desired. What, then, are the remedies?
That, of course, is always the difficult thing. How can we provide
any adequate protection of the milk supply? After talking with a
good many different people and thinking the thing over a good deal,
I have about come to this conclusion: The local board of health
in any city interested in the milk supply has got to make rules that
no milk shall be sold in that city which it has reason to regard as
suspicious. And, in order to determine its condition, it has got to
employ skilled veterinarians and sanitary inspectors to visit the
farms and see that things are done there somewhat as they should
be done. Whether they can add to that successfully chemical and
bacteriological examination remains to be seen. I do not think that
that question can be settled off-hand. But I think it has got to

come down to this: If any community wants to be sure of the excellence of its milk supply, it has got to put in the hands of its own board of health authority to exclude from the city or town all milk concerning the character of which the board of health is not well satisfied upon reasonable scientific grounds. And it has got to provide that board of health with money enough to employ the necessary assistance to carry out such inspection and regulations. Take Cambridge, for instance. That is a case I have in mind. No milk ought to be delivered in the city of Cambridge about which the Board of Health has not a good deal of information. It is simply a question of expense and proper administration to look after the farmers supplying Cambridge. Tell the milkmen, " If you want to send milk to Cambridge, you have got to clean up, you have got to have your cows examined by our veterinary, you have got to satisfy us, from the cleanness and the freshness of your milk, that you are doing your best." It may be that the board of health in question must be able to prove the presence of dirt or decay or some other unsanitary condition in the milk as it arrives; but I fancy it would be sufficient to publish lists of approved dairies, and let the citizens do the rest. Then the dealers must either meet the requirements or send the milk somewhere else. I see no escape at present from something of this sort. It is expensive. It involves further administration on the part of boards of health, but I believe it is a sanitary necessity which is coming upon us now very fast.

THE PRESIDENT.— Before proceeding to the discussion of this very interesting paper of Professor Sedgwick's, I will submit to you the report of your Nominating Committee, Dr. Gage having unfortunately been obliged to leave the room. They present the following names :

President.

HENRY P. WALCOTT, M.D.

Vice-Presidents.

S. H. DURGIN, M.D.   S. W. ABBOTT, M.D.

Secretary.

EDWIN FARNHAM, M.D.

Treasurer.

JAMES B. FIELD, M.D.

Executive Committee.

J. C. COFFEY, ESQ.	W. H. CHAPIN, M.D.
J. A. GAGE, M.D.	H. L. CHASE, M.D.
R. L. NEWCOMB, ESQ.	

What action will you take upon the report of your committee?

DR. DURGIN.— I move that the Secretary be authorized to cast the ballot of the Association for the officers named.

Dr. Durgin's motion was unanimously carried.

THE PRESIDENT.— The Secretary informs me that the ballot cast for the officers of this Association contains the names which I have read to you. The discussion of Professor Sedgwick's paper is now in order. Dr. Chapin may possibly say something to us upon that subject.

REMARKS OF DR. CHAPIN, OF SPRINGFIELD.

It seems to me that the first thing to be done to prevent the contamination of our milk is to educate the people. There never was so good a thing happened to the city of Springfield as the epidemic of typhoid fever in 1892, and the appearance of Dr. Sedgwick in search of the cause, the appearance of the health officers from house to house, asking everywhere about the milk. The prolonged search, which was a great bother to both Professor Sedgwick and myself, was in the end a good thing; for, when we got through with a two months' search for the cause of the epidemic of typhoid fever, nearly everybody in Springfield knew that in some way or other, at some times, milk does make people sick. And they have not forgotten it. And, what is better than that, all milk dealers except the one that peddled this milk believed the same thing, too, and they still believe it. And I have had more than once, and more than ten times, perhaps, in the last two years, a milk dealer come to me personally and say, " Doctor, I am a little suspicious about a case of sickness over in Suffield, Conn. ; and would you mind going down there with me ? "   " Oh, no ; not at all. I should like to go."   And I would go down there, and either condemn the farm as being infected with a contagious disease or pass it by as probably free from such contagion.

Last summer, about the first day of June, I had reports in one day from two physicians. And, by the way, the physicians got educated, too ; everybody took part in that education,— nothing like stirring things up. On one day two physicians reported to me as follows : Dr. A. stopped me on the street. He said : " I have two families in which there is typhoid fever. One has three cases, and the other four. They are both supplied by such a milk dealer." Ten minutes after that I had another report from another physician, that he had a case of typhoid fever which he had found out was supplied with milk by this same milk dealer. They had taken the pains to do the search work for me and to report to me. The result was that in about three hours from the reports of those cases I had the case of typhoid fever which produced an epidemic of about eighteen cases. Within three hours of the first report I had the case located. As I say, the education of the people, of the physicians, and of the milk dealers, is the thing to begin with. But with all sorts of education there will come a case now and then where milk will be polluted, without any possibility of help. For instance, in the epidemic which I have just mentioned, a servant-girl began working on the farm on the third day of May, and on the twenty-first day, or about the twenty-first day, of May, she went away from the place sick, having been on the farm only three weeks. So far as the people on the farm knew, she had malaria. And they were honest about it. I traced the case back to Springfield, where she was then residing, and found her on a sick-bed with typhoid fever, as I expected she would be. I judged from the number of cases that she helped with only one or two cans ; in some way or other she had to do with only one can, I think, and there were about ten families infected with typhoid from that cause. Now, no amount of caution would prevent that, that I know of. But when the people of the State, and the people of Boston particularly, look upon raw milk as being as bad as raw beans, then we shall be a great deal better off than now. I wouldn't drink a glass of raw milk. I have had enough of it. I had four weeks on my back from it. I had typhoid fever. So, I say, educate the people in the city, the consumers of milk, to the belief that milk is a danger; teach them that sterilized milk is better than raw milk, and let them demand of their dealers that their milk shall be properly prepared.

In order to get at the farmer, it seems to me that a better way than to put the matter in the hands of local boards of health would be to appoint a district inspector of dairies. It is not necessary to examine every dairy in one day; and one inspector might cover considerable territory. If he did that, inspecting the cows as regards the health of the cows, particularly in regard to tuberculosis, cleanliness of the stables, and cleanliness on the farm, we might possibly educate the farmer to keep them clean. What time in the morning do you suppose the average farmer washes his hands for the first time? I suspect about breakfast time, after the milking is done. All milk that contains sand, manure, hair, ought to be rejected without any question whatever, as being filthy. And yet people will take that kind of milk without making much fuss about it. They do not look upon a teaspoonful or so of cow manure in the bottom of a [quart-cup as very bad. Possibly they may say something the following day to the milkman about it, but they take the milk just the same. I think that is true,— I know that is true. I was brought up on a farm. The most sensible food that we have upon our tables is produced in the filthiest localities possible. Now, no farmer ever thinks, as far as I know, of ever washing the cow's udder or of washing his hands before he goes to milking. I think there are some cases where they do, but they are few.

THE PRESIDENT.— Dr. Chapin, I hope your namesake of Providence can give us some more assurance of a better condition of things in Rhode Island.

REMARKS OF DR. CHAPIN, OF PROVIDENCE.

When Dr. Chapin said that he did not think the farmers washed their hands until breakfast time, I felt like offering an amendment.

We have in Providence recently established a model dairy farm, which I think *is* a model farm. And near by it is one of the old-fashioned kind. But the man on the old-fashioned farm felt that, if the model farm was going to start in and run competition against him, he would have to do something. So he determined to furnish milk which would be as clean as the other man's. I visited his farm and saw the men at milking time. I had just come from the model farm, and knew how they took care of the cows' udders and sterilized their glass jars, etc. And so I asked him various questions as to what he did. I asked him if they wiped the cows' udders, and if the men washed their hands. And he said yes. And I examined the men's hands, and I concluded that instead of washing them before breakfast they washed them about supper time, the time of the last milking. He told me that they always wiped off the udders with a dry cloth, because a damp cloth was bad for them. I asked him to step to the barn and show me the cloth. He stepped to the barn, and said, " Bill, where is that cloth that you wash off the udders with?" The man said, "I don't know." He said, "You are sitting on it." He said, "No, that is it out there." He got it and showed it to me. It was full of dust; it hadn't been taken down for a couple of months. So I think things are even worse in Providence.

I think you will find that Rhode Island people usually come to Massachusetts to receive rather than give. I came down here to receive information, and I have received a good deal of very useful information in regard to the management of the milk supply. And it seems to me that the difficulties have not been exaggerated. So what we have to do, if we want a milk supply which is clean and free from disease, is to make all the people that handle that milk, from the time that it leaves the udders of the cows until it is delivered to the customers, clean. And that is quite a contract. We have got to make them clean. If they will be cleanly, the dangers of receiving contagious diseases will be reduced to a minimum; though, even if they are cleanly, we cannot get rid of the danger entirely.

The points which Professor Sedgwick alluded to in regard to the different ways in which milk is delivered in different cities impressed me a good deal, as I was thinking of the way it was delivered in

Providence. It is quite different from the way it is delivered in Boston. Most of the milk in Providence is brought from the farm to the customer in a ten-gallon can. Some of it is brought in on the cars and mixed by the milk dealer, but very little of it. Most of it is either brought in in wagons or in cars in ten-gallon cans, and at the door is poured into the customer's measure.

We have not had much contagion due to milk. We have had within the last ten years only two or three epidemics, only one of which could be positively traced to the milk supply. It seems to me the chief way we can guard against this is to secure through the whole district from which the milk comes a thorough control of contagious diseases. When I said that Rhode Island people expect to receive from Massachusetts, I did not mean they expected to receive contagious disease. But it sometimes happens that in Providence we are liable to receive that very thing. I have at the present time a milkman who lives in Massachusetts, who has a case of scarlet fever in his family. He is still delivering milk, because I had a consultation with his physician and found that the case was very well isolated indeed, so that there was no danger in his continuing to deliver the milk. Last fall I learned of a case of typhoid on a milk farm in Massachusetts; and in that case I was not at all satisfied that it would be safe to have the milk brought into Providence, and I notified the man that he should not do it, and he did not do it. I also notified the secretary of the State Board of Health of Massachusetts in order that he might see that the milk was not delivered to customers in Massachusetts. I believe it was fed to a hog.

It seems to me that the only thing that we can do is to do that very expensive thing which Professor Sedgwick has suggested,— that we shall have a constant inspection of the sources of milk supply.

Dr. Chapin, of Springfield.—I should like to mention a fact that happened within the last two years in Springfield. A cow was quarantined for tuberculosis. The farmer was somewhat sceptical. He was obliged, however, to throw away the milk, and fed it to some kittens. The kittens are dead, and the autopsy has shown tuberculosis. And the farmer is converted.

The President.— Perhaps Professor Ernst will help us out.

REMARKS OF PROFESSOR ERNST.

Most of what I should have liked to say has already been said, so that there is very little left for me to add.

In regard to the general subject there does not seem to be any question that there is but one way in which the milk supply can be regulated and improved; and that is, a campaïgn of education so far as cleanliness is concerned. The stories that I have heard, and what I have seen of the surroundings of cows and of places from which the milk comes, are something almost unbelievable. The knowledge upon the subject is at such an extremely low ebb that I agree with Dr. Chapin in the feeling that it is a difficult problem to solve, a difficult matter to bring to a successful conclusion.

There are one or two points that struck me in what Professor Sedgwick said,— one in particular, laying so much stress upon the disadvantages of mixing milk,— that are so entirely contrary to my own feeling that I thought I would speak of them. The fact of mixing milk, it does not seem to me, is a matter of so much importance, provided this question of cleanliness is sufficiently well understood. The advice that I have given to my patients for years, and especially in feeding children, is, if they cannot get their milk supply from a single cow that they know, to be sure not to depend upon a milkman's single cow's milk, for the very reason that, if the cow be affected, for example, with tuberculosis, the chances of infection from a mixed supply seem to me to be very much less than the chances of infection from a single supply,— in accordance with experiments which are so well known, showing that it is not only the variety of the infectious microbe that is used, but the size of the dose that determines the results. So that, if the conditions of cleanliness are fulfilled, it would seem to me it is a little better to have a mixed supply than an unmixed. The forty-quart cans spoken of must contain mixed milk, and it must be mixed somewhere, because no single cow ever gives such a supply of milk; and in the creameries in New York State, outside of the city limits, the milk must be mixed there in order to fill the forty-quart cans.

There is another point of interest to me, from a scientific point of view, but I think Professor Sedgwick has already given the answer to it.   I have been interested to know whether, in any of his investigations, he has ever found in any of these cases the specific microorganism of typhoid fever.   I understood it was distinctly stated that the evidence was circumstantial entirely, but I wished to be sure that there is no direct evidence.

I think Dr. Chapin, of Springfield, insisted upon the use of sterilized milk at all times, which rather roused me, because I believe that the fad for sterilized milk has done more harm than it has good to the digestive apparatus of the coming generation.   I think the use of sterilized milk on all occasions for children is a great mistake. I speak with feeling about it, because, so far as I know, the first sterilized milk that was ever used in this country was given to a patient of mine; but it was used for a definite purpose and with a definite idea of obtaining results in that case.   I agree most heartily with Professor Sedgwick that the campaign of education, as regards cleanliness in the handling of the milk supply, is a necessity; but I believe it to be a great mistake to sterilize milk at all times for healthy babies, because it puts what seems to me to be an entirely unnecessary strain upon the digestive apparatus of those using it, especially of children.   I do not think children should be fed with sterilized milk unless there already exists some disturbance of the digestive apparatus, when the object of the sterilization is to prevent the addition of further ferments to the excess already present.

THE PRESIDENT.— I suppose we shall all have to admit that there really are two sides to this question; that, while there is milk which is not looked after and not cared for and not conscientiously treated, there is fortunately a certain amount of milk which receives everything that conscientious care and intelligent supervision can give to it.   And I am going to ask our guest, Mr. French, to tell us something about that.   No man knows more about it than he does.

REMARKS OF MR. FRENCH.

Mr. President and Gentlemen,— I have been very much interested in the milk question, I might say ever since I was an infant; and I do not know that it is necessary to go back any farther than that.

If I was to take any text on which to speak to-day, it would be some resolutions which I had the honor of offering at the annual meeting of the Bay State Agricultural Society, which was held here on the 20th, and which read something as follows: —

Whereas the object of all laws in relation to contagious diseases in cattle is for the protection of the consumer of meat and the products of the dairy, and whereas a large amount of milk from other States is brought into the State of Massachusetts without any guarantee as to the freedom from disease,

Resolved, That our present State laws are insufficient, so far as they give no adequate protection to the consumer from milk from diseased herds outside of our State;

Resolved, That the Bay State Agricultural Society he 'y offer a petition to the legislature now in session to take such action as will authorize the State Board of Health to make such regulations for the importation and sale of milk as will protect the inhabitants from the consumption of milk from diseased cows.

Now, I am assuming in this, or have assumed, that the State laws now were not sufficient to authorize the boards of health to take action in relation to milk outside of the State. Whether this could be done by ordinance or not, I am not prepared to say. In the city of Minneapolis it has been done by ordinance, and that ordinance has been sustained there in the State of Minnesota by the action of the Supreme Court. I have here a decision by the Supreme Court of the State of Minnesota, sustaining the milk and dairy ordinance of the city of Minneapolis providing for the inspection of dairy herds outside of the city and the use of the tuberculin test. Now, of course it is different in the city of Minneapolis, because a large portion or probably the whole of the milk that is brought into the city of Minneapolis comes from the State of Minnesota. Of course we cannot enact what might be called an extra-territorial law here which would govern the milk supply or regulate the milk supply in other States. But we do know here that as high as 40 per cent.,— it is so estimated by the Dairy Bureau,— as high as 40 per cent. of the milk that comes into the city of Boston comes from outside of this State. It comes from the State of Maine where, until a short time ago, it was supposed there was very little tuberculosis. And now it is estimated as high as 20 per cent. Large quantities come from that State. There are carloads of milk which come from New

Hampshire, and likewise from Vermont. I believe there are two carloads of milk that come from Connecticut. Now, under the general laws, as I understand, of the State of Massachusetts, the State Board of Health has power to inspect milk so far as adulteration is concerned and so far as they can detect disease here. But they have no authority, at least I assume they have not, to lay down laws and regulations in regard to the sale of milk in the city, so far as suspecting disease is concerned. We do not propose to interfere at all in any such legislation as may be desired with reference to what might be called the Interstate Commerce law. We would not say that you cannot bring any milk here. We cannot prevent carloads of milk from being brought in here if you choose. But what we want is that the State Board or the city Board of Health here in the city shall be able to say, if they are not already authorized so to say, that the milk when it comes here is under their care and inspection,— that is all. Of course you can detect adulteration, but you cannot detect disease until some unfortunate victim has been afflicted. Now, what we desire is, if a law is necessary, to have a law that will give the State Board power to say, " You may bring in all the milk that you want here, but, when it gets here, it is under our inspection," and to allow them to lay down such rules and regulations as shall govern it when it is here as they have done in Minnesota. Say to the milk contractors and to the milk dealers, "When you bring your milk in here from outside the State, you must be subject to these regulations."

Here is this great loophole. We pass laws here in regard to our own cattle and our own cows,— pass those laws here at the State House, and say to the farmers here that they must have their herds inspected, and that they must not send milk from diseased cows; and yet we allow this large percentage of milk to come in with perfect freedom without any inspection whatsoever. Now, we want the State Board to be allowed to lay down such regulations that they can say to the contractors and milkmen who bring in milk here from outside of the State, " You must prove to us that the milk that you bring in from outside of the State is not from diseased herds; that the sanitary conditions are likewise proper."

Now, that is the point, Mr. President, that I wish to emphasize, so that the milk from the dairies outside of the State that comes in here shall be accompanied by certificates from the State Cattle Commissioners or from the sanitary inspectors there, or from veterinary authority of some kind, that every dairy that sends milk in here from outside the State shall be inspected at least twice a year, and that the milk shall be accompanied with proper certificates, stating that the herd from which it comes is kept under proper sanitary conditions, and that the cattle are not diseased.

I do not know, Mr. President, that I have anything more to say except, if the boards of health consider this of sufficient importance, and if they have not sufficient power or authority at the present time, as I have assumed they have not, to do this thing, the Bay State Agricultural Society and other societies, I think, will be very glad to co-operate with them in asking for more legislation if it is desired. But it does seem to me that this is a matter that has been overlooked. Certainly I have never heard it discussed or talked of in any of the milk meetings of the milk associations or any other assemblies, in relation to this large amount of milk that is brought in from outside the State without any guarantee as to freedom from disease.

CLOSING REMARKS OF PROFESSOR SEDGWICK.

I might say just one word, perhaps, in the way of closing the discussion. It seems to me that the secret here is, just as it is everywhere else, a campaign of agitation and education. It is not that we are prejudiced against the farmer. Most of us are closely connected with the farming community, and have ourselves, perhaps, as Dr. Chapin says, been brought up on farms. We know the difficulties in the way, and we dislike to put burdens upon people who are little able to bear them. But sanitary science has its requirements; and an enlightened public opinion is going to demand a much more careful supervision of all this matter of milk supply, unless I am very much mistaken, and that in the near future.

Obviously, it would be unwise for any State to enact strict rules for the governance of its own citizens, and then by some loophole allow citizens of other States to bring into the State materials which it would not tolerate from its own citizens, if there is any possible way of preventing it. And I think we are indebted to Mr. French for calling our attention to this side of the matter.

With regard to the whole question, it seems to me we want to take this ground: We have got to be patient. Milk supply is a primitive industry. It goes back to the time when man led a pastoral life and lived with his flocks and herds. The good opinion of milk is based on that long acquaintance and experience with it. We still believe, as Dr. Ernst very wisely says, that, if only we could enforce cleanliness, all things would be well. The secret of modern sanitation is in one simple phrase, " Be clean." It is so in antiseptic surgery, it is so in everything sanitary.

In regard to mixing milk, which Dr. Ernst has referred to, it was not so much that I had in mind the mixing of the milk of different cows in the same dairy — though that of course is objectionable — as the mixing of the milk of the different dairies. So that, if there was a case of typhoid fever or scarlet fever upon one dairy,— I was thinking more particularly of human diseases when I spoke,— there would be trouble; and I meant diseases arising in that particular instance from a human being through the mixing of the milk from different dairies. That seemed to me, and does still, very objectionable, although I see the point, of course, of diluting the germs. However, under the Boston system you must bear in mind that the milk is kept in the little can after it is thus diluted; and the chance is that the germs are going to grow more or less.

I forgot to say, what I am very glad Dr. Ernst stated, about pasteurized milk. Sterilized milk is somewhat under a cloud, as he says, as being comparatively indigestible, besides the reputation which it must bear of, rarely, producing scurvy; and pasteurized milk, probably to a less extent, also. At the same time there are nations, I believe, which live upon boiled milk and are thriving. And it is here, it seems to me, simply a question of choice whether we should have more damage or less by sterilizing or pasteurizing than we now have with raw milk. There are grave dangers no doubt connected with the indigestibility of cooked milk. But those dangers are trifling, it seems to me, compared with those which pertain to raw milk. If we could get raw milk, as Dr. Ernst says, that is in its right condition, fresh and clean, I think I should be dis-

posed to agree with him.   But the human race being what it is, and
the historical development of mankind being what it is, I can simply
say that personally I never think of drinking any milk that has not
been boiled or pasteurized.   The results of pasteurizing, from a
bacteriological point of view, are very striking.   We can reduce the
number of germs from millions down to units by comparatively slight
pasteurizing.   And it seems to me that this is a very great safeguard, although we must always bear in mind, of course, the possible
danger of occasional cases of scurvy, and those other things which
enter into the problem.

Dr. Durgin.— I think this interesting address and discussion this
afternoon must have impressed every one present with the need of
some action.   And, in order that we may pursue this subject farther
and get the best results from it, I want to move that a committee of
five be appointed by the President, who shall draw up a set of rules
for adoption by boards of health within the State, and also a
set of rules for investigating cases and epidemics of disease which
may result from such polluted milk.   I make that motion.

The motion was then unanimously carried.

BACTERIA AND ACIDITY
OF THE MILK SUPPLY
OF BOSTON

REPORT OF THE COMMITTEE.

The committee appointed to consider and report upon "rules for protection of milk supplies from pollution and for the investigation of cases and epidemics of disease supposed to result from such pollution" have not formulated rules, and, if desired to do so, must ask for further time.

The committee prefers to present a plan which may be adopted by the local boards of health for the protection of the milk supply for the locality rather than attempt to formulate rules for carrying such plan into effect. The plan recommended is as follows : —

The object to be attained is *the greater purity of the milk supply*.

The essentials to the attainment of this object are *improvements at the source of supply and in handling the milk*.

The method to be adopted is that all local dealers in milk be licensed by the local board of health; *i.e.*, the business shall not be carried on without such license.

RULES TO BE OBSERVED IN GRANTING SUCH LICENSES.

1. No license shall be issued except on declaration by the proposed licensee of his sources of supply.

2. No license shall be issued unless all sources of supply so declared conform to a certain standard.

(*Mem.*— This standard might well be fixed by a vote of this Association.)

In order to enable each local board to ascertain whether such sources do so conform, information should be at their disposal, and this information may well be supplied by a system of State inspection of such sources, the reports of which inspection should be at the service of all local boards; and, in the absence of such system, such information may be supplied by the co-operation of local boards.

The great result which may be obtained by a system of licensing the local dealer or distributor is that, in case he fails to satisfy the local board that the milk he proposes to supply will probably be free from objectionable impurities or conditions he will be unable to carry on his business; and, if this inability arises from the shortcomings of the milk producer, he will bring pressure on the producer to make his conditions conform to those which are indicated as likely to produce cleaner and safer milk, and that, unless this be done, he will buy milk only from those whose conditions do so conform.

By the requirements the following points should be covered : —

1. *Cleanliness of stable and wholesome conditions of keeping animals.*

Among tests of cleanliness which may be applied is that of observing dirt indicated by separator slime or sediment of tube, also excess of bacteria. Cows, being sources of food, should be tended and kept with as great or greater care than horses used only for burden or pleasure. Barns should be well ventilated.

2. *Health of the animals.*

The best and most approved methods of determining the existence of tuberculosis or other disease, such methods to be determined upon by each board for itself, should be employed, and the sale and use of milk from a tuberculous or otherwise diseased cow prevented so far as practicable.

3. *Cleanliness and freedom from disease of the milkers.*

The operation of milking should be looked after with special care. Above all, the hands of the milker should be carefully washed just before he begins to milk, his own personal cleanliness being even more important than that of the cows.   No person should be retained as a milker who, or any member of whose family, is affected with typhoid fever, scarlet fever, diphtheria, or any other infectious disease.

4. *Cleanliness of milk-cans.*

Before a can is used, it should be thoroughly sterilized by the use of steam or boiling water.

5. *Prevention of pollution of source of water supply used in washing cans, etc.*

6. *The milk should, as soon as possible after it has been drawn, be filtered, placed in a clean receptacle, thoroughly chilled or cooled, and started on its way to the consumer.*

HANDLING.

Points to be covered as above : —

1. Length of time consumed in transit between source of supply and consumer.

This time should be the shortest practicable necessary to secure an adequate supply.

2. Temperature of milk in transit.

The milk while in transit should be kept ice-cold, or as nearly so as practicable.

3. Method of delivery to consumer.

The preferable method of delivery is one in which the milk is poured from the large can directly into a vessel which does not leave the consumer's house.

4. The practice of returning uncleaned cans and stoppers from the dealer to the producer is to be condemned.   Before so returning them, the dealer should be required to see that they are thoroughly cleansed and sterilized by the use of steam or boiling water.

Inasmuch as milk is one of the best culture media for micro organisms, and is always liable to become infected with the organisms of disease, and, further, inasmuch as the process of Pasteurization is known to destroy such organisms, it is recommended by a majority of the committee that, as far as possible, all milk be Pas teurized before it is sold.

In the case of epidemics supposed to be due to polluted milk the usual methods of epidemiology should be followed, so far as locating the cases, fixing the dates of attack, and seeking for a common bond are concerned. If it then appears that the milk supply may be at fault, every endeavor should be used to connect the epidemic in question with one or more cases of disease on the farm supplying the milk or among the persons handling it. It is not enough to discover cases of the disease in question among those producing or handling the milk: the dates of such case or cases must be such as to allow a reasonable probability that the epidemic is secondary to the cases discovered. If such cases are found, it is important to discover the precise connection between the person or persons affected and the milk supplied. Such connection will usually be found to consist of milking, washing pails or cans, or testing or handling the milk in milk-houses. Contact by the hands or fingers of persons diseased with milk or milk utensils, is a ready method of infection.

THE PRESIDENT.—The next business in order is the paper, rather incorrectly stated in the programme, upon the " Milk Supply of Boston." The title should properly be " Paper upon Bacteria and Acidity of the Milk Supply of Boston," by Professor William T. Sedgwick, prepared with the assistance of Mr. H. W. Marshall; and Professor Sedgwick will kindly read it.

BACTERIA AND ACIDITY OF THE MILK SUPPLY OF BOSTON.

A FAMILIAR TALK.

BY PROFESSOR WILLIAM T. SEDGWICK.

Mr. President and Gentlemen of the Association,—When this matter came up in the shape of a paper which was read at the meeting before the last on the " Protection of Public Milk Supplies from Pollution," it was brought out at the discussion that it was very desirable, if possible, to have some tests or some methods by which it should be possible to discover from the actual condition of the milk itself the sanitary condition of that milk. That, for example, would be of great service in treating such a problem as the control of milk from another State or from one town into another town on its journey; and I had long had in contemplation an investigation of the relation between the fermentation of the milk — the ordinary sourness and the like — as produced by bacteria and the acid actually produced, believing that, if that were worked up, it might possibly give us some such method, or at least might be an aid looking in that direction. And, accordingly, I invited one of my students who has recently graduated, who was then about making his thesis, to work under my direction upon the milk supply of Boston, studying the numbers of bacteria present, and correlating them with the development of acidity or growing old of the milk; and another was put on the question of the influence of dirt in milk upon its aging and acidity. Of course, it was firing more or less in the air, as investigation of that kind always must be. We did not know how we were coming out when we began. We only knew that the Boston milk supply, like all public milk supplies, contained a great many bacteria. We also knew that this was not the fault, as a rule, of the contractors and milkmen, but that in spite of them it does frequently sour, and that all milk necessarily sours as it grows older. In fact, it might be said that one problem, and a most serious problem, of the milk supply is to get the milk to the consumer without its souring; and the results of the investigations have been, to me at least, quite interesting.

In the first place we took careful pains to confirm the older results as to the actual pollution of the milk by bacteria. In company with a former student of mine, Mr. John L. Batchelder, in 1890 I made the first investigation that had ever been made in this country — one of the first, I think, anywhere — upon the bacterial condition of the public milk supply, and showed that, when the milk arrived in Boston, it contained on the average a million or more of bacteria per cubic centimetre, and when it got on the tables of the people, and into the groceries especially, it contained a good many more than that; in other words, that it was a fluid very rich in bacteria. Ever since that time, and also since this spring, I have had the hope that these results, if confirmed, connected with the acidity, might not only throw some light on the possible means of detecting the actual sanitary condition of milk, but also might throw a good deal of light on the causation of cholera infantum. Cholera infantum is a reproach, of course, to sanitation. Our great cities in the summer see children mowed down by this disease, and we know very well that it is not merely the hot weather. That has been proved time and again, yet it is something that goes along with the hot weather; and I had hoped that, if we could show that milk was full of acid and rich in bacteria, it would throw great light on the causation and control of cholera infantum.

Now, without saying more of what we undertook to do, let me say what Mr. Marshall has found. In the year 1890 experiments began with the cow and with what I call, and would like to have generally called, normal milk. Normal milk is milk as its flows from the teat of a healthy cow or mammal. Such milk is, of course, warm, free, or nearly free, from bacteria, clean, and sweet. The first thing that we did, then, was to find out just how sweet it is, in order to be able to trace its souring, its progressive growing old; and for that purpose Mr. Marshall visited farms to draw milk directly from the teat of the cow into bottles carefully prepared for the purpose, and tested the acidity and the richness in bacteria. In the first place twenty samples of such normal milk drawn from different cows gave, on the average, an acidity indicated by the figures 1.66. I need not give you the chemical significance of that. It would take us too far into technicalities. I will ask you to bear in mind that figure,— that normal milk, as drawn from the cow in the neighborhood of Boston, has an acidity such that it will neutralize under certain conditions the amount of alkali represented by the figures 1.6, those being standard conditions.

You will see that normal milk is not quite sweet; that is to say, it already contains a little acid, but, as the figures especially in these analyses would show, it is very little. To go to a very extreme sour milk, I tested the milk; and it contained, on the average, 7.9, had an acidity of 7.9, as opposed to 1.6, or 16, if you choose, of normal and 79 the sour milk. Now the whole process of the aging of milk is the passage from 16 to 79 degrees of acidity, and right here I would like to mention a very interesting fact.

In 1891 a German investigator, an assistant physician at the University of Breslau, published a paper on the reaction of cow's milk and human milk, using precisely the same methods that we have used, and getting results, on the whole, very well agreeing with these, his average having been 1.9 for the normal milk, while ours was 1.6, 16 as opposed to 19. In other words, Boston milk compares with Breslau milk as 16 to 19 in acidity,—a very little bit sweeter; but we do not know exactly how he took his samples, or the numbers of cows used, or the time of year, or period of lactation. All these things have their influence. So I think it is perfectly fair to say that the results agree remarkably.

Now the further history of the souring of the milk, or its growing older, further fermentation, consists simply in passing from 16 to 79. The problem for the milkman is to keep it from so passing. The problem of the sanitarian is the same, so far as the supply of sweet and normal milk is concerned. In the case of this normal milk, to part company with that, no particular attention was paid as to whether it was the first or last part of the milking. The German investigator found that the milk was almost the same in the first and last portions, but not quite. It was a little bit more acid in the first portion than the last. The cows in those cases were mixed breeds, and were fairly clean. At the time of milking there was no bedding on the floor: the cows were quiet and peaceable. Other precautions, such as washing the hands or washing the cows, were not observed. In this case the milk passed through a two-inch sterilized funnel into a sterilized bottle.

Now milk contains bacteria under ordinary conditions, as milk is drawn by the ordinary milkman: it is seeded with bacteria. It is still an open question whether in the teat of the cow there are resident a few bacteria. It is claimed in a recent article of the bureau of animal industry that there are some such. It has been claimed by almost all investigators,— I perhaps have no right here to say it, but I personally do not believe that it is true,—all the observers who get this result got occasionally sterile samples; and I believe, if they took precautions enough, they would nearly always get sterile samples, and that, in cases where they did not get them, it would be either due to disease or to accidental introduction of bacteria from the air. By passing a sterile catheter up into the cow, I have frequently got sterile milk from the cow. That does not, however, exclude the possibility that fore milk, as it is called, milk in the duct of the teat at the beginning of milking, may contain a few bacteria; but, personally, I believe that is very unlikely, although many investigators claim that the duct is more or less charged with bacteria. At any rate, the number is low; that is, dozens or hundreds or units even instead of thousands or millions in freshly drawn milk.

This sweet and comparatively bacteria-free milk then proceeds to grow old or ferment by virtue of these same bacteria, and the process is a gradual one under ordinary conditions: in hot weather, a rapid one; when the milk is refrigerated, a very slow one. We have been very much aided in this investigation by milk contractors and their agents. They have put at our disposal every possible facility, and we are very glad to return them our heartiest thanks for all their kindness.

Now it will be interesting to see how the milk arrives in Boston after it has started with an acidity of 16 or 1.6, if you prefer, and a very low charge of bacteria.

The average of thirty-seven samples taken from various contractors was 1.71,—that is, instead of 166 it was only 171 in acidity when it arrived in the city,— as it seems to me, a really fine showing, proving that milk when transported on the trains is very thoroughly protected *en route* from souring; and, if you will look for a moment, you may see that this must necessarily be so. The one danger that threatens the contractor or the ordinary milkman is souring of his milk, because people won't buy sour milk. They will buy dirty milk, they will buy old milk, anything except sour milk. Milk that is sour is sent back to the farmer. By the process of testing I shall describe, I would like to have the dealer or contractor determine whether it is sour or not, and, if it is sour, send it back. If the milk actually taken into the city and distributed by the great contractor was hardly richer in acidity than normal milk, if it was a little richer, as may be expected, the reason, as we know from experiments, is it is so well refrigerated, because by icing milk you can keep acidity down; but I should say you cannot keep bacteria down by ordinary icing. That is shown by these facts. While the acidity is 1.71 as against 1.66 of normal milk, bacteria, instead of being dozens, hundreds, or units sometimes per cubic centimetre, are over seven million per cubic centimetre. In other words, those bacteria that produce the acidity are kept down by refrigeration, but a lot of bacteria that do not produce acidity were able to grow at that low temperature to the degree that milk was really aged seriously, although it was not damaged seriously by acid. From a sanitary point of view it was damaged very much, but from the chemical point of view it was not; and nothing is more natural than that might be the case, because the milk supply involves the question of getting milk to the people without its being sour. In this milkmen have done admirably in aiding us, and are entitled to our thanks for it. That, however, is milk as it arrives in the city; and, if any one could go and get that milk, it would be comparatively sweet, but it would be very high in bacteria. I should like to say that I repeated these counts on bacteria because we have more decidedly improved methods over those of seven years ago, and I was anxious to see whether my results there came within or outside the limits of error. I found that they were well within, that the numbers were really much larger than we used to find, and that by the modern methods we got a good many more bacteria. The contractor sells to the dealer: the dealers take it to their milk-house, ice it, keep it some time, and then finally deliver it; and, to go to the other extreme, probably the worst condition we shall find any milk in, in the city of Boston, is to be found in the groceries, especially in the tenement-house district, — groceries to which the people send for a cent's worth of milk. Mr. Marshall has been to the North End, Charlestown, and Cambridge, and all through the city, and has done it all through the spring; and up to the present time he has found a very unsatisfactory state of affairs in these groceries.

It may not be known to all of you, although it must be to many, that a good many cheaper stores will advertise milk below the regular rates,—"Pure milk, four cents a quart!" "Pure milk, five cents a quart!" That means they do it at a loss, in order to get people to come to their shops and buy other things. And those people, since they lose on the milk, are not very careful about it. The cans will not be very thoroughly iced. They stand upon the counters and behind the counters, and in hot weather there might be very serious results from bacteria. Up to June 8, or, I will say, July, we had a very cool season. We have not had the usual hot weather through the spring; and it is also to be noted we have not had the usual cholera infantum. so far, and the milk is particularly good this year, giving better results than we should get in the ordinary season. Up to June 8 the average of one hundred and four samples taken from these cheap groceries gave an acidity practically normal, 1.6, the numbers of bacteria hardly above ordinary, eleven millions, whereas the ordinary, when it arrived in the city, might average seven millions. That means that, with the cool weather we have had through the spring, the treatment was so good that we got nothing very bad; but now, during June, the thirty samples gave an average acidity of 1.7. It had gone up a tenth; and bacteria had gone up two millions,— nine millions. During July, when, you remember, we had some very hot weather, there was a tremendous jump in acidity, the average of seventy-nine samples giving 2.11 acidity,— a very large amount comparatively,— and the number of bacteria per cubic centimetre nineteen millions, the amount previous to June 8 having been 16 as against 21 in acidity, and twelve millions as against twenty millions, during this hot time and the rest of July to date; but to this company it means that, as the season goes on, the bacteria are increasing in those groceries, and the acidity is increasing, so that people who are buying that milk are buying sourer and more decayed, fermented milk. What it will amount to in August, if the thing continues, we do not know; but we are having a very cool season, and we are probably not going to get as high results as in the ordinary season. It will be interesting to see, too, if cholera. infantum follows the same rule, as I think very likely it may.

Some tests of buttermilk were made. The average of five samples showed an acidity of 7.9. I spoke of the effects of refrigeration, and the excellent work that is done in that direction by the milkmen; but, to show that test and the effect upon acidity and upon bacteria, we got results like these. Some normal milk — that is, milk with an acidity of 1.6 — was put in the refrigerator, at a temperature of from four to sixteen degrees Centigrade; and at the end of one hour the acidity was normal, 16. The bacteria were 475 ; and at the end of 288 hours in the refrigerator, or more than ten days, the acidity was only 19 as against 16. The acidity remained low, but the bacteria were ten billions per cubic centimetre. In other words, while the refrigerator is an economical device of great merit, as a sanitary device it is a very serious failure. This milk was not soured, but it was most disagreeable and rotten : it was nauseous. It had ten billions of bacteria in it; and it was milk that nobody could possibly have drunk, and yet it was not sour and was not clotted. So the refrigerator has a very valuable effect in preventing souring, but it is only a very imperfect instrument in keeping milk, from a sanitary point of view.

We have other results of the same sort. Here is one with a very low acidity, 1.1. At the end of 288 hours it was 1.8 in acidity, but the bacteria had risen from eleven thousand to eight billions. Milk like that, of course, is not at all fit to drink; and nobody could drink it as a matter of fact. It is very disagreeable, really rotten, though not sour, due to fermentation ; and this we regard as quite a discovery,— that the growth of the lactic acid bacteria can be checked by refrigeration, but other bacteria, which are possibly more dangerous from the sanitary point of view are not to be so checked.

Then, in order to see what can be done by Pasteurized milk, we have examined ten samples of Pasteurized milk. The actual acidity of such milk is slight. Normal milk is 1.6 : this had an acidity of 1.7. The normal number of bacteria is units, dozens, or hundreds : this had about seven thousand. That is very low indeed for any milk. It proves this : that Pasteurizing not only keeps down the acidity, but that it also keeps down bacteria. Refrigeration prevents milk from souring, but does not keep it in a strict sense. It keeps it in an economical sense, but not in a chemical or sanitary sense ; while Pasteurizing keeps it in every sense.

The moral of all this, it seems to me, is as follows : we know now far more accurately than we have known before the value of a bacterial examination of milk, and that the high numbers of bacteria in that milk mean either dirt or age, — in either case highly objectionable,— and wherever there is an excess of bacteria it can be therefore said that milk is not in the normal or even in the approximately normal condition, no matter whether the acidity is high or low. If, however, the acidity is high, that is evidence of bad refrigeration ; and we found some samples of milk during the hot spell that, instead of being 1.6, gave 6 of acidity. It is well known that in a prolonged hot spell it is very difficult to supply the city with milk, because so much of it sours. It is very difficult then to carry out effective refrigeration. Therefore, while I think I cannot claim that these results have shown all that I hoped,— namely, a method which would enable us to examine milk and learn a great deal more with it directly,— both of these methods are very easy of application, the test for acidity and the test for bacteria; and I believe that the time will come when every well-regulated local board of health will have some one at its laboratory,— I mean in every city of any size, or large towns,— who shall make an examination of milk that is sold, not only in respect to the amount of water that it contains, that being probably the least damaging of all things, but in respect to dirt and its age or staleness, and that in such examination counting the numbers of bacteria and determining the acidity will be of very great value.

THE PRESIDENT.— The report presented by the chairman of the committee and the paper read by Professor Sedgwick are now subjects for discussion or question. Dr. Chapin, you have had a good deal to do with milk in one way and another. What do you think about it?

DR. CHAPIN.— I have had the pleasure of speaking with the committee that formulated this report, and what I think has already been read. The point that seems to me to be of the utmost importance is that the raising of milk to a temperature of say 160 degrees will exterminate bacterial life in that milk. We know that, when suffering from time to time from epidemics of all sorts of contagious disease, some of those epidemics are distributed through the milk supply. I think there can be no question that many of our epidemics — scarlet fever, diphtheria, and, I speak without knowledge, but I presume that measles and various other diseases which owe their existence to some form of bacterial life — are transmitted by milk. We absolutely know from sad experience that that is true of typhoid fever, and I think some cases of diphtheritic epidemics are known to be due to milk. That certain animals may distribute tubercles from their milk I have no doubt. It appears, then, that milk is an excessively dangerous thing to drink; and, while everything that we can do to get clean milk and normal milk in the beginning is good, yet it seems to me that the heating of milk to a temperature of 160 or 165 degrees is a great deal better. I cannot state too strongly my opinion that the only safe milk to drink is milk that has been at least Pasteurized. That is all, Mr. Chairman.

MR. GAGE.— I would like to ask Professor Sedgwick if I understood him to say he found seven thousand bacteria per cubic centimetre in Pasteurized milk, or was it commercial?

PROFESSOR SEDGWICK.— Commercial: it had been through the hands of several people. It was hardly giving it a fair show.

A MEMBER.— I would like to ask what was found in the laboratory with Pasteurized milk as regards bacteria.

PROFESSOR SEDGWICK.— I do not know what the number in such a case would be; but it is a hundred or two,— something like that or even fewer. I think done in the laboratory, you can get it down to dozens or units; but I mean, done on a large scale by an intelligent man, you can get it down to a hundred or two. It is well known that all germs of typhoid fever or tuberculosis are killed by proper Pasteurization; but there are some forms of bacteria, as there are some human beings, that resist more than usual. It depends very largely on the milk that is Pasteurized. If you go and buy some milk that already has millions of bacteria in it, and a lot of dirt and all that, and Pasteurize that milk, you will undoubtedly have rather a hard time. *Milk ought to be Pasteurized at the latest very soon after it is drawn from the cow, and then it would be much cleaner and better taken care of;* and, when it is treated in that way, it is almost perfect. I should like to second what Dr. Chapin has said. *I really believe the time is coming when it will be regarded as a very unusual and uncivilized thing to drink unpasteurized milk; and I think, if I had brought in some Pasteurized milk and passed it around here, and said nothing about it, nine out of ten of those present would not have known but they were drinking ordinary sweet milk,— that is most people, having had no sweet milk in their lives, have got used to a commercially sweet milk, and, when they get hold of sweet milk, they think something is the matter with it.* But anybody who has ever squirted milk into his mouth from the teat of a cow, as all boys have done who live in the country, knows that milk that has been Pasteurized tastes like that he used to get when he was a boy,—practically, normal milk. I believe in cities especially we have got to come to that sort of thing; and I believe that, unless we do come to that, we shall see cholera infantum and epidemics of typhoid from milk. I really believe, if we could put Pasteurized milk into Boston to-day, and let nothing else go into the tenement-house districts, the number of cases of cholera infantum we should have would be too trifling to mention.

DR. MILLER.— I would like to ask the professor how high he would have to raise the temperature, in order to be sure he would destroy those germs he spoke of?

PROFESSOR SEDGWICK.— That is a very difficult question to answer, for boiling does not kill all of them in all cases. As a rule, boiling will do it,— boiling for a few minutes only; but there are spores sometimes present which will withstand even considerable boiling, and one would really need to put the milk in a retort and give it superheated steam, or something of that kind, to be perfectly sure he had destroyed the last one of all.

THE PRESIDENT. I hope Dr. Russell may be able to say something to us on this subject.

DR. RUSSELL.— Mr. Chairman, I count it a matter of great good fortune on my part that I am here to hear this discussion. I came down from my home this morning by special appointment to go before the Cattle Commission on this very subject, and I imagine our interview would have been very interesting. I will tell you of an experience I have had, which you probably have all had in your work, but which is new to me.

Two years ago, as the chairman of the Board of Health in my own town, I looked up the matter of the milk supply, and at once stumbled on one of the most wretched condition of things which I believe could exist in any civilized community. The members of my board were not in sympathy with me, which sometimes happens in local boards of health. So I had to shoulder the whole responsibility and do all the work myself; and in the summer I went with the official inspector of animals, appointed, as you know, by the select-men, who represent the State Board of Cattle Commissioners. His business was to inspect all the animals in that town,— a visual inspection. Not being an educated man, he could not make a physical examination. He also had to inspect the condition of the barns, the size of the rooms, the water supply, whether hogs were kept in the same barn, etc. The first place I went to or the second we found the man kept his milk in a little room six or eight feet wide, and had a well underneath where the water stood six feet deep, close to which there were half a dozen hogs,— as filthy a place as could be imagined. In this room were harnesses, blankets, bags of phosphate, and other things, besides some old rubber boots.

The next place I went to the man had a new barn, quite clean; but he said he had had to give up the water from a certain well, it had become so bad he could not use it any longer. I said, " You have continued to use that until quite recently? " " Yes, until within a very few days." The water was positively rotten.

The third place was a farmer's barn. When we entered this barn, we were completely upset. The odor was simply horrible, and we spent fifteen or twenty minutes trying to find out what the odor came from. We found three cows in this barn and four or five hogs on the same floor, without any possibility of drainage; and there was something else — we could not find out what it was — that made the most infernal odor I think I ever knew.

The fourth place I went to there were seventeen cows. The place had not been cleaned, the same condition underneath, a damp cellar. There were lots of rotten pumpkins in the same room with the cows, and cobwebs hanging down two feet long, and about everything as unsatisfactory as it could possibly be. I then went to the farmer's own house, and asked him to show me the milk-room. This was as dirty a place as you can imagine. There were piles of food on platters and sour milk in wide-open pans and articles of clothing in this room; and the place where the mother of the family was washing the pans and cans was the ordinary sink, in which was piled up, I think, the accumulated dishes of at least two or three days, which had not been touched.

I went to another place, after this, and found the same condition so far as the barn was concerned. I went into the house, and asked where they took care of the milk. They said it was a very nice milk-room, where they kept the milk with great care. I asked if I might see it. He hesitated a moment, and consequently I pushed in; and here in this milk-room were particles of food, part of an old ham, a tub of old clothes, and on the top was the monthly wash of the females of the family. That is a fact, gentlemen. It does not seem possible.

After I finished this investigation, I began to correspond with the Board of Cattle Commissioners, and not to my satisfaction, however. I then went to work to see what I could do about the matter. I found that my board would not join with me, but I was determined that some of these animals which I had seen and knew to be diseased should be killed. I had one killed from a herd of six. I was at the *post mortem* myself. That cow was driven in; and, although I have no knowledge of cows, of course, in a practical way, I saw at once it was diseased. Milk had been sold in my village all that summer from that cow. As soon as it was killed and the lungs removed, I made an incision with a knife, and held the lung up like this, and pus ran out of that lung by the spoonful. I had two others killed, and they were found to be riddled with tubercles from head to foot.

Some of these statements I made known, in order that I might wake up public sentiment. One milkman said he had just as lief drink milk from a cow that showed this diseased condition as from any other cows. The tubercles were not found in the milk, therefore the milk was just as good as ever. I woke up a lot of public sentiment on the matter, and then began on the regulation of the milkmen themselves. My board would not aid me, and I thought I would stop for a while; but I very quietly got myself appointed milk inspector,— an unusual position for a man to take that had my work to do, but I was bound to see the thing through. I went to work, and of course was the recipient of all the curses that can be imagined. All the milkmen in the town got after me, and there were not words enough in the dictionary to give a statement of their ideas of my conduct, the money I had, the clothes I wore, and everything else; but I stuck to it, and I refused to give any man a license who did not conform to the regulations.

I might mention here, however, that in that first paper the recommendation of the committee was made that boards of health license the milk inspector. As I understand it, now, in the country towns at least, they cannot do that. The license must be given by the milk inspector. He is appointed by the selectmen. There may be one or more. He then appoints a series of collectors, one or more, subject to the approval of the selectmen. Well, I got myself appointed as inspector, and went to work with one person. I told him what I wanted done and why I wanted it done. We went to a certain barn, and had it thoroughly swept with a coarse broom. That got the cobwebs, lice, etc., out of the way. Then I had the stalls washed with hot water, with one per cent. of corrosive sublimate solution wherever the animals could reach with their tongues, the sides of the stalls, and front of the place in which the animals stood. Then I had the whole whitewashed thoroughly. This was in accordance with a State regulation put out by the Board of Cattle Commissioners, but not insisted on only under circumstances of this nature wherever they find an animal which is diseased with tuberculosis and condemned. Then they will not pay the man for his cow unless he has done this. I went still further, law or no law in this case, and insisted that I would not grant a license to any man who did not put his barn in this condition. Now I have licensed about fifty men in my town; and they have carried out these recommendations very thoroughly indeed, and only two refused to do so. One of these was an elderly man, quite broken, and the other quite eccentric; and these two men positively for the last three months have stood on the street corner three or four hours a day damning me.

Now the issue is between them and me as to these last two licenses, and I may get beaten. I cannot tell how that will be. One of these gentlemen has the dirtiest of barns. It has never been cleaned. The man himself wears a suit of clothes that has not been changed probably for ten years. The second man I mentioned has the dirtiest barn I ever saw. It has not been cleaned out for twenty years. The hens have their dust piles, in which they shake themselves to get the lice out, in the place where the cows are.

Now, gentlemen, you who have not been through an experience of this kind have no conception of the dirtiness and filthiness of that barn. Last week I cleaned the barn of a poor man in whom I take a great interest, who cannot work, and who has the worst of all afflictions in his family. I went up myself to his barn, and where the cattle stood there were millions of live lice. You could not put your hand on any part of that stable where you could not cover thousands of them. The man that did the work was so disgusted he wanted to give up the job. Said he, "I never thought such a thing could exist"; but by persuasion I got him to finish the work. I tell this, so that others who have not had this experience can look around, and see what they have got in their own towns. I do not think it is possible to have a decent supply of milk unless you have honest and honorable milkmen.

The President.— I will call upon Dr. Davenport.

Dr. Davenport.— The paper which has been read upon this subject has been interesting to me. I have had some little experience for the last fifteen years in the examination of milk, having been milk inspector of the city of Boston and chairman of the Board of Health in one of the suburban towns. The recommendations of the committee are most excellent and very desirable, but I think the gentleman who starts in to carry them out in the city of Boston will have his hands full for some while. I wonder if the committee have any idea what would be the expense of carrying them out. The present appropriation of the city of Boston for milk inspection is some $12,000, I believe; and in regard to the licensing of milkmen I do not think the inspector has any authority to discriminate between whom he shall give a license to. I think the statute, as I remember it, says he shall license whoever apply; but, if he is on the Board of Health, he has ample authority to complain of a milkman as a nuisance. He can cover it in that manner.

In regard to the regulations of the Cattle Commissioners about using corrosive sublimate upon the walls of barns and then using whitewash, I do not exactly see the object of that contention. One would tend to destroy the effect of the other, and the other is not chemically economical.

Dr. Russell.— They require the corrosive sublimate to be washed off before the whitewash is put on.

Mr. Davenport.— Many of the recommendations of the committee are such as would have been carried out if we had been able to learn how to do it. There were many practical difficulties.

The President.— The Association, fortunately, has as its guest this afternoon Mr. Burns, of the Boston Dairy Company; and I hope we may hear something from him.

Mr. Robert Burns.— Mr. President and gentlemen, I have thought this subject over, and our company has given it some attention. Last summer we sent what we considered an extremely experienced man to visit our dairies. He was a man whom we thought competent to talk to the farmers, and tell them how they should take care of their milk and everything in that line. This year, some ten weeks ago, we started him out again on a different plan. We wanted him to go to different farms, and inspect the place and make a report; and we furnished him with the means to make a report of the conditions of each dairy. That is, he made a note of the number of cows a certain man kept, the breed as near as he could, and the kind of water, whether well water, running water, or a windmill. Now he has found this year a great improvement over last year. In fact, we have some twelve or fifteen hundred dairies; and he has found that the large majority of these dairies keep their places as cleanly as can be under existing circumstances. Of course, in a good many places the farmers milk their cows, and strain into cans directly behind the cows; but the majority of them do not do that. He has discovered some very crooked places. It seems to me it would be a good thing, if it could be done, to have a law passed, so that the boards of health of the different towns could inspect the farms, and prohibit the sale of milk from those farms, if the conditions were not satisfactory.

Now one particular case. This man, going to a certain town, before he got to this farm, people said to him, "I wonder what you are going to do when you get to so and so's place?" Well, when he got there, he found,— what? This man's barn was filled with apples from last fall. Of course, they had all rotted; and the juice was running all over the floor. The cows were being fed on those apples. Of course, such cases are exceptional. We find very few of them in that condition. Of course there can be improvements; and it seems best, as I say, that a law should be passed, so that inspection by the boards of health may do a great deal of good. We have a law, you know, on the statute books concerning brewers, dealers, and contractors; but that is inoperative, and does not amount to anything. If a law could be passed that gave power to the board of health to prohibit these things, then I think the trouble would be minimized to a certain extent.

Now as to sour milk. Professor Sedgwick says this has been a very good season. It has been a majority of months; but, as a matter of fact, during this hot spell there was more sour milk in Boston proportionally than was ever know before. Perhaps the idea was given to you that the milk soured on board the cars coming to Boston, but, as a matter of fact, probably ninety per cent. of that milk was sour before it was ever set on board the cars; but the time of receiving it is so limited that it has to be put on board the cars, and brought to Boston. I know one of our men who tasted three hundred cans of milk to get one hundred, during this hot spell. That milk came from Connecticut Valley, as fine a farming neighborhood as there is in New England; and the milk of one of these particular dairies was soured every day. That particular farm probably is as fine a place as there is in New England. The cows are a fine breed of Jerseys. The conditions are as perfect as under the present system they can be. The man has ice, nice water, everything as clean as possible; but there was not a day that that milk came to Boston it was not sour when it was set on board the cars. We sent our inspector to this place immediately. The farmer's wife said that she did hope her husband would find some other place to dispose of his milk instead of sending it to the milk car. The milk was found to be sweet at the farm, but sour when it reached the car in the morning.

Now, personally, I do not think that it is much trouble tasting sour milk. The worst trouble we have is with what we call rotten milk. Its taste or smell, too, is simply awful. A man can taste sour milk all day, it won't affect him at all; but just one whiff of that milk would affect the whole business. Now that kind of milk, as far as sweetness is concerned, is perfectly sweet, and probably would keep. I do not know any reason why it should not keep as long as milk that has no odor whatever. Now, of course, the argument here is to do away the conditions that generate bacteria. Of course, farmers set their milk in troughs to cool, and leave their bungs out. I do not see any way now to take care of milk under those conditions without leaving the bungs out. As a matter of fact, milk will not taste properly if it is stoppled up before cooled; and, if it is left open, of course bacteria will generate in there right straight along, and you cannot help it; but that is the way milk has to be put up to come into Boston properly.

Now the samples that Professor Sedgwick has compared may not be samples of the very best dairies. I cannot say. I gave him one sample of a very fine dairy, I know; and I doubt if he has got samples of the very best dairies. We have customers that have practically never returned us a can of sour milk. This year I know one has not returned us a can of sour milk: that milk is put up properly; but there are other dairies where we have had to run two extra carloads of milk to make up for their sour milk.

The report of the committee said something about washing cans and sending them back to the farmers. Well, we have been all through that; and I think we got conditions that proved that that, from a health point of view, was the worst possible thing that could be done,— not only upon health, but from a financial point of view. The financial part of it is that milk has a preservative effect upon the can. A can will last for years simply with milk in it, whereas with water in it it will rust out in a few months. We have always considered that. In fact, we would not buy of farmers or dealers of that description, who rinse their cans in cold water and return them to us. They may stand a day or two a certain amount of water left in there, but that is going to rust the cans. That is a good deal worse than sour milk, to our minds.

Now, as for washing the cans clean and sending them back to the farmer, of course, perhaps the majority of the gentlemen present would take these cans as they came back clean, wash them out thoroughly, and let them air out; but I am very much afraid the large majority of farmers would never stop for that or never would rinse those cans out before they put milk in them, and cans in that condition, stoppled up in the hot season, present what is perhaps the worst condition possible.

Now as to sterilizing the cans with steam. I do not know just exactly what you mean by that,— whether you wash the cans first and then sterilize them or wash them and boil them right out with steam. But I can give you a few facts on that subject. We in our factory have a large pump, fitted up with a four to six inch pipe, which is used for raising milk from the lower story to a higher one. We commenced by cleaning the pump with boiling hot water. After a short while we found there was a very offensive odor coming from them, and we discovered that the sour milk would cake on the inner lining of the pipe and inside the pump; and that, of course, was the source of the odor. Now we have built a tank, and we pump cold water through the pipes, then rinse them through with a solution of sal-soda and boiling hot water; and we find there everything is clean and sweet as far as smell is concerned, and as far as we know, of course, it is all right. We use up our surplus milk by making cheese of it after it goes through the pump.

The worst trouble is sour milk. There is no doubt about that. The ordinary milk supply of Boston, the ordinary amount that is brought in, would be perfectly sufficient to supply Boston if there was no sour milk. There is no possible need of a single can of sour milk coming into the city of Boston, if proper care is taken. We have an extra car come to Boston in a hot period from our cheese factories in Vermont. and there is practically no sour milk; and, if one can do it, there is no reason why others cannot do it. Of course, farmers say they are short of cans, and have to wash them and fill them immediately with milk. That is true; but that is a condition that no contractor ever solved yet, and certainly cannot solve with the ordinary can used to-day. Possibly, if a forty-quart jug was used, we could solve that question; but contractors all know that something ought to be done, and are willing to co-operate with the authorities whenever occasion requires, but it involves an enormous expense.

THE PRESIDENT.— Mr. Jordan, of Boston, has had a very useful experience in this matter. Possibly he will say something to us on the subject.

MR. JORDAN.— Mr. Chairman and gentlemen, I do not know that I can add anything to what has been said. I was very glad to hear the report of the committee to-day, that they had not suggested the adoption of any rules. I think that is a good idea, because I think this subject will bear a good deal more discussion before any rules are adopted. I think we can afford to wait, and that it will be a good idea to adopt the report of the committee merely as a progressive report, and refer the matter back to the same committee to see if they cannot add something more to their report at the next meeting. As far as large dairies in Boston are concerned, for the last two or three years I have had occasion to visit them very frequently; and I can say that the majority of those dairies have been very good in adopting any suggestion the board made to them, and trying to do everything they possibly can. There has almost been a complete revolution in such dairies in the last three or four years. I have in mind now a dairy which is undergoing a complete revolution in the manner of conducting business. And, in regard to Professor Sedgwick's remarks about the grocery stores down at the North End, I think that it is a very good idea of his in making that report, and making those inspections in those places. That is a condition of affairs which we are very frequently called upon to interfere with. Down in the crowded part of the city they do not have any idea at all what the conditions should be. We very frequently have to inspect those places, and call them to account for the manner in which they carry on their milk business. Very seldom we find the cans washed at all. They are left around the floor in a filthy condition, and very frequently we have called their attention to the condition. At the present time, but more especially this year, the board has closed up quite a number of cow stables in Boston, the conditions not being at all fit to carry on the milk business. There have been quite a number of places closed entirely. In other cases the owners have agreed to written conditions, to make certain changes before going on trial again in the fall. I think, if this discussion is carried on further, extended to the next meeting, it will prove to be of great benefit.

THE PRESIDENT.— Hasn't Cambridge something to add to this discussion, Dr. Farnham?

DR. EDWIN FARNHAM.— Mr. President, Cambridge last fall had an outbreak of typhoid fever that was due to the polluted milk supply of one milkman. The Cambridge Board of Health thought they would send around some inquiries to the different towns from which milk was obtained, to see if they could find out what the conditions were of the farms, or their barns, and other places where the cows and milk were kept,— not with the idea that they could do anything themselves, but possibly to help along by finding out just what these conditions were. The large milk companies and contractors very willingly supplied me with the names of the places from which they obtained their supply; and the board then sent round this circular, which I will read to the Association. This was Feb. 2, 1897.

CITY OF CAMBRIDGE, OFFICE OF THE BOARD OF HEALTH.
CITY HALL, Feb. 2, 1897.

To THE BOARD OF HEALTH:

We have adopted and are enforcing in Cambridge certain regulations regarding cow stables, a copy of which regulations is for your information herewith enclosed.

The object of these regulations is to insure that the cows from which the milk supply of our city is in part derived are kept under wholesome and sanitary conditions.

We are desirous of ascertaining how far this is the case with those cows not kept within the city of Cambridge whose milk is, however, brought for sale therein; and we ask that you will kindly aid us in this investigation by furnishing us with the information respecting the farm of ——— in your town which is sought by the questions printed on the next sheet, that farm being one of those from which milk is brought for sale in this city, and, if your investigation of this farm discloses conditions which should be changed, we ask your assistance in bringing about an improved state of affairs.

Believing that through the co-operation of local boards of health much sick ness, of which milk may easily become the vehicle of transmission, may be prevented, and thanking you for such aid as you can afford us in this matter, we are, Very truly yours,

E. EDWIN SPENCER,
EDMUND M. PARKER,
CHARLES HARRIS,

Board of Health of the City of Cambridge.

TO THE BOARD OF HEALTH, CITY OF CAMBRIDGE:

In response to your circular letter of Feb. 2, 1897, we send the following information respecting the farm of ———— on ———— Street in this town : —

1. How is the privy vault constructed ? *Answer :*

2. How far is the privy vault from the well ? *Answer :*

3. Is the drainage of the ground from the privy vault toward the well or away from it ? *Answer :*

4. How is the well constructed? (If no well, state how water is supplied.) *Answer :*

5. Is the well protected from surface pollution ? and, if yes, how ? *Answer :*

6. How many cows are kept in the cow stable or barn ? *Answer :*

7. What other animals are kept therein with the cows ? *Answer :*

8. What is the cubic contents of that part of the stable or barn where the cows are kept ? *Answer :*

Is there a privy in this stable or barn ? *Answer :*

9. How is the cow stable or barn drained ? *Answer :*

How ventilated ? *Answer :*

How lighted ? *Answer :*

10. What is the condition of the cow stable or barn respecting cleanliness ? *Answer :*

11. Have the cows been tested with tuberculin ? and, if not, what veterinary examination has been made of them, and when ? *Answer :*

12. What changes, if any, should be made in the premises to put them in wholesome and sanitary condition ? *Answer :*

13. Is the foregoing information furnished from personal inspection of the premises by some member of the Board of Health ? If not, by whom is informa- tion furnished, and from what inspection ? *Answer :*

(Signed) ———— *of the Board of Health of* ————

I sent one of these to nearly every town in the State of Massa- chusetts where I knew that milk was obtained which came to Cam- bridge for sale. Of course, the answers were of various descriptions. Nearly every one answered: there were very few exceptions. One man said "it would be too much trouble: we have just been all over it with the Cattle Commissioners "; and he sent me their blank, which, I must say, did not give us the information we wanted. Another man wanted to know how much we would pay him for doing it. Still, a large number of answers were received. I have selected a few showing what I thought the needs were.

The chief ones seemed to be these. In the first place, very few barns have any drainage, as far as I could make out from the replies. They seemed to let urine and everything else soak into the cellar. That is almost the universal condition to-day,— to let it run down and soak away somewhere in the ground. The privy vault in a very large number of cases was quite close to the well.

In a number of cases it was simply a hole in the ground, and in some few cases there appeared to be no privy vault at all. I do not know what occurred there. The well in a certain number of cases needed to be protected more than it was ; that is, there was no protection at all. It was level with the ground, quite near in a large number of cases to a manure pile. In some cases there was no ventilation: in other cases it was manifestly inadequate. The air space, to which one question referred, was quite often deficient. The stable barn was built probably for a certain number of cows, and the person who built it may have had some idea of how much air was needed; but many more cows had been put in than was at first intended. As to cleanliness, of course, I had to take the report just as it came to me from the persons who made it, not knowing what their idea of cleanliness was: that is a very variable factor; but quite a number mentioned that the stables might possibly be improved if they were kept a little cleaner.

I have not sent any outside the State. It was quite an expense getting these printed, and the board simply went into this for a feeler to see what could be done ; but it showed, I think, pretty conclusively this,— that a great deal needed to be done. I do not know why the local board of health should not be able to regulate these various things. We drew up a list of regulations, compliance with which is required by the Cambridge Board of Health before it licenses keeping cows in the city. I will read these regulations.

REGULATIONS REGARDING COW STABLES.

1. Every building used as a stable for cows shall contain at least one thousand cubic feet of air space for each animal kept therein.

2. The lighting and ventilation, and the condition of the roof and floor, shall be satisfactory to the Board of Health, and shall be so maintained. There shall be a sufficient supply of pure water, and such other means for maintaining the health of the animals in said stable as the Board of Health may deem necessary.

3. The stable shall be drained in a manner satisfactory to this board, and, wherever practicable, shall be connected with the public sewer by a good and sufficient particular drain.

4. The manure shall be kept in a pit constructed of brick laid in cement, with a concrete floor at least three inches thick, and ventilated as required by the Board of Health; and no more than one cord of manure shall be allowed to accumulate.

5. The animals shall be examined by a veterinarian approved by the Board of Health, whenever directed by the board.

6. The premises shall at all times be kept in a condition satisfactory to the Board of Health.

The foregoing is a true copy from the records of the Board of Health of the regulations adopted at the meeting of said board, held the twenty-sixth day of October, in the year eighteen hundred and ninety-four.

Attest: JAMES B. SOPFR,

Clerk of Board of Health of the City of Cambridge.

CAMBRIDGE, Nov. 3, 1894.

We have had no trouble so far in enforcing these regulations, and I think the cow stables in Cambridge have improved very markedly.

If the city of Cambridge can make those regulations and enforce them, I presume any other city or town in the State of Massachusetts can do the same thing and protect its own interests.

THE PRESIDENT.— Dr. Durgin, shall we hear from you?

DR. SAMUEL H. DURGIN.— It seems to me the report of the committee has given us a great deal of light on this subject, and will be of the greatest use hereafter in formulating rules and in making regulations to control our milk supply. There is one part of this report which refers to sterilization which seems to me of very great importance; and while we are not yet ready to deal with the farmer until these regulations shall have been formed, and while we cannot prevent the milk reaching us in this poor state, there is one thing which we might advise the people to do, and that is by sending out little circulars to mothers, who may fairly well sterilize this milk before using it, especially for babies. The Boston Board of Health has issued a little circular of this sort, in which it tells the mother how she may sterilize the milk by placing it in bottles and boiling it for twenty minutes, giving specifically what may be done. It seems to me that this has some value immediately to families.

DR. J. A. GAGE.— Mr. President, in reply to what Dr. Durgin has just said I will say this: That, when I have had to answer the question that a mother has asked me, what she could do to be sure that her child was getting proper milk, I formerly advised her to boil the milk, as he has suggested, and sterilize it. But it has been my observation, and I find others have made a similar observation, that children do not always thrive well on milk that has been heated to a high temperature, 212° F.; and Pasteurized milk, I find, is not always easily obtained by uneducated people. One of my professional brethren asked me to advise him in regard to a baby he had. He had lost two children. I urged upon him to be very careful and Pasteurize the milk, went into details with him. It was some time before his wife could be persuaded to carry out all the details of Pasteurization, but, once she had learned the method, she was satisfied; but that was an intelligent family, whereas among the poorer classes it is very difficult to obtain those results. I do not like milk which has been heated to a high temperature.

Formerly I was a member of the Board of Health of Lowell. We got our milk very largely from farms immediately surrounding the city. Some of them were in New Hampshire. There is no inspection of those farms, and I know that recently a great many of them are in a very poor condition. There has been some tuberculosis with us, as the slaughter at Dracut has testified. That town supplied milk to the city of Lowell, and I know from my own personal observation and experience it is a very fruitful source of danger to us there. A recent case may illustrate. A man, who had been out of work on account of illness, thought before he went back to his regular work he would go out on a farm and get strong. I had had the man under observation some time, and there was no indication of tuberculosis; but after being on the farm awhile, and drinking two or three quarts of milk a day, he came home, and I found tuberculosis. The cow was killed. The man who lives on that farm is a fairly intelligent farmer; and, if he knew positively, and was convinced that he was feeding his family on tuberculous milk, he would not do it. I do not think he is convinced thoroughly.

This case bears upon one point I wanted to make with reference to the whole question of milk supply. I do not know that there is anything in the report in relation to giving these milk producers information. I knew one place where a man was starting in the milk business, and the first thing he did was to start a well in the barn yard. That was due to ignorance. I certainly feel we ought to have some inspection. I myself am afraid to drink milk without knowing the source from which it comes; and, when I go among my poor families, I hardly know how to tell them to Pasteurize their milk, feeling sure they will get the best results. We want to get the source pure, and as fresh as we can, and get it as soon as we can from the supply into the hands of the consumer; and it seems to me, while restrictive laws are very necessary, and I thoroughly agree with the suggestions of the committee, that something might be done tentatively in the way of education, certain suggestions as to measures that they could take without great expense, which, I think, would help the matter.

DR. MILLER.—It seems to me something might be done in this direction. I think the majority of milk producers would like to do just about the best thing if they knew what to do. Certainly, they would if it was made clear to them that it would be a financial benefit. Now it seems to me, if the State Board of Health, or some authority would send a circular free to anybody in the State, that produces milk, giving them directions how to care for their cows and cans and the like of that, that we might in this way educate farmers and milk producers, so that they would give us a better quality of milk; and these gentlemen who deal in Boston, to a very large extent, could give their milk producers to understand that their milk would be more likely to be received if they conformed to certain rules. Now I have paid some little attention to this subject, and I am inclined to think that the fault is due to the kind of can in which the milk is conveyed from the producer to the dealer in the city. I have tried this experiment, taking milk from some milkman and letting him bring it to the house in his can, and then furnishing a can of my own and telling him to fill that can instead of leaving it in his; and I find that milk would keep a great deal better, when I furnished the can, than it would if the milkman brought it in his own can. I always cleanse the can with boiling water thoroughly, and then I find the milk will keep a great deal better. I am inclined to think the great fault is in the condition of the can in which the milk is conveyed; and I think, if the proper information could be given to the dealers in the Connecticut Valley, so that they would see their milk would be more likely to be received if the farmers could be educated on that subject, they would do better, because you can touch every farmer through his pocket, surely. And, if you can make him believe his milk will have a larger sale and will bring him a better price if he will do so and so, he will be more likely to do it. And say to these dealers, " We will give you something more for your milk if you do so and so: we will pay you more for your milk." I think in that way the farmers might be educated, through their heads and pockets, so that we can get a better quality of milk.

Mr. Burns.— In regard to this circular business, telling the farmers how to care for their milk, I will say we sent our man right there to inspect everything. He has gone right into the kitchen, and inspected everything on the premises, and told them how to do it; and, if that is not telling them how to do it, I do not know how we can do any better. We ought to have a law that we could make some complaint to the local board of health that we do not think the conditions are right in a certain place, and then it could send an inspector there without bringing us into it, and tell them the place was not right. Inspect it again; and, if they do not attend to it, take them into court, and prohibit their selling milk. I think that would be a great improvement. In some places, in the city of Boston, people put rotten eggs and cheese and things of that kind in cans. Where a man has a customer taking two hundred cans a day, he cannot say, " You

must stop putting that stuff into my cans." We ought to have
authority in the city of Boston to send an inspector to such places,
and prohibit it; and, if it is not stopped then, bring the man into
court.   Then I think cans would be in better condition than they are
now.   The bad condition is due to rotten eggs, molasses, and that
kind of things being put in the cans.   We ought to be able to prevent that.

There is another matter I will speak of; that is, this cheap selling
of milk in the North End,— selling for four cents a quart.   In fact,
that was rather a high price.   I think milk was sold there for two
cents a quart.   As near as we could find out, the method was this:
In the morning they would sell milk of good standard quality; and,
when the collector of samples came round to these stores, they would
get that milk.   The minute they went out they would take skim milk,
and sell to these ignorant people.   It cannot be sold to a nice family;
but it is sold to these ignorant people.   I am happy to say that they
do come into court, and pay a fine sometimes.

Dr. Miller.— I did not intend to find any fault with the dealer.
I would have this circular issued by the State Board of Health, or
some authority backed up by the power of the State; and then it
perhaps might be made easier for some member of local boards in
each town, so appointed, to look into the matter.   If he was backed
up by the State, it would be universal over the whole State.

Mr. Burr.— Mr. President, I have been much interested in
Dr. Farnham's remarks in regard to the condition of the farms in
New England from which his milk comes; that is, of the farms from
which he obtains milk.   It seems to me it would be a good plan in
this State if every board of health could have a record of each
farm from which milk comes, whether it is in the State or out of the
State.   In that way we might have registered farms; and we might
make regulations that these barns should conform to, and refuse to
grant permits unless the barns did conform to the regulations.   For
instance, I think the storing manure in the barn cellar has come to
be quite an objectionable feature; and the method of handling milk,
after it has been drawn from the cow, needs attention.   Now in a

good many farms the milk is handled directly in the same barn. It seems to me that is quite an objectionable feature, and, as the committee reported, that milk ought to be handled outside of the barn, and also outside of the dwelling-house, and also that the milk-cans, if washed upon the farm, should not be washed in the kitchen of the house. So much for that.

Now I am a little interested in the method of the transportation of milk. I do not know whether that has been touched on or not. It seems to me that the milk supply has got to be improved from all points, not only its production, but its transportation and handling also. The Board of Health of Boston sent out a few questions to the different dairies or contractors in the city of Boston, delivering milk in the city of Boston; and among them were questions asking the maximum time that it took the cars to come from the country milk-station, the minimum time and the average time. I do not think, with but one exception, the maximum time was given over three and one-half hours. Now I know we have some milk contractors here to-day who perhaps can correct me in what I say. I was interested the other day in a reply that came from a farmer in New Hampshire, in which he reported the route of a certain car. That car left Claremont (I will give the towns: perhaps I may be corrected in it), we will say, on Monday morning, containing Sunday night's and Monday morning's milk. It went through Claremont to Bradford, arrived there some time Tuesday morning, and took on Monday night's milk and Tuesday morning's milk. It went from Bradford to Hillsboro, N.H., and arrived some time during Wednesday, and took on Tuesday night's milk and Wednesday morning's milk, arriving in Boston on Wednesday about ten o'clock. Now that car contained Sunday night's milk, Monday morning's, Tuesday's and Wednesday morning's milk. It seems to me that is quite a serious condition; and, if that is the case, certainly the transportation should be improved. While that car was iced, as all cars are, considerable milk is stored on the floor of the car; or I might say, further, that milk which arrived here, we will say, on Monday or Tuesday, was put into the closet for these cars, which are probably iced; and, as the milk came on later, it was stored on the floors and about the doors. The ice stays in among the mass; and, as the cans come along, different layers

were made.   So a great deal of that milk, it seems to me, was not
probably iced.   I have no great doubt but all those cans put in the
closet were properly iced.   It seems to me that transportation could
be considerably improved, as well as all other sides of the question.

MR. DAVENPORT.— Mr. Chairman, the improvement of the milk
supply of the city of Boston, when it comes to the hands of the consumer, has shown the advantage of having the appointment of the
milk inspector under the charge of the board of health, as it has
now come to be in the city of Boston.   It is also so in the case of
the city of Lynn, but I think those are the only two cities in the
State where the inspector is appointed by the local board of health.
In the case of Cambridge he is, I think, appointed by the mayor;
but the inspector, as a health officer, ought to be really under the
appointment of the board of health.   An attempt some years ago was
made to accomplish that for the State at large, but it was defeated.
It would be a great improvement, and I think, if this Association
should make a concerted effort, it could be brought about; for, certainly, it should be considered as a health matter, and not, as it generally is, an appointment made simply for political purposes.

DR. FARNHAM.— I would say the list of regulations drawn up by
the city of Cambridge required cow stables to be kept in a condition
satisfactory to the Cambridge Board of Health.   There was one
dealer in Cambridge last year who kept his cow stable in a very
unsatisfactory condition.   I wrote to him about the matter several
times without effect; and, when he applied for a license this year, he
was given leave to withdraw.   He applied successively for three
weeks, and each time was given leave to withdraw.   He was then
prosecuted for keeping cows without a license obtained from the
Board of Health.   That case is now in court.   When it is decided,
we shall know just what we are able to do with cow stables in
Cambridge.

THE PRESIDENT.— It seems to me there is a sufficiently con-
tented expression on the faces of gentlemen here,— an expression
which certainly ought to be there.   It is that expression which

shows the successful digestion of an exceedingly good dinner, and I am therefore going to introduce another subject, which should be in harmony with such an occasion; and that is reminding you that Dr. Field is anxious to take a dollar and a half, the annual assessment, out of every member here who has not already paid it. Mr. Gove, have you anything to add in closing this discussion?

MR. GOVE.— I think, Mr. Chairman, instead of my saying anything at the present time, it will be much better to have the discussion closed by Professor Sedgwick.

PROFESSOR SEDGWICK.— Mr. Chairman and gentlemen, I think there has been a very full discussion. I have been particularly gratified to see the breadth of the discussion. It won't do to narrow the question of polluted milk down to a question of tuberculine or anything of that kind. It is the whole question of getting more normal milk in the city; that is, the question of cleanliness in the barn, cleanliness on the part of the milkmen, cleanliness and rapidity of transportation, and care of the milk after it arrives. It seems to me those various points have been touched upon, and a good deal of valuable matter has been elicited. The only way to bring about improvement in this matter is the old one of keeping everlastingly at it; and it is very encouraging to have these statements that some of the inspectors have made, that there has been a very decided improvement. For instance, in the speed of transportation I think the idea of education is a very important one. I think that wherever the farmer is given to understand what it means to have sour milk, why it is a bad thing to squirt milk on his hands when he sits down to milk and lets the drippings run into the pail, why it is a good thing to wash the hands, and that it is a good thing to wash the hands even before sitting down to milk,— if a campaign of education in that direction can be had, the better it will be for the whole city. Personally, I feel very much gratified at the interest that has been expressed, and I believe we have now reached this conclusion: first, that at present the milk supply is not satisfactory; second, that it can be made much better; third, that, in order that it shall be made much better, the farmer must be informed, and, if the necessary pressure is to be brought to bear upon him, the milkmen themselves must be informed, and led to deliver the milk as rapidly and as fresh as possible; fourth, when the consumer demands a cleaner and better article, when he objects to dust in his milk, when he objects to a black sediment in a glass of milk, then we shall get a better supply.

I have been particularly gratified with the breadth of the discussion, because it seems to me that is exactly what the whole thing needs. If the Association sees fit to recommit the subject to the committee or to require further elaboration of this matter, that would be well worth it, only I think we should be in no great haste about it. We do not want to wear the Association out in talking about milk; but, for instance, if at the meeting after the next one there should be a further report, it might be well, and I think the committee would very cheerfully undertake to do what they can, and be very specific, and state that a cow should have just so many cubic feet of air, although that is not the most important thing. The first things to be understood are the principles underlying the milk supply. The danger is to-day that the public will get so frightened about milk that they won't drink it at all, and it is better they should not unless it is improved. I never do drink a glass of raw milk; but, as soon as the public become sure that there is care on the part of the farmer and milkman to be clean, and the milk-cans are all clean, we shall get ahead. I do not know that I can personally agree with the idea that it is best to let these cans go back with the drippings of milk in them after standing round in that hot store that has been mentioned. It seems to me it leads the farmer into dirty habits, because he has got his can home in a very unsatisfactory condition; and he might say, "The people in the city don't take any pains to clean the cans," and then he will be apt to take no pains. It is a new point to me, and so in regard to other points I am sure the Committee have learned a great deal; and I only hope the Association has learned something from the committee.

Dr. Durgin.—I move, Mr. Chairman, that the report of the committee be recommitted with instructions to further consider the matter, and report such rules as can be adopted by the boards of the State and put into practice. I think a report in October would be far better than a report in January, if it could be completed, on account of the possibility of further legislation being needed for getting the best effect of the regulations. In January it would be rather late for any new legislation for the present year; but that matter might be left with the committee if it is able to report in October.

(The motion was seconded and adopted.)

A MEMBER.— I would like to suggest that Mr. Burns or Professor Sedgwick take particular notice of the treatment of cans and of transportation,— the treatment of cans before they are sent back from the consumer,— that that might be embodied in the next report.

THE PRESIDENT.— It is understood the committee will consider the various topics which have been introduced at this meeting.

The meeting was then adjourned.

[RULES . . . FOR THE PROTECTION
OF MILK SUPPLIES]

Professor Sedgwick.— Mr. President, those who were present at the last meeting will remember that the chairman of the committee on this subject begged for more time than would be given if a report were to be brought in at this meeting, but that the committee were instructed nevertheless to report to-day. It has been found very difficult, however, for some, at least, of the committee to give any attention to the matter; and the report which I have the honor to bring before you to-day is not, therefore, as complete as might be wished.

Before actually proceeding to the rules which we have undertaken to prepare, and more especially as some members of the committee who are coming here in a few minutes have not as yet come in, and ought to be here, I should like briefly to bring up to date, as it were, this whole subject. The Association is now sufficiently informed — and, it seems to me, very well informed — on the general question of the needs of a sanitary control of milk supplies.

It is only a few years since we had to say that such safeguards as were placed about milk or were called for by any one were safeguards in regard to the addition of water. And to put good pure water into milk is probably, from a sanitary point of view, one of the least harmful things that could be done. A position like that, however, was not, and is not, consistent with modern sanitary science. If that were our position, there would be no occasion on the part of an association like this for making any rules, or for this Association to deal with the matter. But I believe that every member of the Association feels, as I do, that the time has now come when something more has got to be done. And, as I understand it, it is because the association feels so that this committee was requested to look into the matter, and actually prepare rules which could be adopted, with such modifications as each city or town should need, for the better sanitary protection of milk supplies.

The reason for this change of view is obvious. It is that sanitary science now holds, and holds rightly, that milk is one of the most easily contaminated articles of food, that many and serious epidemics have been traced to milk; and, now that we are looking into it, it is found that cow stables are not what they should be, and that there are opportunities — very numerous, altogether too numerous — for the serious incrimination of this most fundamental food product. That is the reason why this Association feels it its duty to take hold of the whole matter. The advancement of sanitary and medical science has obliged persons having the care of the public health to give their attention with renewed energy to the matter of the sanitary control of milk supplies. It is no longer sufficient to watch against adulteration and fraud: we must now begin to take care that milk does not contain the germs of disease. And I believe that in that respect we are as far on as anybody in the world. I visited England this summer, and looked into the milk supply question there somewhat; and I hold in my hand a copy of the regulations of London County Council in regard to dairies, cow-sheds, and milk-shops. Many of the rules and regulations which we shall propose are — in spirit, at any rate — foreshadowed in this older community of London. As has happened so often in sanitary endeavor in this country, we find that it has been foreshadowed by sanitary endeavor in some older country. Nevertheless, I do not find that they are any further on there, practically, than we are here; and I believe that this Association and the people of Massachusetts whom we represent have an opportunity to lead the world, as it were, in this matter. To do so, however, we must of course be sure of our ground. We must be as reasonable as the circumstances will allow, while watching over the safety of the people, must be careful not to trespass any farther than is absolutely necessary upon individual initiative or individual rights.

The one fact which the committee has sought to bring out in this particular report, and make very strong and clear, is that a local board of health should have, first, knowledge, and, second, control of the sources of milk supply and the character of the milk distributed within its particular district. And to that end the committee, and more particularly one member of the committee — not the chairman — who has been able to give more time to it than the others, has put together a number of articles and sections which the committee would recommend to this Association to be considered, and, if approved, adopted, and recommended to boards of health as the basis for legitimate and reasonable sanitary protection of public milk supplies.

The present situation those of you who are connected with boards of health know very well. It is simply one in which the board has little or no knowledge of the actual sources of the milk brought into its district, and little, if any, control over the milk after it has got in. It is possible, we believe, to remedy this condition, and along the lines now to be indicated.

I will now read, if you please, the actual rules which we would propose; and I will read them all through, as far as we have them, without comment or remark, in order that the general bearing of them may be obvious and the general effect clear. Then, if it is your wish, I will read them over one at a time, or in any other way that you like, so that they may be discussed in open meeting. We are not at all sanguine about their acceptability. It is a good deal easier to order a committee to get up some rules than it is to get them up or to approve them, when got up; for we have found, as of course was to be expected, that what would appeal to a citizen of Boston or be useful to the Boston Board of Health is not, without considerable amendment and modification, likely to be useful to the board of health of a smaller city than Boston or of a town. In making general rules, therefore, it is difficult to hit all needs; and these which we offer are not to be regarded as iron-clad or as adapted to all localities or conditions. It is presumed that each board of health will modify them to suit its own needs, and they should be heard by you now with that fact in view. It should not be supposed that the committee for a moment imagines that the following rules are as applicable to North Adams and Greenfield, we will say, as to Boston and Fall River, or to Fall River just the same as to Boston.

Now, with so much of preface, I will proceed to read the rules which have been drawn up, and which have met the general approval of those members of the committee who were present. One member of the committee was ill, and unable to be with us in our debating of the proposed rules; and another was not notified in season.

RULES SUGGESTED BY A COMMITTEE OF THE MASSACHUSETTS ASSOCIATION OF BOARDS OF HEALTH FOR ADOPTION BY THE BOARDS OF HEALTH OF THE STATE FOR THE PROTECTION OF MILK SUPPLIES FROM POLLUTION.

ARTICLE I.

SECTION 1. All persons engaged in the production of milk for sale, or in the sale, delivery, or distribution of milk in the city or town of ——, shall annually, on or before May 1, make written application, on forms prescribed by the board, for a permit or license.

SECT. 2. No person shall engage in the business of producing milk for sale, or in the sale or distribution of milk, in the city or town of —— after April 30, 1898 (?) without a permit or license to do so signed by said Board of Health, and under such conditions as said Board of Health may impose, revokable at the pleasure of said board.

SECT. 3. The conditions under which every cow is kept, whose milk is brought into any city or town, or kept, delivered, distributed, sold, or offered for sale, in such city or town, shall be made known to the local board of health in such detail as the board may require, and shall be approved thereby; and no milk except that delivered from such cows shall be so brought, kept, delivered, distributed, sold, or offered for sale.

SECT. 4. No milk shall be sold, offered for sale, or distributed in any city or town, unless the cows from which it is delivered have within one year been examined by a competent authority, and shown to the satisfaction of the local board of health to be free from disease.

SECT. 5. All persons having a permit or license to sell, deliver, or distribute milk in any city or town, shall keep a copy of the same constantly posted in a conspicuous place on premises and vehicles from which milk is sold or distributed or in which milk is kept or delivered.

ARTICLE II.

SECTION 1. No milk shall be kept for sale or distribution, or handled, transferred from can to can, or stored in any stable or similar place, or in any room used in whole or in part for domestic or sleeping purposes.

SECT. 2. Milk shall be stored or regularly mixed, cooled, or poured from can to can only in a room not directly connected with a stable or stables, provided with a tight floor, and kept constantly neat and clean, the walls of the room being of such a nature as to allow easy and thorough cleansing. The room aforesaid shall contain proper appliances for washing and sterilizing all utensils actually employed in the storage, sale, and distribution of milk in said building, and all such apparatus and utensils shall be washed with boiling water or sterilized by steam regularly after having been so used.

SECT. 3. No urinal, water-closet, or privy shall be in the aforesaid room or any room directly connected therewith.

SECT. 4. All milk directly after it is drawn from the cow shall be at once taken to, and be at once filtered, cooled, and stored in a room such as is described in Article II., Sections 1 and 2.

ARTICLE III.

SECTION 1. Milk kept for sale in any store, shop, market, bakery, or other establishment, shall be always kept in a covered cooler, box, or refrigerator, properly drained and cared for; and while therein shall be kept tightly corked or closed, and only in such location and under such conditions as shall be approved by the local board of health.

ARTICLE IV.

SECTION 1. All cans, bottles, or vessels of any sort used in the sale, delivery, or distribution of milk to the consumer, must be cleaned and sterilized by the milk dealer before they are again used for the same purpose.

ARTICLE V.

SECTION 1. Every person engaged in the production, storage, transportation. sale, delivery, or distribution of milk, shall immediately, on the occurrence of any case or cases of infectious disease, such as typhoid, scarlet fever, or diphtheria, either in himself or in his family, or amongst his employees or within the building or premises where milk is stored, produced, sold, or distributed, take care that the local board of health is notified of such case or cases, and at the same time suspend the sale or distribution of milk until authorized to resume the same by the local board of health.

SECT. 2. It shall be unlawful for any person suffering from a contagious or infectious disease, such as typhoid fever, scarlet fever, or diphtheria, to handle, transport, deliver, mix, taste, work over, or distribute milk, or in or about places where milk is stored, sold, or distributed, or to serve as a milker or milkman. No vessels which have been handled by persons suffering from such diseases shall be used to hold or convey milk.

In addition to these, which we propose to the Association to recommend or to adopt as guides, the committee have certain recommendations to make, and also certain forms of application blanks suitable for the carrying out of the rules here proposed. In preparing them, we have been much guided by the blanks now in use in the city of New York ; and Dr. Burr, who has had much to do in the drawing up of these rules, and given a great deal of time and trouble to the whole matter, has with him copies of the proposed application blanks which we would recommend, or which we would submit as typical of what might be kept on file and filled out by persons seeking for permits or licenses.

But, before proceeding to this part of the subject, I may briefly recapitulate what I have read, with a comment or two. In the first place, the idea of the rules is to make the people who deal in milk responsible to the board of health,— not merely responsible to a milk inspector, however excellent he may be, but to make them, if possible, feel their responsibility to, and to bring them under, a definite sanitary authority.

In the second place, while I believe it is a fact that the ordinary licensing of milkmen is largely a matter of a small fee and of routine, so that any one can get a license, the milkman of the future, if these rules are adopted, or anything like them, will be made to feel that he must show cause why he should be allowed to sell milk, and should be made to feel the serious sanitary responsibility of the work in which he is engaged. It is not desired to be unduly severe upon him, but only so severe as the necessities of the case and the health of the people absolutely require. He will therefore on this plan make application for a permit annually. And this is done simply to make sure that in his application blank the facts shall be brought up to date, as to the people from whom he gets milk, as to the location of the farms upon which the milk is produced, as to the sanitary condition of those farms as far as it can be determined, and so forth and so on. The great point, the whole point of this matter so far, is to make milkmen realize that they are engaged in a business which requires sanitary supervision. And, to make them do that, it was felt that no better plan could be adopted than to require them to have and to keep posted a permit to carry on what might almost be called a "dangerous trade," though I do not wish that term to be applied in this connection, because it is too harsh.

In the next place, the second section forbids any one to sell milk without such permit.

The third makes it certain, as far as such a thing can make it certain,— of course, all this depends on the way on which it is carried out by the boards,— that the board shall actually have information, of a rather concrete kind and specific nature, of the conditions under which the milk is produced. They shall not merely publish certain conditions, and let the man certify that the farms from which he gets this milk do conform to certain conditions, but they shall require him to actually report where the farm is, and how many barns it has, and what sort of a stable, and all that sort of thing. And my own idea is, though I do not know that I am supported in this by the committee, that, as boards of health are able to do so, they shall send inspectors to see what the actual conditions on these farms are. Of course, that is an easy thing for a small city; but it is a very difficult thing for a large city, like Boston. It would not be easy, off hand, to send inspectors all over the States of New Hampshire and Massachusetts, and a considerable portion of Maine, Rhode Island, and Connecticut, to see what the actual condition of the cow stables is. But, until we do reach that point, we shall never wholly solve this problem.

I should like to say, by way of parenthesis,— and I appeal to farmers and milkmen themselves,— that the public is getting very sensitive on this question. I had a good illustration of it while I was in England. Danish butter is very much sold in England, and very much liked by the people. The English farmer, of course, is not specially in favor of it, because it cuts into his market. And the whole subject was thrown into a ferment, while I was over there, by an article, in the *North British Agriculturist*, describing the serious sanitary condition or unsanitary condition of the Denmark cow stables and methods of keeping cows. The fact is that at last, after all the talking and begging that we have been doing for some time, people are beginning to turn their attention toward cow stables and farmers. And it has got to come to pass before long that farmers who wish to sell milk, and sell it successfully, and to sell butter successfully, have got to take such care of their cows as would be taken by a breeder of horses; and cows have got to be looked after, and not allowed to have their udders and sides caked with manure. And the milk farmers will not be allowed to have the milk come from their farms tasting " cowy," as it is called. Now this third section of Article I. is an attempt to enable and to encourage boards of health to look into these matters; for we say that the conditions under which every cow is kept whose milk is brought into any city or town, or kept, delivered, distributed, sold, or offered for sale in such city or town, shall be made known to the local board of health in such detail as it — that is, the local board of health — may require, and must be approved thereby, and that no milk except from such cows shall be brought, kept, sold, delivered, etc., in that town.

The next section refers to the health of the cows. A critic writing on the English law has said, and very well said, that it makes good provision for the physical condition or health of the people, of the human beings, employed about the milk industry, but pays no attention to the cattle themselves. That is a sound criticism, unquestionably; and, having that in view, we have undertaken to go a little further than they have gone, and to require, but still in a way which we believe will not impose any serious hardship, that, " unless the cows from which this milk is derived have within one year been examined by a competent authority,"— and no one knows better than the committee how loose that term is,— " and shown to the satisfaction of the local board of health to be free from disease," its sale shall not be allowed. The committee felt that, while that was not saying much, perhaps, it was pointing in the right direction ; and if any particular board of health sees fit to make that stronger, and to require an examination by a particular authority defining it, the committee would be very glad. But it was felt, in the present state of the art, if so it may be called, it was not possible to go much further.

The next article requires the keeping posted of a permit to sell the milk. I can say from personal experience that is an important thing. You go into a little milk-shop on some side street in a city, and you cannot tell at first whether it is a milk-shop or not. You have to inquire around, " Do you sell milk ? " And, if a woman is in charge, as is often the case in these little places, and she happens to say no, you go out ; and you may miss a milk-shop in that way. They are not registered in any public manner which you can easily get at ; and it is no more than fair that they should have something posted, so that an inspector, learning of an epidemic and looking at the milk supply, should be able to know at once whether that is a milk-shop or not.

The next section deals with the question of the room in which the milk is to be handled. Now there is a certain moral reason in this,

— the requiring of a decent room, a separate room. Of course, in good dairies, those rooms have existed for many years. This is no hardship on them. But there are many farms where the milk is taken from the cows, and emptied into the cans right in the stable or in some dusty barn or in some undesirable adjoining room, used perhaps also for a horse stable, it may be. And it is very common in this city to have the apparatus for putting up milk, or, as it is called, mixing milk, in places where the horses' tails are not very distant. It has seemed that it would be well to require, if possible, that milk shall be handled only in a decent room, not directly connected with anything objectionable. Every one knows that the manner of handling will improve the quality of it. Every one knows that the uniform put on the street-cleaning employees of New York improved their tone at once, as it has improved the tone of our railroad service and everything else where used. A man in uniform feels more responsible. Now we do not propose to put these men in uniform. Bnt we do propose to put the business, as it were, in uniform; that is to say, have the room worthy of this important industry. We should have liked to say the building, a separate building, where milk could be treated as a delicate food product, which it is, and taken care of as it should be. But we felt that the best we could do was to require that it should not be handled in any room used in whole or in part for domestic or sleeping purposes, or any place directly connected with a stable or stables, and that such a room should have a good tight floor. We wanted to say an impervious floor, a concrete floor or cement floor. But some members of the committee did not feel that we ought to do it, because, while that would be all right in Boston, it would be a hardship on some of the milk dealers in some of the little towns; and of course we are anxious, as far as possible, to do something which shall be of universal application throughout the State, though I am not altogether sanguine that it is possible to do that. The conditions are so different in a big city, like Boston, and in a small country town that I am not at all certain but we are undertaking to do something that it is not possible to do. And I would have it borne in mind by this Association that this was not voluntary work on the part of this committee. They had no desire to sit down and draw up these rules, knowing the difficulties involved, but were ordered to do it at the last meeting, and cheerfully accepted the duty.

Obviously, no urinal, water-closet, or privy should be in the aforesaid room or in any room directly connected therewith. Obviously, also, the milk, after it is drawn, should be at once taken to some such room, filtered, cooled, and stored in it.

Then comes the subject of milk-shops and stores. Some members of the committee felt that it would be very desirable to take the milk trade out of the grocery stores and meat markets if we could. And, if you go to the people who sell milk in those places, they will always groan, and say that they do not want to do it, that they only do it to accommodate their customers; and some members of the committee thought we should relieve them of that trouble by making a rule that they should not do it. But other members thought that what they say is only talk, that they really do want to sell milk, and that it would be regarded as a hardship if we proposed a rule that markets and butcher-shops should, under no circumstances, sell milk. Nevertheless, we felt that it was not requiring too much to have the milk, when so sold, kept under decent conditions. And it was desired by some to require that it should be kept in separate refrigerators, coolers, or boxes. The committee, as a whole, finally decided that it would not be well to do that under all the circumstances; and so a more general rule was made,—that it should be kept in a covered cooler, box, or refrigerator, and while there kept tightly corked and closed, that this refrigerator should be properly drained, and that the whole thing should be under such conditions as should be approved by the local board of health. It would be a very simple matter for the inspectors of the local board of health, as they are going about, to visit these milk-shops,— not all in one week, perhaps, but on their rounds,— and see where the milk is kept, and see if it is decently kept. And, if the board has good inspectors, as all Massachusetts boards are supposed to have good inspectors, that would be a matter quite easy to carry out. They could report information which would be passed on by the local board of health, and rules governing the subject could easily be made.

With regard to the cleaning of the cans, bottles, vessels, and all

that, it was thought that a rule was certainly of fundamental consequence, and that these should be cleaned, and not only cleaned, but
sterilized. We have got to rise to the point of sterilization. It is
a high point to reach, I know; and I do not suppose it will be faithfully carried out for a long while, but that is the goal toward which
we are striving. If you say the cans shall be cleaned or thoroughly
cleaned, they will be cleaned, as very many of them are now, in
warm or warmish water. They will not be thoroughly cleaned from
a bacteriological point of view, or even a sanitary point of view.
And so we have said "must be cleaned and sterilized"; and by
that we mean treated with really scalding water in abundance or
with live steam. That may or may not meet your approval.

With regard to the contagious diseases there can be, it seems to
me, very little question that every person actually engaged in the
sale or distribution of milk should, as soon as he has an infectious
disease himself, or has it in his family or among his employees or
within the building or premises, report it (of course, it is the business
of the doctor to report it; but then it is his business, too, so as to
make the thing doubly sure), or see that it is reported, and should
suspend the sale of milk until he is authorized to resume it. Also
it seemed desirable to have it stated that it should be unlawful
for any person suffering from contagious disease — and of course
whether he is so suffering would have to be determined by a physician — to go on working over the milk, and distributing it, and so
on. We have sometimes had cases where a man who was pronounced by the physician to be probably in the early stages of
typhoid fever has refused to knock off work about milk, but has
persisted in going on, saying he felt all right and was all right.
Those cases are not as rare as some of you may think. Very naturally, a man, laboring in that way, is desirous not to lose his place
just because he is a little feverish, and does not wish to knock off
work until, perhaps, he is so sick he cannot ride on his wagon or
something of that kind. And it should be distinctly known that the
handling of milk under those conditions is not only undesirable, but
is unlawful. So, at least, your committee thinks.

So much of the report we have prepared, and would submit to
you to-day. But I think that, before the discussion is opened, it

might be well, Mr. President, to ask Dr. Burr to give us the outlines at least of those blanks,— that is, the application blanks which he has ; and I think he has also in his pocket, somewhere, outlines of certain recommendations which we might make, but which it was not intended should be embodied in the ordinances or definite laws. Possibly, he is not ready to do that part of the matter ; and, possibly, you will wish to give the committee more time to report at some future meeting on matters which still remain to be touched upon. The committee is well aware it has not covered all the ground ; but it felt that it was important to strike first at the root of the evil, and to correct it by making sure that the milk trade, the milk industry, shall come to be recognized by those who deal in it as one legitimately under sanitary authority. That is the fundamental idea, it seems to me ; and, so much, at least, we have tried to cover in these proposed articles and sections.

THE PRESIDENT.— The Association would be very glad indeed to hear from Dr. Burr.

DR. BURR.— Mr. Chairman and gentlemen, as your committee has reported, it seemed best that we should get up certain application blanks which should be filled out by those applying for permits to sell milk. We divided those blanks into three forms, one of which applies mostly to the milk dealer. We speak of the milk dealer, meaning the milk pedler, the man who goes to the railroad and gets his milk, takes it home to the barn and there mixes it, puts it into the small cans and into the ice chest, and delivers it the following morning.

Then we have a second blank that is made out for the store people, those who simply receive the milk at the store and sell it.

The third is a blank which both the store seller and the wagon milk seller shall fill out when they apply to the board for permits.

In regard to the barns and the cows where milk is produced, whether it be in this State or in any other State, as Professor Sedgwick said, we copied the New York laws to a certain extent.

I have here the application blanks which are used by the Board of Health of New York, and I will hand those about. We have added,

I think, considerable to those. [The blanks were then passed about the room.]

Now, in regard to application blank number one, which is used by the milk dealer, who goes to the station and gets his milk, and carries it to his barn: —

Name and business and location and district in which the milk is sold. That is, in a large city like Boston, one man may be selling entirely in Dorchester, and another man in Roxbury.

The amount sold per day?

Do you keep cows? If cows are kept, he fills in special blank number three.

From whom do you purchase your milk? And, if he purchases milk, he also fills in blank number three.

Time when the milk enters the city, over what road, and from what depot? In that way we will know over what road it comes.

Marks on the cans?

Where is the milk stored and cared for? That is, of course, at his place of business, which would be, in these cases, mostly in the barns.

Is the milk-room or building in direct connection with the stables, sleeping room or rooms used for domestic purposes?

Of what material is the floor of the milk-room?

How is the milk-room drained?

Is there a urinal or water-closet in this room or room opening into the same?

Means of cooling and storing the milk? In an ice-box or refrigerator?

How drained?

Do you wash and sterilize all utensils in this milk-room, and the method of sterilization?

Application blank number two, which is confined to the store milk dealers: —

Name, business, location, quarts sold per day, from whom purchased? If purchased or obtained from farmer, milk agent, or farm belonging to the applicant, he also fills in blank number three.

Location, time of delivery, marks on the cans, is the milk kept in a separate cooler during sale? Is the cooler or refrigerator drained?

What is kept in the immediate vicinity of the milk? We mean by that, in provision stores, we want to know whether the meat and vegetables are in close proximity to the milk refrigerator.

Do you wash and sterilize all measures and utensils?

Where are the utensils washed and sterilized? The reason we ask that is that in a great· many of these smaller stores there may be a kitchen or sleeping-room off from that store. We want to know whether they are washing the cans in that kitchen or not.

Method of sterilizing?

Is there a urinal or water-closet in this store or room opening into the same?

Does the store open into a sleeping room or rooms used for domestic purposes?

Special blank number three : —

This is the blank that is filled out by each applicant for the sale of milk. That may be filled out through the contractor, or it may be sent direct to the farms where the milk is produced and filled out there, or it may be obtained through an inspector or agent of the board of health receiving the name of the milk agent or contractor.

Business address? Name of producer of milk. Oftentimes the contractor, of course, and not the producer.

The city or town, county and State, shipping station, railroad?

Number of cans per day? Marks on the cans?

What milking is shipped? Time of arrival at the country railroad station? That is, we want to know at what time the milk is delivered to the railroad station. In that way, we will find out the age of the milk and the length of time after it has left the farm; in other words, the time in transit while in the hands of the contractor or railroad.

The time in transit?

The number of cows?

Are the cows regularly inspected?

Is the stable well lighted and ventilated and drained?

Condition of floor?

Where is the manure stored? If in cellar, what is the condition of the cellar?

How often are the cows cleaned?

Average amount of air space per animal?

Condition of cow yards?

Where is the milk stored?

Is the milk-room or building in direct connection with the stable, sleeping room or rooms used for domestic purposes?

Of what material is the floor of the milk-room?

Is there a urinal or water-closet in this milk-room or room opening into the same?

How is the milk-room drained?

Means of cooling and storing the milk, whether in an ice-box or refrigerator? How drained?

Do you wash and sterilize all utensils in this milk-room?

Methods of sterilization?

Water supply for cows? Water supply for cooling milk?

That completes the three blanks. I will send these blanks about. I think, Mr. Chairman, that is all I have to submit.

MR. COFFEY.— I would like to ask Professor Sedgwick to read again that section in Article I. which empowers the boards to provide a test or examination.

PROFESSOR SEDGWICK.— Of the cattle, do you mean?

MR. COFFEY.— Of the cattle, yes.

PROFESSOR SEDGWICK.— "No milk shall be sold, offered for sale, or distributed in any city or town, unless the cows from which it is delivered have within one year been examined by a competent authority, and shown to the satisfaction of the local board of health to be free from disease."

MR. COFFEY.— Is it contemplated, in that, to exact the tuberculin test?

PROFESSOR SEDGWICK.— That is for the local board to decide. That was not defined.

MR. COFFEY.— Are these resolutions to be incorporated in a statute, or are they suggestions to local boards?

PROFESSOR SEDGWICK.— I think they are merely suggestions. That was my idea of the thing. I do not remember, at the moment, the exact wording of what we were told to do.

MR. COFFEY.— How are you going to get around the fact of the statute already in existence, which puts it in the hands of an inspector of milk to be appointed by the mayor, and does not give it to the local boards at all?

PROFESSOR SEDGWICK.— Does not give what?

MR. COFFEY.— The authority over licensing the sale of milk.

PROFESSOR SEDGWICK.— Well, we had a lawyer on the committee, — Mr. Gove, of Salem; and, I believe, while he did not wish to say positively that he was certain the thing could be done, he was sufficiently so to go on with the work. He felt that it was within their power for the local boards to make these ordinances, if they saw fit. That was my understanding, at least, of his position.

MR. COFFEY.— As I understand it, there is a general statute law now that provides that inspectors of milk shall be appointed by the mayor and confirmed by the board of aldermen.

PROFESSOR SEDGWICK.— It is not intended to contravene any statute or anything of that sort. It is rather to make rules in addition to these.

MR. COFFEY.— What authority has the local board over inspectors appointed by the mayor?

PROFESSOR SEDGWICK.— None whatever, I presume; but it has power to appoint its own in addition to those.

MR. COFFEY.— In addition to those?

PROFESSOR SEDGWICK.— Yes, not in place of those, of course.

DR. DURGIN.— As I understand it, this is to be a regulation made and adopted by each local board of health. Under the general law the boards of health are empowered to make these regulations, which become in themselves a law; and, unless they conflict with the statute law, they are in full force. And I do not understand that anything drawn up in this way will conflict with the present statute law on the inspection of cattle.

MR. COFFEY.— I do not clearly understand that. It seems to me that the board of health, if these rules are adopted, could refuse a license to a milk dealer. Now suppose the regular inspector appointed by the mayor and confirmed by the board of aldermen approved that license: would there not be a conflict at once? Now you know the statute law. Lynn has a special statute, empowering the Board of Health to license milk dealers. Boston, in its charter, has authority in the Board of Health over the milk business; and I think at Lowell, through an understanding with the city government, the Board of Health there have appointed a milk inspector, or at least the mayor appoints an inspector whom the Board of Health nominates. And, as far as I know, those are the only three places in the State that have that authority. At Worcester, for several years, in addition to being health officer, I was milk inspector. There the inspector receives $150 or $200 for his services. It is merely routine work, and very little inspection is done. Most of the work is simply the issuing of licenses. Of course, it stands to reason that a man cannot give a great deal of his time for $150 a year; and consequently his other duties, which may take up most of his time, for which he receives the greatest recompense, are attended to, to the detriment of that. So that it would become there simply a matter of routine. He issues licenses, occasionally he takes some samples and makes a rough test, looking for adulteration; and that is all. And that system has always been in force there. And it does not seem to me that, unless you change the statute law, putting it in the hands of the board of health, the mere adoption of the rules while that statute remains in force would amount to anything. It would simply precipitate a conflict between the board of health and the mayor and aldermen.

Dr. Simpson.— Mr. Chairman, this subject is one I am considerably interested in. I represent a small city, of about 23,000 inhabitants only, in the north-west corner of the State,— North Adams. And coming, as we do, in direct contact with the milk producers, it occurred to me that, if anything is to be done for the purity of milk, it must be done largely through the representatives of the smaller towns, who, in cleaning up the premises from which the milk is sold in their own cities and so setting the example, shall clean up the premises of the larger cities and towns. The milk in Boston, and in a number of the large cities,— in all the large cities,— comes primarily of course from country towns. Now, if the board of health in each town could control the purity of the milk in that town, whether the milk is sold in its own town or whether the milk is exported from that town, why, that would give you pure milk in the large cities. And, in order to give ourselves pure milk, I have been for a year now trying to get either some rules passed by our board or an ordinance by our city, to control the sale of milk. And I have succeeded thus far,— that I have myself drawn up some rules; and I came here to-day, knowing this report was to be made, to determine, upon my return, whether these rules shall be embodied as the rules of the board or whether I should try to get our city to pass an ordinance to this effect.

Now the point that the gentleman brings up, of the legal authority, I have looked into pretty carefully. I first went to our city solicitor. He took into the conference with me another lawyer, who is a good man. Our mayor is very much interested in the subject. I took the matter to him. He is in close touch with a very prominent firm of lawyers here in Boston, and they have been consulted; and the result seems to be this: that there need be no conflict with the public statutes. Because the way they put it to me is this: that, broadly, boards of health may make such rules as they see fit, to govern their towns and the health of their towns, and to protect the inhabitants from disease, from whatever source it may come. The statute gives that broad power to boards of health. Now suppose we have a milk inspector. We have one in our city. This will not interfere with him in any way, because the city may make this ordinance. We get some of our milk from Vermont. We will control that in this way. While we cannot say any man shall have his premises inspected, provided he lives out of the State, we can say to him that he shall not sell his milk in our city until he has complied with the rules that we see fit to make or that our city makes, and passes into an ordinance. Now that will not interfere with the milk inspector. The milk inspector may give him a license if he chooses, but that will not interfere with our power to prevent him from selling milk until he allows us to inspect his premises.

In Pittsfield, I understand, they commenced this thing last year, and made a rule that all cows from which milk is sold in their city shall be examined by the tuberculin test; and they carried it out, and they did so under the statute. Now I wrote to the State Board of Cattle Commissioners, and asked them, as they have had considerable experience in the past two or three years, what their opinion was as to the advisability of my putting into our rules or into our ordinance the clause demanding that all cows shall be examined by the tuberculin test. And there, again, we could not compel the Vermont farmer to have his cows examined; but, if he did not have them examined, we could prevent him from selling milk in our city. They made this reply: that it has been their experience that, the premises from which milk is sold being often in bad condition and the farmers not taking particular pains in replacing cows that have been condemned, it hardly seemed to them that a wholesale tuberculin test was necessary. But I was going to, and shall, put this into the ordinance: that all cows must be examined and pronounced free from disease,— and that covers the point Professor Sedgwick brings up,— that all cows must be examined and pronounced free from disease by a veterinarian appointed by the State Board of Cattle Commissioners. I thought, anyway, I would put that in, and let him pronounce on it. Then, if he says the cow is free from disease, it will be all right. If he says the cow is under suspicion, she will be immediately quarantined; and then the State will pay if such cows are condemned. But they said they thought that it would be sufficient if such cows as he finds, from a critical examination, have inoculated udders or other symptoms of tuberculosis, are thrown out. I have spoken with several veterinarians on this subject, and they all say that a physical examination is very, very uncertain; that it is difficult, even in some cases where the disease is considerably advanced, to tell whether it is tuberculosis or not.

Then, in regard to the premises, I was going to put this in our rules: that all premises, all dairies, all places from which milk is sold, shall be under the supervision of the board of health. Then that inspection shall be made at certain times. We can set this to suit ourselves; and we shall compel them to sweep down the cobwebs and clean up the barns,— some of them have never been cleaned,— and ventilate and light properly, and clean up the barn yards. We see so many barn yards that have never been cleaned, where the cows wade through manure to their udders; and we shall stop that.

Now I am going to do this; and I shall be very glad to let this body of men know, if they care to know, a year from now, how we come out,— whether we succeed in getting pure milk and cleaning up the premises and vehicles and barns and utensils. And I do not think we shall have any trouble with the law part.

I would like to know whether any one else has had any experience and can say anything to help us. Our rules will go into operation very soon.

DR. PETERS.— Mr. President, as chairman of the Board of Cattle Commissioners, I have had a little correspondence with the gentleman from North Adams recently ; and I have had a good deal of correspondence with members of other boards of health in various parts of the State,— in Fall River and Pittsfield and Waltham and various localities. They are all very anxious to have the cows tested with tuberculin. Now, when a cow is but slightly diseased, she will often react more, to a higher degree, than cows that are quite badly diseased. And it seems to me that at the present time, in order to protect the public health, it is sufficient if boards of health in various cities and towns will appoint, or if the selectmen shall appoint, or the mayor and aldermen,— if pains are taken to get competent ones,— inspectors of cattle, who shall make a careful physical examination, and report to us all the cattle that have inoculated udders or symptoms of tuberculosis, and put them in quarantine, sending duplicate orders of quarantine to us ; and we will send some one to test them. But, if all these cities and towns are anxious to have a wholesale tuberculin test, and should insist on it, I think it would take $500,000 or $600,000 at least to do it. As our annual appropriation is only about $250,000, I do not see how we could possibly do the work. At the present time we are trying to do all we can with the means at hand, and to do as good work as we can. I think if these cattle that show physical evidence of disease or have inoculated udders are quarantined or killed, that is all we can do, for the reason that, if the owner of the premises does not thoroughly disinfect (and some premises cannot be disinfected unless you set them on fire and burn them down) or if he is not very careful in buying healthy cows, in six months from now there would be just as many cows that would react to the tuberculin test in this State as there are to-day. You might just as well throw money into the Atlantic Ocean as to buy cows very slightly diseased, and kill them and destroy them, and do the work in that way. And, therefore, with the means at hand and the present condition of the farmers' premises, it seems to me that the only thing to do is to take the cows with diseased udders, those that are badly diseased; and there may be a day coming, somewhere near the time when the millennium approaches, when tuberculosis will be so rare among cattle that we can insist upon a compulsory tuberculin test of all the cows in the State. But we are not in a position to do it yet. What we want is to do the best work we can with what money we have. And, if we try to do more than that, we shall run into debt, and be discredited with the legislature, the public, and everybody else.

To show how little importance the farmers attach to disinfection, and how much importance has been attached to simply testing the cattle with tuberculin, I will say that this year we have put on a man to go around, and inspect all the stables where cattle have been taken that are diseased. And I was looking over his reports, and I got a few figures from them before I came down; and, very briefly, I will say that he examined 583 stables. And, at the time of his first visit to these stables, only 109 people had taken any pains to clean up and whitewash and disinfect in any way. On his second visit to these places, when he told them they had got to clean up their premises, 283 more had cleaned up the second time. On the third visit to the same places, about 18 more had cleaned up. So, of 583, only a little over 400 have disinfected their premises properly so far. Under the law we do not seem to have any power to make them disinfect their premises, so far as enforcing our request by any penalty goes; but we have a clause in the law that says, "Whoever by his wilful act or negligence contributes to the spread of tuberculosis shall not obtain any more compensation from the State for animals killed." And we have held that out over the farmers; and we tell a man, "While we have not any power to pull you into court, if you do not comply with our orders and regulations, yet unless you do clean up and disinfect, if you have any more cattle taken, we won't pay you a cent for any that are killed." And that seems to be a sort of bugbear that makes them clean up. And I think it has done a great deal of good.

Another point in connection with a healthful milk supply, I think, is the water that the cows get. A great many of the reports of our inspectors show that the cows get well water; and the well is generally under the barn or in the barn yard, where the surface drainage runs into it. And it seems to me a very important matter that something should be done for the water supply of these farmers' barns. As it is now, in some instances the water that the cows drink actually has a terrible stench.

I think another very important thing, from the producers' and consumers' point of view, is to bring the producer and consumer as near together as we can. I think we have too many middlemen. The milk is produced by the farmer, who only gets two or three cents a quart for it, and is brought here to Boston by a middleman. The pedler buys it from the middleman, and perhaps a little green grocer buys it from the pedler. Now there has to be a little profit made by two or three people in bringing that milk from the producer to the consumer; and it seems to me a very important thing, and a thing that ought to be worked for, to bring the producer and consumer in as close contact as possible. Then the farmer will get a better price for his milk, and the consumer will get it purer and fresher. At the present time, when a farmer only gets two or three cents a quart for milk, it is a question whether he can afford to produce milk under the Utopian conditions asked for. He does not make much of any money now; and, if it costs him much more to produce the milk than it does at present, why he won't make anything.

MR. COFFEY.—I haven't any doubt at all of the authority of the boards of health to prescribe certain rules regulating the care and distribution of milk. But I do think that with the present statute in force, giving the authority to appoint inspectors of milk to the mayor and aldermen, there would be a conflict between the city council and the boards of health in a short time. And I am firmly of the opinion and firmly of the belief that this matter of handling milk and the licensing of pedlers and distributors of milk ought to be in the hands of the boards of health. I have held that opinion for seven or eight or nine years, since I was a milk inspector myself. And I think, if you go to the legislature and ask for an act enabling boards of health to license milk pedlers and distributors, an act that is not too radical in its provisions, you will have the aid and assistance of the farmers. I have reason to believe that. If you leave it so that this tuberculin test can be exacted, and if the present law allows of the exaction of that examination, you will probably find that the farmers of the State will go to the legislature and have the law changed, so that you cannot have that power. Any one who is at all familiar with the legislation of the past two or three years, in relation to tuberculin and the power of the farmer, knows that they have gone to the legislature, and have so changed the laws there that tuberculin is no longer required; and they have materially altered the law in relation to it in the past two or three years. And I think, if they find out that boards of health have now authority to exact that test, they will seek to get legislation that will prevent it. I know, or at least I have reason to believe, that the farmers are willing to co-operate with this organization in the obtainment of an act that will put the care and licensing of milk pedlers in the hands of boards of health; but I think they would ask that the tuberculin test be not included in that act. If something to the effect that an examination by a competent veterinarian should be required was put in there, I think they would be perfectly satisfied with it. We know how powerful they are in obtaining legislation, and I think they would exert all their power to prevent it if you asked for or had an act that would allow of the use of tuberculin and making that a necessary test.

DR. BURR.— I do not think that the committee considered tuberculin in any way. I am sure that hardly a word was said of it in any of our meetings. It never was intended that the examination of the cows on farms in this State or other States should be made with the tuberculin test.

MR. COFFEY.— If you will pardon me, that section I had read empowers the board of health to require that. It says a test satisfactory to the board. Now, if the board deemed the tuberculin test desirable, it can exact it.

DR. BURR.— If the section referred to was so worded that it would be possible for a board of health to call for the tuberculin test, I must say I am not in favor of it. I cannot speak for the rest of the committee; but I am very sure the committee did not consider tuberculin in any way, and did not mean that tuberculin should be used or required.

Now, with regard to the examination made by qualified veterinarians, it seems to me we can hardly exact that at the present time, because the Board of Cattle Commissioners in this State do not call for it. If we go into an examination of the cattle through inspectors appointed by the mayor and board of health and confirmed by the Board of Cattle Commissioners, we are not going to get qualified veterinarians: we are going to get anything from a cobbler up. It seems to me it is going to be pretty hard work to call in a qualified veterinarian. Many of the towns and cities have no qualified veterinarian within twenty miles. I want to emphasize the fact that the committee did not call for, and did not intend to call for, the tuberculin test in any way.

DR. MILLER.— In order to expedite business, I would suggest that the gentleman read the articles, beginning with the first one, and we discuss them and adopt them as we go along; and then whatever is left unfinished we can discuss at some other meeting. By the present method we are scattering over a good deal and finishing nothing. It strikes me it would be better to have the first article read; and then we can approve of it, or dispose of it in some way, and go along in that way, and finish up as far as we go.

Dr. Miller's motion was then put by the President, and unanimously carried. In accordance with the motion Professor Sedgwick read the first section of the first article.

PROFESSOR SEDGWICK.— I will say in regard to that, "persons engaged in the production of milk for sale," it was not intended to make it necessary for the man who keeps a cow for his own use and produces milk, not for sale, or who gives it away to his neighbor, or anything of that kind, to come under this,— simply men who enter the market of public milk supply.

DR. RUSSELL.— I am glad the gentleman put that word in,— "public" milk supply. That leaves out most of the sources of trouble we have. The milkman who makes a business of selling milk, for instance, in my own town, does now keep his barns in reasonable shape. I have licensed between fifty and sixty men this last year, but only ten or twelve of them are milkmen; and other men all about town have cows,— one, two, or three, or even half a dozen,— and sell milk, at least fifty of them. And those are the men who make trouble. I do not see how it is fair to say that the man who carries milk around in his cart for ten families shall have a license, while the man who does not have a cart shall not have.

PROFESSOR SEDGWICK.— I beg pardon. "All persons engaged in the production of milk for sale." That would include every one.

DR. RUSSELL.— Go on, and read the rest.

PROFESSOR SEDGWICK.— "Or in the sale, delivery, or distribution of milk in the city or town."

DR. RUSSELL.— You also added to that the word "public."

PROFESSOR SEDGWICK.— That was not in here. I think the doctor misunderstood me, or at least I did not make myself clear. What I meant to say was, it was not intended to make it necessary for the man who keeps one cow for his own use, or who keeps a cow and gives milk to his next-door neighbor, to take out a license. But the moment he begins to sell milk, even if he sells only a quart, then he is included.

DR. RUSSELL.— I am glad you make that explanation. In my own town we have the trouble from these people who sell to one or two persons, and many of those people sell to eight or ten. Then the men who are recognized as milk dealers, who go out with the carts, go to the inspector of milk,— and, by the way, please remember the inspector of milk is not an inspector of cattle: they are two distinct officers,— they go to the milk inspector, and say, "This man is selling milk." The inspector goes to that man, and says, "You are selling milk." He says, "Well, I only sell to two." The answer is, "There is no difference between selling to two and ten." The man gets angry, and says he is not going to take out a license for selling to two people; and we have a great deal of trouble with him. Another man goes, and says his neighbor across the way gives the milk away; and so the poor milk inspector is in hot water all the time.

THE PRESIDENT.— What is your pleasure in regard to this section?

Dr. Miller.— I move it be accepted and adopted.

Dr. Miller's motion was put by President Walcott, and unanimously carried ; and the section was declared adopted.

Professor Sedgwick then read Section 2.of Article I.

Mr. Coffey.— Now, Mr. Chairman, that goes back to the original point I made. Is it clear that boards of health have the right to license milk pedlers, when that right is distinctly conferred upon an inspector of milk appointed by the mayor and confirmed by the board of aldermen ? Now, supposing that we had that right, and that the milk inspectors did not license until after the board of health had licensed, both acting in concert, and that the board of health for some reason or other revoked that license, as this section gives them the right to do, and that the milk inspector refused to revoke. Then where are you ?

The President. — I do not know ; but I have assumed that the object of these regulations was simply to obtain an ideal set of rules, and that this Association would subsequently ask an appropriate committee to obtain legal advice as to the limitation of the powers possessed, and, if any additional power was needed, to secure it by an application to the legislature for legislation. I should think that would be absolutely essential, whatever we do.

Dr. Miller.— Mr. Chairman, I move this also be adopted.

The motion was unanimously carried, and Section 2 was declared adopted.

Professor Sedgwick then read Section 3. Mr. Coffey moved that it be adopted. The motion was unanimously carried, and the section declared adopted.

Professor Sedgwick then read Section 4, and Dr. Miller moved that it be adopted.

Professor Sedgwick.— Dr. Smith makes a valuable point, which I will ask him to state himself.

Dr. Smith.— I simply wish to say that the statement " free from disease " is rather broad, because a cow may be suffering from some local disease which does not affect the milk supply. I should say " any disease dangerous to human health."

PROFESSOR SEDGWICK.— I will see if I can work that in,— "and shown to the satisfaction of the local board of health to be free from any disease dangerous to man."

DR. SMITH.— There is some objection to that, because a cow may be affected with incipient tuberculosis which is not in that stage dangerous, because the cow does not shed tubercles in that stage. It is only in the later stages that it is dangerous. It is only a question whether " free from disease dangerous to the public health " would not include all cows that are slightly affected, but not under those circumstances dangerous to human health.

THE PRESIDENT.— Why not say " not now dangerous " ?

DR. SMITH.— It may be a full year, according to that statement; and during that time she may have died of tuberculosis.

MR. PARKER.— There is a very interesting point that bears on this subject. Of those animals quarantined by the local inspectors on physical examination, and tested and condemned by the board, the cases of generalized tuberculosis which might be considered the dangerous cases have been enormously reduced upon physical examination, so that, from somewhere about 32 per cent. in 1895 and 25 per cent. in 1896, it had been reduced somewhere to — I won't say exactly, but in the neighborhood of between 2 and 3 per cent. this present year. It seems to me that is a very important point.

MR. COOK.— It seems to me this annual inspection of cattle is already provided for under the statute. The local inspector, under the statute, by order of the Cattle Commissioners has to make an annual inspection. And in relation to any conflict between local inspectors and the local board of health, so far as our experience has gone, it has been entirely free from any friction whatever. Early in the year our board determined upon a thorough inspection of every cow stable in the city of New Bedford. They had some sixty applications for licenses to keep cows. And, before issuing those licenses, the entire board, together with their local inspector, who is appointed by the mayor and aldermen also,— for he is a cattle inspector and milk inspector,— went to every stable throughout the city, and examined it, and the cows were also examined; and the inspector and the board were in perfect unison in the matter, and had no difficulty whatever. The result was the New Bedford Board of Health drove ten cow stables out of existence. Whether they had authority or not, they did it. And there are ten less cow stables in New Bedford to-day than there were early in the year. They finally did that, and they assumed that they did have control of the milk; and, if it came from localities that were not what they should be in the opinion of the board, the board would not hesitate to prevent the sale of that milk; and, if those who felt aggrieved by it wished to carry it further and test it, it was their privilege to do so. The board felt they were able to cope with it. The result was, all the cow stables in New Bedford that were not properly ventilated or were not large enough were made to be enlarged, and new windows put in; and they were made to put in fresh sawdust, and to keep the stables in suitable condition at all times. And our inspector goes around very frequently, and visits all these stables now, and sees that they are kept in that condition. And we have so far this year had no trouble whatever. And the condition of the cow stables in New Bedford to-day is vastly superior to what it was six months ago, and I cannot see why the matter is not entirely within the scope of the authority of the board of health. At least, we have tried it; and we intend to go still farther with it.

PROFESSOR SEDGWICK.— Dr. Smith has made a suggestion that may meet the difficulty or may not. He proposes that it shall read something like this: "No milk shall be sold, offered for sale, or distributed in any city or town unless the cows from which it is derived are considered by the board of health, for practical purposes, free from diseases dangerous to the public health." That leaves out the part about examination by competent authority. But it was assumed that the board would have to get some examination from some source to show that they were free from diseases dangerous to the public health. I do not know whether this will meet with approval or not.

THE PRESIDENT.— The section as originally presented to this Association was this: "No milk shall be sold, offered for sale, or distributed in any city or town unless the cows from which it is derived, have within one year been examined by a competent authority, and shown to the satisfaction of the local board of health to be free from

.disease." It is proposed to amend this, so that it shall read, " No milk shall be sold, etc., unless the cows are considered by the board of health, for practical purposes, free from diseases dangerous to the public health."

MR. COFFEY.— I would like to amend that still further, Mr. Chairman, by adding, " provided, however, that the tuberculin test shall not be exacted except with the consent of the owner of the cattle."

DR. PETERS.— I think, in the general law covering the work of the Cattle Commission, that is provided for. In the law it says that tuberculin shall not be used for diagnostication without the consent of the owner, unless the animal is first said to be diseased by a competent veterinarian. So I think the owner is already protected.

THE PRESIDENT.— The question is, first, in regard to the amendment introduced by Mr. Coffey. Is it your pleasure that the amendment should be adopted ?

MR. COFFEY.— If you will permit me to say a word ? The gentleman from North Adams said they exacted that test in Pittsfield, and he proposed to exact it; and I have rather the feeling, if the doctor says he will do it, he will do it.

DR. SIMPSON.— I wrote to the Board of Cattle Commissioners,— I did not know Dr. Peters was here until a moment ago,— and asked them whether that was advisable. They wrote to me, and said they did not consider it necessary. Now, as they do not consider it necessary, I shall of course drop that. And I do not think there is any board of health that could exact it, or would exact it contrary to the wishes of the State Board of Cattle Commissioners. I should have exacted it if they had considered it necessary ; but, as they did not, that will be dropped out.

MR. COFFEY.— I withdraw the amendment, Mr. Chairman.

THE PRESIDENT.— The question is, then, with regard to what the committee chose to submit.

PROFESSOR SEDGWICK.— I should prefer, rather than to have this carried through hastily, that it be referred back to the committee for further investigation.

THE PRESIDENT.— It is moved that Section 4 be referred back to the committee for further consideration. Is that your pleasure ?

The motion prevailed, and Section 4 was referred back to the committee.

Professor Sedgwick then read Section 5.

Mr. Pilsbury.— I move that all these sections, unless objection is made, be considered adopted.

Mr. Pilsbury's motion was seconded, and unanimously carried.

Professor Sedgwick then read Section 1 of Article II.

The President.— Is there any objection to this section? If not, you will signify its acceptance by saying aye.

The section was adopted by a unanimous vote.

Professor Sedgwick then read Section 2 of Article II.

Mr. Ellis.— I would suggest a slight change, that instead of "the room" a different provision shall be made. This makes it obligatory that this sterilizing be done in a certain room, and I suggest that provision should be made that it should not necessarily be in that room.

Professor Sedgwick.— The committee thought it ought to be done in this particular room. I should like to ask why not.

Mr. Ellis.— In my own case, my milk-room and my provision for sterilizing bottles, etc., are independent one of another. Why should I be obliged to do it in the same room? If I have provision for that, is not that sufficient?

Professor Sedgwick. —"Or in some room satisfactory to the board of health" I should suppose that would be all that was required. I think, if there is any debate, that had better not be accepted, but referred back.

On motion of Mr. Coffey, Section 2 was referred back to the committee.

Professor Sedgwick then read Section 3 of Article II.; and it was adopted, there being no objection.

Section 4 was then read by Professor Sedgwick.

Professor Sedgwick.— The idea is that the milk should be taken after milking right away from the stable or cow yard, and handled, cooled, and stored in the regular milk-room, as it is in many cases now.

Mr. Coffey.— I think that ought to go back also with the other one, because my idea of the first one was the impracticability of the adoption of this for the small dealer.

The President.— If there is any objection, I think it will be referred back without question.

Mr. Coffey.— A large number of milk producers have only a few cans.

The President.— This section will be referred back to the committee.

Professor Sedgwick then read Section 1 of Article III.

The President.— Is there any objection to this?

On motion of Dr. Durgin the section was adopted.

Professor Sedgwick.— It was suggested that this section should contain the word "ice,"— that the refrigerator might be used without ice. That may be introduced if there is no objection.

Professor Sedgwick then read Article IV.

The President.— Is there any objection to this article?

There being no objection, the article was adopted by a unanimous vote.

Professor Sedgwick.— There only remain the two articles on contagious diseases, which I hardly think there can be any objection to; but I will read them. [Reads first section.]

The President.— What is your pleasure in regard to this section?

On motion of Dr. Farnham the section was adopted by a unanimous vote.

Professor Sedgwick then read the second section.

Mr. Cook.— I would like to ask if the boards of health through-out the State are not already carrying out that same idea?

The President.— I hope so.

Mr. Cook.— It seems to me that is already being carried out by the local boards.   I am sure it is in New Bedford.

Mr. Ellis.— Its adoption, then, can do no harm.

Mr. Cook.— It surely can do no harm, but I am surprised that it should be deemed necessary to suggest it.

The section was then unanimously adopted.

The President.— Will you authorize your committee to obtain proper advice, if necessary, upon the legality of the rules that they have proposed?

It was unanimously voted that the committee be authorized to get proper legal advice upon the constitutionality and propriety of the rules.

The President.— Is there any other business?   If not, we still have a few minutes of time.   The Association has present certain gentlemen who are interested in the production of milk, and I wish we might hear from them.   Mr. Ellis, haven't you anything to say upon this subject?

Mr. Ellis.— I doubt, Mr. Chairman and gentlemen, if I could say anything that would be of service.   The question, as it touches me, is somewhat different from that touching most producers and sellers of milk.   I am in direct communication with my own consumers.   And about the only thing I would say is that I think the general public appreciate, and will appreciate, the efforts of boards of health, of producers, and of dealers in milk, to furnish a pure article, to an extent that they have not been fully credited with. My own experience has indicated that people in general are willing to pay a higher price for milk that they are reasonably sure is pure and is well cared for.   I happen to be so situated that I am within easy access of nearly all the consumers to whom we supply milk,—some fifteen hundred quarts a day; and we have adopted, as far as possible,— with the exception of Pasteurization. which I believe Professor Sedgwick considers not only important, but essential,— most of the new ways of handling milk. In our case the milk is drawn from the cow, and almost immediately cooled to a temperature of between 38 and 40 degrees, and bottled. My own theory — not being a scientist — is that such milk is better — at any rate, I would rather have it — than Pasteurized milk, if properly taken care of after it leaves my place. And that milk is in the hands of consumers within three hours. I cannot well contribute — in a moment, at any rate — to this discussion with anything valuable, because, as I say, my own experience is different, necessarily, from that of most producers.

DR. DURGIN.— I would like to ask Mr. Ellis whether or not it is possible or practicable to have the cow so cleaned before each milking as to avoid a large amount of this filth which is continually dropping into the pail during the process of milking.

MR. ELLIS.— As to that, I will only say that last Sunday a lady came to me at church, saying that the day before she had visited our farm, and had been greatly pleased to find in our strainer cloth, through which the milk from one hundred and twenty cows had been strained, less filth than she had seen, in her old days on the farm, after one cow's milking.

DR. DURGIN.— How do you obtain that, Mr. Ellis?

MR. ELLIS.— By care of the cows, sir.

DR. DURGIN.— Well, particularly?

MR. ELLIS.— In my case the cows are groomed every day. Most of my cows — seventy-six of my cows — are kept in pens, 7 feet by 9, never tied. They have before them water all the time. They are carefully cleaned. The pens are carefully cleaned every day; the manure carried off the farm. They are bedded with sand. There are no floors in these pens. The bedding is sand and planing-mill shavings. Our building is a one-story building with a dome roof; and I would not undertake to say how many square feet or cubic feet of space our cows have, or how many windows there are, but they are plentiful.

DR. DURGIN.— Would you regard it as unreasonable, Mr. Ellis, if the committee or this Association required in each instance that the cow should be so cleaned before milking as to avoid this large amount of filth dropping into the milk ?

Mr. Ellis.— I think we have got to come to that. We have got to work toward it. I do not know that you could at once adopt rules that would compel all farmers to do that.

Dr. Durgin.— To my mind, it becomes a very important part of our work; for, do as much as we will, there is more or less dropping of dust and filth from the cow into the pail which contains the milk. There ought to be such grooming or cleaning of the cow's teats before the milking as will avoid very much of this filth getting into the milk. It seems to me also that, in the pasturage of the cows, we ought to so regulate that cows shall not be allowed to wade in filth, which soils the teats and becomes a serious means of polluting the milk.

Mr. Ellis.— My own theory would be that that would be impracticable, particularly in hot weather. Cows too much enjoy getting into the water and in the edges of rivers, and so forth.

Dr. Durgin.— I think we shall try it in Boston.

Mr. Ellis.— I think it would be impracticable.

Dr. Burr.— Mr. Chairman, I would like to say just one thing, in addition, that this committee did not touch on or did not report on it. It was well considered, but we hardly knew how to report upon it; and that is, in regard to milk transportation. Milk is transported now from the farms by the railroads and contractors. We have made no rules and regulations governing the contractor or the railroad. We have believed that at times our milk is very old on arriving at the railroad station in the city or town where it is consumed, and it seems to me that something ought to be done in regard to that. As you all know, in the city of Boston the milk arrives at a late hour in the morning, about eleven o'clock; and that milk may be this morning's, in some instances last night's or yesterday morning's, possibly. And I think, in a good many instances, that of the day before. On arriving at Boston, at ten o'clock, it is taken by the milk dealer to his place of business, and there cared for during the day, and delivered the following morning, which makes it at least thirty-six hours old. I think that must be pretty near the minimum. It seems to me that it would be a good plan to limit the age at which milk should be received in Boston or in any city. Supposing we limit it to twenty-four hours. It would then be at least twelve hours older before it reached the consumer. If milk should arrive in Boston or any large city in the evening from ten to twelve o'clock, it might be this evening's or this morning's milk, and then be delivered immediately by the dealer the following morning,— in that case not to be over twenty-four to thirty hours before it was received by the consumer. I know, from a few questions that were sent out from the Boston Board of Health, that in almost all instances it does not take over four hours to get the milk into Boston. If that is the case, if it does not take over four hours to get the milk into Boston, it seems to me we can get this morning's and last night's milk delivered in Boston to-day. If it arrives in Boston at night, we might have this evening's and this morning's milk delivered the following morning. It seems to me that question ought to be considered by this Association. I will say that the committee hardly knew how to fix it.

A Member.— I would like to say that, if all milk farms were in the condition of those managed by Mr. Ellis, there would be no occasion for any rules either by this Association or by the legislature.

Mr. Ellis.— Mr. Chairman, I will extend an invitation to this Association to hold its next meeting at Wauwinet Farm. It is very easy of access on the Commonwealth Avenue line of the electric road. I should be glad to extend that invitation.

The President.— I hope I may call to Mr. Ellis's attention the fact that this Association will have to hold its next meeting in Boston; but will this invitation hold good for the meeting after the next?

Mr. Ellis.— Certainly. Yes, sir.

Dr. Osgood.— One thing I would like to say. In order to bring about any great results in the line of the purity of the milk supply, one thing we ought to consider; and that is, the price the farmer is getting for his milk. The average farmer to-day is getting about three cents a quart for his milk. Now we are requiring him to conform to a great many rules and regulations, increasing the expense of the production of that milk. In my past experience with the farming community, I found that a large part of them thought that by having their herds subjected to a test, assuring their customers that they are furnishing a pure milk supply, there would be a disposition on the part of the consumer to give a little more for that quality of milk. Now I think this Association can do a good work in encouraging their clients to be willing to give a living price for a pure article. I think that is a fundamental step; and I think it is the duty of every physician and of every one connected with this Association to encourage the people, first educating them to the idea that we need a better article than the farmer can furnish at the price he is getting to-day, and then encouraging them to be willing to pay a living price for that product.

Mr. ELLIS.— May I add one word? This last summer, when Mr. Whiting,— who is, I suppose, one of our largest milk contractors,— was visiting at my farm, he dropped the remark that, if the contractors could buy from the farmer milk properly taken care of, they, the contractors, could well afford to pay a higher price for that milk, if they sold it at no higher price. I presume Mr. Hood will bear me out?

Mr. Hood.— Yes, I think so.

Mr. ELLIS.— If the milk coming from the producer were of such quality and of such character that the contractor would lose less, he could easily pay a higher price for his milk. Mr. Hood, I think, agrees with me.

THE PRESIDENT.— Mr. Hood, haven't you something to say on this matter? We should be very glad to hear from you.

Mr. HOOD.— Mr. Chairman and gentlemen, I do not think I ought to take your time, though I am very much pleased to be here, and say a word. I have been much interested in what has been said; and it is very interesting to us, as dealers, to hear such a discussion, which should be interesting to every consumer and producer. The producers, first, have got to be educated,— no, not first. We should be educated first. Then we can help to educate the producers. Most of our producers are willing to do what they can to furnish the best article for the market. And, if we ask them to do anything that they can see for themselves will improve the milk, they will do what we ask. But, if we tell them that the milk tastes of clover, which fact they cannot themselves detect, and ask them to take their cows up at two or three o'clock in the afternoon, they are not willing to do that; and they may say to us: "We ought to know something about it. We sold milk before you were born." Yet we think the producers, as a whole, are always willing to do their part in helping us to get the best. Many of our farmers feed turnips, and we find that they can be fed without harm immediately after milking; but, if fed before milking, they affect the milk.

Mr. Ellis.—The same is true of ensilage.

Mr. Hood.—Yes, the same is true of ensilage. Now, to come to the question of the transportation of milk, we are all anxious to get the milk off the farm as quickly as possible, because we lose money by holding it. Large milk contractors have chemists; and the next thing for them to do is to have bacteriologists, and I think that is a move that will be made very soon.

After transportation, we come to the milk dealer, but just a word in regard to the middlemen. In New York there are no middlemen; and every farmer is a shipper, and is therefore a competitor with his neighbor. When he loses a customer, he goes to New York, and tries to place his milk. Then the other farmer, who has lost the customer, goes there also to place his milk again, and, as a rule, has to place it at a still less price. Then the next farmer goes, and, finally, all the farmers. The result is, the price paid for milk within one hundred miles of Boston is 20 per cent. higher than in New York, where there are no contractors, and has been for the last few years. The contractors keep up the price in the country, and they are the ones that can help bring about the improvements which you recommend. They are the ones who must provide chemists, who must help the boards of health in the country towns and in the cities, who must provide men to test for bacteria, and who must do all they can to educate the farmers.

Now we come to the milk dealers here in Boston. They judge milk almost entirely by the sense of taste; and some, of course, become so expert in tasting milk that they can detect the difference between milk flavored with turnips or ensilage or cabbages, can distinguish the taste coming from a dirty stopper, wormword in the pasture, or clover, when fed in excess. They will detect the bad effect caused by mixing warm and cold milk, and a good many other things, which perhaps, cannot be detected by any other means. The milk is taken by the dealers to their stables; and, of course, in some instances, it is handled in a very poor way. Yet many dealers take pride in the neatness of their milk-rooms.

About the price of milk in the city. The milk dealers are selling a great deal of milk delivered up several flights of stairs, in pint cans, for three cents a pint, the year round. They cannot afford this, and pay the prices they do for the milk. But they are compelled to do so, because there are stores in town that are selling milk for four cents per quart, and perhaps less. And they say, "We must hold our business." They do it by using cans badly jammed, cans that are not fit to use, washing them, but not sterilizing them, and furnishing the cheapest stoppers. They must deliver milk at an early hour, between one o'clock and six. They cannot deliver it in the daytime because their customers might wish to speak with them, and they have no time for that. To improve the milk supply, we should do something to stop the sale of cheap milk. No one should be licensed unless he will sell at a fair living profit. But we find it is said to the storekeeper: "Sell your milk cheap, because you will sell a lot of it. Don't try to make any money on it, but sell it as a leader." If he drops a cent on beef, nobody will know it; but, if he drops a cent on milk, everybody will know it. These stores can cut the price on milk, and make money on something else; while the milk dealer has only one article to sell; and, furthermore, he is poor. That is, he is running along, and doing the business in the cheapest way possible. Some storekeepers have no suitable ice-chest in their store, and handle the milk in the most careless way, and perhaps do not thoroughly wash the measures used for the milk from one week's end to another.

As to who shall wash the cans. Perhaps they should be washed twice, once in the city as near the consumer as possible, and once in the country by the producer; but the consumer or the person who empties the can in the hotel dining-room or store should immediately wash the can. That is just the time and place to have them washed; for it could then be done most easily, and it would remove all the milk on which the bacteria so thrive. Let them be washed and sterilized again at the farm, for that will be found quite necessary.

I will say, in sterilizing the cans, I think it is quite important that the can should be sterilized and stopped up dry; that is, the water, the draining water, should be out before the cans are stopped up.

To go back to the farm again, I should think that the interior of barns should be whitewashed twice each year. The lime costs practically nothing, and the producer has plenty of time in the fall and spring to whitewash the barn; and those who have it done are very well pleased, and take pride in the changed appearance. The stables should get plenty of sunlight, and the cows should be on the sunny side as much as possible.

I am very glad to have had the opportunity to be with you, gentlemen, and to enter into this discussion.

THE PRESIDENT.— Dr. Durgin inexorably moves that we now adjourn, because our places are needed by others. If that be your pleasure, you will manifest it by saying aye.

The motion was unanimously carried, and the meeting was adjourned.

[THE PROTECTION OF MILK SUPPLIES]

PROFESSOR W. T. SEDGWICK.— Mr. President and gentlemen of
the Association and our distinguished guests, you are all aware
that this Association has been for some time trying to formulate a set
of rules which would look to the betterment of the milk supply of
our larger cities and towns. As is often the case, when people undertake improvements, it is easier to undertake them than to carry them
out; and that has been found so here. Nevertheless, your committee,
after considerable hesitation and a good deal of advice freely solicited
and sometimes freely volunteered, has arrived at certain preliminary
conclusions. These were stated in the rough at the last meeting,
and in the main were adopted by this Association as expressing its
desire; but I am sure that I am voicing the feelings of the Associa-

tion, as I know that I am the feelings of the committee, when I say that we realize fully that these rules are tentative and experimental, subject still to criticism and amendment. It should also be borne in mind that they are only suggestions and recommendations to boards of health, and that each board of health may, if it chooses, neglect them altogether, carry them out in part, or adopt them in full.

At the last meeting certain sections were referred back to the committee for amendment and, if possible, improvement; and the committee was also instructed to inquire whether the steps already taken were in line with the statutory law. These things have been looked into, and certain results reached. Before proceeding, however, to state precisely what the results are, I wish to repeat what has been said already several times as to the object of these rules. The object is a very simple one. It is to endeavor to bring the milk supply of modern cities and towns as far as is practicable up to the present standards of sanitary science; and in this respect, as the Association well knows, our ideas have changed within the last fifteen or twenty years very materially. A standard which was good twenty years ago is inadequate to-day; and it is our duty as representatives of the various cities and towns on the sanitary side, and as in a measure guardians of the public health, to endeavor to make action fit theory as far as is practicable, and only so far as is practicable.

The one main object which the committee has had in view all through has been the bringing about of greater cleanness. Everything, I think, may be reduced to that greater cleanness, because greater cleanness is going to mean a better sanitary condition, fresher milk, safer milk. With that in view everything else has been set aside. For example, as you will see, when I proceed to read the amended rules of the committee, it has not been deemed wise or necessary to introduce or attempt to introduce anything which is still seriously under debate,— such, for example as the tuberculin test, believing that, if we undertook to do that, in the first place, we should not be, perhaps, perfectly sure that all members of the Association would agree about the rules providing for the use of tuberculin, and, in the second place, that we should be trying to do something that we have not set out to do. What we are after is to get cleaner, fresher, purer milk, and not to get milk that is beyond any of the modern reasonable requirements of any city or town or, as we believe, beyond the reasonable ability of any set of people supplying milk. To carry this out, we believe that all licenses for the sale of milk should be brought under the authority of the boards of health. The sale of milk is henceforward to be regarded as a sanitary matter. It is a matter of food supply as much as any other food, perhaps more than any other food, that man has; and it is believed that the boards of health are able to attend to that, and pronounce as to the sanitary condition of the milk, and not, as still is the case in some places, the so-called inspector of milk, not answerable to a board of health in any way.

It was pointed out at the last meeting that, in undertaking to do this and in recommending that boards of health should license milk dealers, and should look after the sanitary condition of dairy farms, the methods of handling milk *en route* and after its arrival in the city, there was danger of a conflict of authority between the inspector appointed by the mayor and aldermen and the boards of health, having separate authority. That fact was pointed out by Mr. Coffey, of Worcester; and your committee was instructed to look into the matter. On looking into it, they find that there is, in fact, danger of some such conflict. We have consulted eminent legal authority, and have been led to believe that there is probably the necessity in some cases — that is, in cases where the inspector is not already connected with boards of health — that there should be special legislation bringing inspectors under such authority. That is not the case in Boston, which has its special statute, but it is the case, I think, still in many cities and towns of the State; and so one recommendation of your committee to-day is that your Committee on Legislation should look into this matter, and endeavor, if possible, to secure the proper legislation, in order that boards of health, the proper and recognized sanitary authority, shall have power, if they choose to do so, to grant licenses for the sale of milk in their respective cities and towns. And, of course, that committee will have to act promptly, because the time for the admission of new business at the State House is limited.

With regard to the other point that was raised, as to the power of the boards of health to make ordinances such as these, and bring them in line with the ordinary ordinance-making power, there seems to be comparatively little doubt. It is granted that, if there is any conflict between boards of health and the inspector of milk, the power of a board of health to establish these rules governing the milk supply is sufficient. But, before that conflict arises, perhaps it would be well for the Committee on Legislation to look into it.

There are certain verbal changes and errors in the rules as printed in the report, which, I believe, most of the members of the Association now have, as it should have been distributed to them, and I dare say has been.

For instance, in Section 1 it was stated toward the end that application "on forms prescribed by the board, for a permit or license," must be made. It was not said what board. It should be the "Board of Health of said city or town."

The same correction should be made in Section 3. "Local board of health" should be "Board of Health of said city or town." In other words, the conditions under which cows are kept should be made known to the local board of health of the city or town in which the milk is to be sold, not the local board of health in the town or village where the milk is produced.

Section 4 was one which made a great deal of trouble at the last meeting, and your committee is not altogether sanguine that it has got it in good shape now; but the form in which it is presented to you to-day is this : —

"Section 4. No milk shall be sold, offered for sale, or distributed in any city or town, unless the cows from which it is derived"— that word is "delivered" in the printed form — "unless the cows from which it is derived have within one year been examined by a competent authority, and shown to the satisfaction of the Board of Health of said city or town to be free from diseases dangerous to the public health. But this shall not be construed as forbidding the sale or use of milk from cows not tested with tuberculin."

In order to prevent all possible misunderstanding, the committee believed that we should exclude the tuberculin test from this set of rules. If the Association desires to take that up later, well and good; but, as I have already said, the object of these rules was primarily to secure greater cleanness and care of the milk. It was not to prevent the use of milk from non-tuberculin-tested cows ; and, therefore, it was thought that, in order to make it perfectly clear, we would say so. I will reread that section, and the Association can then adopt it either now or later. [Section 4 was then reread.]

Then one or two other sections were referred back, and we have taken the liberty of changing Section 2 of Article II. Although it was not referred back to us, we had no right to do so, perhaps ; but, as now proposed, it reads as follows : —

"Section 2. Milk shall be stored or regularly mixed, cooled, or poured from can to can only in a room not directly connected with a stable or stables, provided with a tight floor, and kept constantly neat and clean, the walls of the room being of such a nature as to allow easy and thorough cleansing." The committee felt that this might be too severe upon some small farmers, so they have qualified it as follows: "or in some room approved by the said Board of Health." So that, if a man came and said that it would be a hardship for him to make a room such as is described, the committee thought it would be reasonable to qualify the rule as suggested,— that the room could be left for the approval of the Board of Health ; and, if they should approve it, no undue hardship would be brought about. "Such room shall contain proper appliances for washing" — the former word was "*and* sterilizing"; but, as it is felt that people won't sterilize and cannot sterilize under ordinary conditions, it would be better to say "for washing *or* sterilizing"—"all utensils actually employed in the storage, sale, and distribution of milk in said building, and all such apparatus and utensils shall be washed with boiling water or sterilized by steam regularly after having been so used."

There are two versions proposed for Section 4,— one just as it is, and the other which amounts to leaving it just as it is ; namely, "some room other than the stable, and not containing any urinal or privy, nor used for sleeping or other domestic purposes." Beyond this the committee was not instructed to go, and has not gone.

I will simply tell you, to repeat what I have already said, that these rules are intended to secure, in the first place, greater care, in the second place, greater cleanness, in the milk supply. The committee felt it very undesirable to bring in any elements which would interfere with those primary and fundamental objects. If we can secure this, we shall be taking a great step in advance.

Finally, I think the committee feels that, after this matter has been disposed of, the Association may well address itself to the preparation of a circular of information which may be distributed to the farmers and others interested in the milk supply, showing how milk becomes contaminated and what sanitarians regard as proper care of milk. It is found that there is a good deal of ignorance on that subject. Sanitarians are thought, on the one hand, to require many things they do not require; and, on the other hand, they are not known to require some that they do ask for. And so in this form I think the committee may safely leave these rules with the Association. Stated somewhat roughly, there is need of more legislation in order to prevent confusion in granting licenses; and, second, there is need for the preparation of a circular of information.

I should like to say, personally, that, after thinking over this thing a good deal, I believe there might well go as a verbal statement from the Association — not to be printed with these rules, of course — the understanding that whatever improvement is made in the milk supply is to come along three lines. In the first place, from the producer, who should clean up, and see to it that the milk is more thoroughly cared for, to start with; in the second place, from the middleman or contractor, who should see to it that the milk is as safely and quickly transported and delivered to the consumer as is possible; and, in the third place, the consumer, whose milk supply has been based hitherto upon a low standard in all these matters, should do his part, and be prepared, if necessary, as I believe it will be necessary, to pay a higher price for safe, pure, and sanitary milk. I think it ought to be very distinctly understood by the Association and by our guests that in all these matters the one desire of this Association is the improvement of the public health. If these rules seem to some to bear hard upon some, it may be due to a misunderstanding or it is inevitable on account of the growth of the science. If it is a misunderstanding, we might hope to clear it up; but the fundamental object of the whole thing must, in any case, be constantly kept in view, and that is to bring the present system of milk supply in Boston and in Massachusetts up to the very highest standard practicable, and to keep it in line with the best sanitary science of the day.

THE PRESIDENT.— The Association has listened to the report of the committee. I presume that the only way in which this Association can intelligibly and intelligently enter upon this discussion would be article by article of this report, but it is simply a suggestion. What action will you take? Possibly, for the information of the Association, it will be well that all the rules should be read. If it is desired, we could then discuss each singly.

PROFESSOR SEDGWICK.— The heading, I think, is very important here,— "Rules suggested by a Committee of the Massachusetts Association of Boards of Health for adoption by the Boards of Health of the State for the Protection of Milk Supplies from Pollution."

ARTICLE I.

SECTION 1. All persons engaged in the production of milk for sale, or in the sale, delivery, or distribution of milk in the city or town of——, shall annually, on or before May 1, make written application, on forms prescribed by the Board of Health of said city or town, for a permit or license.

THE PRESIDENT.— Is it your wish to discuss this report article by article or to have the whole report read to you?

A MEMBER.— Article by article.

THE PRESIDENT.— The first article, then, is before the Association for discussion. I shall be very glad to hear from anybody who has anything to say upon the subject or to ask questions.

DR. MILLER.— Mr. President, I would like to ask one question. Some of these articles were adopted at the last meeting, and some were referred back to the committee. Now, if the chairman of the committee, as he reads these, if he is going to read the whole right along, would tell us which ones he desires the present meeting to act upon, or if there are any changes to be made, I think we should act more intelligently. Of course, those that were adopted at the last meeting do not need to be touched now.

THE SECRETARY.— Article I., Section 1, was accepted.

PROFESSOR SEDGWICK.— Article I., Section 2, Article I., Section 3, Article I., Section 4, were referred back to the committee.

DR. MILLER.— Then Article I., Section 4, would be the first one to consider, wouldn't it?

Professor Sedgwick.— Mr. President, we have with us to-day a number of guests representing farmers and representing contractors; and it seems as if so rare a chance were too good an occasion for us to lose to hear from these gentlemen, and to learn whether they have any fundamental objections to any of these rules. And, although we have expected to meet objections, and it is very likely shall continue to do so, yet we should be glad to hear if there is any sound criticism of them, because our one object in all this is, as I have said, the real benefit of the public.

The President.— I presume it is the wish of this Association to get all the information that it can upon the subject, and we shall be glad to hear anything that may be said upon this matter.

A Member.— Mr. President, it might be that, an article having been adopted, some one present might have some valuable amendment to offer; and, if the articles are not too long, I for one would like to hear them read.

The President.— We will proceed to do so. Is there anything to be said upon this Article I.?

A Member.— Mr. President, as I understand it, the law distinguishes between milk, buttermilk, and skim milk. Now would it be any object to insert in Article I. "in the production of milk, butter- r " or skim milk," or add the word "cream"? I ask this question because there are some practical troubles with this matter. Certain ones who sell buttermilk say they are exempt, or would say so; and others who sell skim milk would say the same, and some who sell cream would say the same. It seems to me it is of equal importance to have all these places kept clean.

Professor Sedgwick.— That has not been considered. We are very glad of the suggestion.

Dr. Charles Harrington.— Mr. President, I would suggest that the Supreme Court of Massachusetts has decided that cream and skim milk are milk, so that is not necessary.

A Member.— Mr. President, at the same time the law tells what we should do to protect dealers and those that sell; and in this case it seems to me just as desirable.

Dr. Harrington.— Mr. President, that question I have had occasion to ask many times, and I will simply say that those are varieties of milk. It is all milk.

THE PRESIDENT.— As I understand it, there is no motion made to amend.

DR. CHAPIN.— Mr. President, I should like to ask if this includes condensed milk.

THE PRESIDENT.— I do not know how it is in Rhode Island, but condensed milk is covered by special legislation in Massachusetts.

DR. BURR.— Mr. President, there has been a question raised in regard to this section concerning the wording in "the production of milk for sale." I think that there are some of the representatives of the milk producers here who perhaps can give us their view on that particular point; but the question is whether the producer of milk should be obliged to obtain his license for simply producing the milk? As I understand it now, a producer does not have to have a license. The one who sells is obliged to obtain a license: the producer does not have to.

PROFESSOR SEDGWICK.— Mr. President, the intention there was simply to affect a man who produces milk for sale; and I cannot myself see why it is not right to say "all persons engaged in the production of milk for sale,"— that is, not the production of milk for their own families or to supply their neighbors, but in the production of milk for sale. It seems to me that is perfectly clear. If it would make it any clearer to say "all persons engaged in the sale of milk," I think it would cover the same idea, because the man who raises milk and sells it would then be covered by it.

A MEMBER.— I would suggest that it be those "who are engaged in the business,"— let the business be the thing,— "who are engaged in the business of " thus and so.

PROFESSOR SEDGWICK.— The committee does not see that that makes any material difference. It is hard to see how anything can be clearer,— "all persons engaged in the production of milk for sale, or in the sale," and so on. If the Association think that ought' to be cleared up, it can be done. It should be understood that this has already been adopted, and the chairman is now simply inviting criticisms. Unless there are pretty sound reasons for change, it seems unwise to depart from it as adopted.

DR. W. P. BOWERS.— One of the prominent producers in our section is here, and he has raised the question where he should get his license. He wants to know whether, if anybody sends milk to Boston, he should get a license in Boston or in the place where he lives.

PROFESSOR SEDGWICK.— I think that is covered by the words "in the city or town." "All persons engaged in the production of milk . . . in the city or town of" blank. That is, for instance, if a man in Hillsboro Bridge, N.H., if there is such a town, is producing milk for sale in Boston, he does not have to get any license; but, if he is in West Roxbury, which is a part of Boston, he has got to get a license just as much as the man who delivers milk from the railroad station. This does not mean that farmers have not got to pay for a license at all,— nothing of that sort: that would be absurd of course,— but simply, if they are engaged in the production of milk for sale in such a town or in the sale of it in that town. Perhaps the punctuation might be improved, but that was the idea.

MR. GEO. H. ELLIS.— "All persons engaged in the production of milk for sale." I do not see why the Hillsboro Bridge man, who is producing milk for sale, has not got to get his license under that. I think, if the words "production of milk for sale to a consumer" were inserted, that would cover that; and, if the Hillsboro Bridge farmer is producing milk for sale, he has got to get a license.

PROFESSOR SEDGWICK.— It was not the intention of the committee at all. I think a comma after the word "milk" would fix the whole thing. It would then read, "any person engaged in the sale, delivery, or distribution of milk, in the city or town," and so on. The idea is not to license the farmer, but to license the man who sells milk in the city, and then to make him report what the condition of the farms is up in the country; but those farmers are not to be licensed. I do not think that was ever contemplated by the committee.

THE PRESIDENT.— As no motion has yet been made, the chairman of the committee will read the next article.

PROFESSOR SEDGWICK.— "Section 2. No person shall engage in the business of producing milk for sale, or in the sale or distribution of milk,"— and here the comma is in,— "in the city or town of" blank. It seems to be understood that there are farmers as well as milk pedlers in the city of Boston, and this was aimed at them as well as at the pedlers; that is, if there is a farm in Dorchester or Roxbury producing milk, that farm within the city limits should come under this just as truly as the pedler who takes it from the railroad station. And I think that is covered by this clause,— " in the city or town of —— after April 30, 1898," or any other date, " without a permit or license to do so signed by said Board of Health, and under such conditions as said Board of Health may impose, revokable at the pleasure of said board." That, it seems to me, is perfectly simple,— no person shall engage in a city or town in the business of producing milk for sale, or in the sale or distribution of milk, without a license.

The legal member of our committee says it would be well to have the word " continue " inserted, so that it shall read " shall engage or continue in the business of producing milk," etc., in that city or town ; but that was adopted at the last meeting of the committee, and, unless there is a motion to do so, it cannot be changed.

THE PRESIDENT.— Is there anything to be said upon the section just read to you?

PROFESSOR SEDGWICK.— " Section 3. The conditions under which every cow is kept, whose milk is brought into any city or town, or kept, delivered, distributed, sold, or offered for sale, in such city or town, shall be made known to the Board of Health of said city or town in such detail as the board may require, and shall be approved thereby; and no milk except that delivered from such cows,"— " derived " that should be again,— " derived from such cows shall be so brought, kept, delivered, distributed, sold, or offered for sale."

Now that, of course, is the attempt on the part of the Board of Health to get control of the conditions on the farm, but not by licensing. It is simply by requiring a statement or report to be made by the person selling milk in the city or town as to the conditions of the farms from which he derives his milk. That seemed to the committee, if this was adopted, to be without any question a perfectly rational and proper thing to do,— a very different thing from licensing a farmer, simply a means of getting information. Then, if the information shows that the farm is in a wretched condition, very unsanitary, the license of that particular dealer in the city can be cut off; and he would have to get his milk somewhere else.

THE PRESIDENT.— Is there any question to be asked with regard to this section?

A MEMBER.— There is one point I would like to ask about in the first section, where the producer of milk sells to a contractor. Some of the members do not quite understand how, if the producer of milk sells to the contractor, that is to be controlled. If he should sell to the contractor, how is he to be affected?

PROFESSOR SEDGWICK.— Well, so far as it appears on the face of it, it would be like this. The contractor would be a person defined here as selling milk in the city of Boston. He would therefore be required, as a condition of his receiving a license, to make known to the Board of Health, in such detail as that Board of Health might require, the conditions under which every cow supplying him with milk is kept; and he would practically, I suppose, have a blank with which the Board of Health would provide him, which he would mail to every farmer supplying him with milk in the town of Sterling. That farmer would fill it out, giving a statement, for instance, of the position of the privy with reference to the cow-barn, the condition of the stables, how the milk is handled, whether the cans are set just behind the cows while milking is going on, and so forth and so forth. A lot of simple facts like those could be easily filled out by any intelligent producer. The producer would send that back to the contractor, then, as a matter of course, the contractor would return it to the Board of Health, the Board of Health would look it over; and, if they felt it needed inspection, they would send one of their inspectors up there to see if the farm was really what it pretended to be. Of course, at first they could not send an inspector to every farm; but they would go at random to just a few farms, and raise the whole standard. The immediate practical effect would be at first very little; but the ultimate practical effect would be an intelligent inspection by the Board of Health, the inspector from the Board of Health saying to the farmer: "You think you are doing everything nicely, but here are such and such things that are not as they should be. You can see this won't do, and I shall have to recommend that your farm be cut off unless you do so and so." That is only my idea. That is the way I should do it if I was on the Board of Health; and I presume my friend, Dr. Durgin, would do it a great deal better and more reasonably than I should.

The next section is one which occasioned a good deal of debate at the last meeting, and very likely will at this, and was referred back to the committee for improvement. In its original version it was this : "No milk shall be sold, offered for sale, or distributed in any city or town, unless the cows from which it is derived have within one year been examined by a competent authority, and shown to the satisfaction of the local board of health to be free from disease." Then the suggestion was made by Dr. Smith — and it seemed to meet with considerable favor on the part of the Association — that this should be changed so as to read in the form given in the report. It was amended to run like this. It was suggested, also, by Dr. Theobald Smith that it should run in this way : "No milk shall be sold, offered for sale, or distributed in any city or town, unless the cows from which it is derived have within one year been examined by a competent authority, and shown, to the satisfaction of the Board of Health, to be free from diseases dangerous to public health." I think I have not got that quite right. I think he left out the clause about having been examined within one year. The committee, on going over it, recommends this instead of either of the others, — that it should stand as printed in the report, and go on as follows, the whole reading in this way : "No milk shall be sold, offered for sale, or distributed in any city or town, unless the cows from which it is derived have within one year been examined by a competent authority, and shown, to the satisfaction of the Board of Health of said city or town, to be free from diseases dangerous to public health. But this shall not be construed as forbidding the sale or use of milk from cows not tested with tuberculin." In other words, we set aside the tuberculin matter altogether. Not but that we have our ideas about it, but we did not think it worth while to raise the question of the tuberculin test in connection with this matter of cleanness. We realize there is a strong feeling on the part of farmers against tuberculin. We realize that tuberculin is not such a condition that it is best to put it in here. At least, that is my opinion. Some members of this Association may not agree with us, and think it is best to put it in ; but that is the feeling of the committee. We had no other object in view in this matter than the protection of the milk supply, and cleanness in the methods of handling it. So we said we would not go into the tuberculin test, and therefore added this last clause: " but this shall not be construed as forbidding the sale and use of milk from cows not tested with tuberculin." This section is now presented to you by the committee in that fashion.

A MEMBER (MR. ELLIS).— Mr. President, I agree exactly with the idea set forth by the chairman of the committee, and disagree entirely as to the last paragraph of that section. You do interfere with the tuberculin test by putting that clause in there. Its effect is to say to the boards of health in the local towns that they shall not adopt the tuberculin test in their own town. It seems to me that is just exactly what this Association does not wish to do. It should leave that matter wholly to the boards of health; but, in thus referring to that matter at all, you are introducing the tuberculin question. If you leave that clause out, it gives the board of health an opportunity to adopt the tuberculin test, if it desires to do so.

A MEMBER.— Mr. President, as one member of the committee, it was my understanding, when this clause was originally drafted without the test, that that was intended,— that, while we did not feel like providing explicitly for the tuberculin test, we proposed to allow local option in the matter, and let the local boards of health require it or not, just as they saw fit. I think the question of making this amendment is a mere question of expediency. If it is necessary to say explicitly that this is not to condemn the requirements of the tuberculin test, in order that it may have the support of those who do not like the tuberculin test, and object to it as a matter of expediency, then it is well to adopt it. If that is not necessary, I should prefer to let it stand as it was originally, so the boards may use their own discretion in the matter.

DR. BURR.— Mr. President, I should like to read a bill which has just been presented to the legislature, which gives each town the right to call for tuberculin, and under which each town can prohibit the sale of milk within its limits excepting from cows which have been tested with tuberculin. I think it is pretty safe to say this bill will be defeated. At any rate, I think within forty-eight hours there will be a bill in opposing that; and I have no doubt, if this Association leaves out that last clause, that there will be a bill in a very short time which will prevent boards of health using tuberculin.

THE PRESIDENT.— This section apparently brings in a very wide view of the whole question; and the Association, fortunately, has among its guests to-day a number of gentlemen prominently connected with the production of milk, and we shall be very glad to hear from them. I shall be very glad to hear from the Hon. C. A. Gleason, chairman of the Cattle Owners' Association.

HON. C. A. GLEASON.— Mr. President and gentlemen of this Association, I received the invitation to be here this afternoon with a great deal of pleasure; and it gives me especial pleasure to say a few words, although I do so with some hesitation as I meet this learned and distinguished gathering from all parts of Massachusetts. I have been interested in the milk question all my life. I have taken quite a large part in its production and in its sale here in Boston. I have listened with a great deal of interest to the remarks of Professor Sedgwick, and I have admired the candor and ability with which he has discussed the subject. I should agree most fully with all things that have been said. I believe that I represent an Association who would be heart and hand in delivering Boston pure, clean milk up to the legal standard. I presume a large number of, this Association fully comprehend that, in order to do that, there is considerable effort and some skill required on the part of the producer. I presume most of the members, or many of them, understand that under existing circumstances, with the price of milk netted the farmers, it is a struggle for them to maintain an existence in many of the hill towns, and produce milk for the Boston market. Many of you know that there has been a good deal of agitation, a good deal of dissatisfaction, with the price obtained; but they all thought, "We stand here as an Association, believing that a good article of food is the only article that should be produced and sold here in the Boston market."

Now it seems to me that it is only reasonable that all due care in cleanliness should be used on the part of the producer to send such an article to the Boston market. So far as I know, a large majority of the producers are men who send good goods here. I am just as well aware that there is a certain per cent. that is produced among the producers of New Hampshire, Massachusetts, and Connecticut, that finds its way into Boston, that is not produced and cared for under the best conditions. I have seen nothing in this bill so far, until this discussion arose on the tuberculin question, that I should object to, and nothing that the producers of Massachusetts, either the New England Milk Producers' Union or the Farmers' and Cattle Owners' Association, would object to. I might say that for seven years I have been president of the New England Milk Producers' Union; and my place has this last week been taken by an able representative of the producers from Concord, Mr. Patch, who is here, and, I presume, would be glad to say a few words on the subject. That is an association that represents nearly all of the producers that send their milk into the Boston market. The Association that I represent more particularly here to-day is a much smaller Association, confined entirely to Massachusetts, but representing a large number of cattle owners; and we are deeply interested in this milk question, because our profit largely comes from the production of milk. We are a large company of producers, and we are working hand in hand, so far as we can, with the contractors of Boston to make a better quality of milk; and I want to say right here that the quality of milk that the consumers of Boston are receiving has improved very largely within the last ten years. The public demands it, and the conditions must be improved. The contractors insist upon it, and they are a greater power in carrying it out than any board of health can be. The cutting off of a dairy by the contractors will induce improved sanitary conditions better than any rules that can be passed here to-day. I think the contractors are the greatest power for the improved quality of milk that we can have; and I am glad to say, as they will say to you to-day,—they will bear me out in this statement, I am sure,—that the milk which was furnished in Boston ten years ago would not be received, much of it, to-day. I think that this, as has been suggested by the chairman of the committee, can be largely done by education. I am glad that these rules that have been presented are mild, because I feel that, if there was anything that seemed to be arbitrary, there would be so much opposition shown and manifested that it would be unpleasant, if not difficult, to enforce them.

But I would be glad to say one word here on the question of

tuberculin. I suppose that there is a wide difference of opinion upon that; but I think it would be very unwise, from my view of it, representing the large number of farmers that we do here to-day in the Association, to leave it an open question at least whether the Board of Health of Boston and other cities were to insist upon the tuberculin test. There is a very strong feeling, and it is getting stronger every day, that it should not be insisted upon; that the cattle that are producing milk for the Boston market should not all be tested with tuberculin. I can safely say, and I feel sure, as has been intimated here, that, if it was felt that this meeting to-day was going to insist upon it, this question would be carried from this room at once to the State House; and I think that there would be an increased interest over the question compared with what there was three years ago, and I should hope that these rules might be adopted by this Association in the form that they have been presented rather than the tuberculin test should be left in dispute.

Thanking you, gentlemen, for this opportunity, I am very glad to have met you here this afternoon.

The President.— The Association would be very glad indeed to have Mr. Patch address us upon this subject.

Mr. Patch.— Mr. President and gentlemen, I do not think I can add very much to what the Hon. C. A. Gleason has already said; but I believe that the milk producers of New England are hand in hand to produce a good article of milk to be delivered in the city of Boston, without going to any unreasonable expense in so doing. I believe, if they could feel that they would be compensated for producing a better article, they would be ready and willing to do it, a large majority of them; but I do not think that they would be willing to be compelled to have all their cattle tested with tuberculin, and I for one would hope that this resolution might be adopted as it has been read instead of leaving it open for discussion.

The President.— The honorable ex-president of the Cattle Owners' Association has called attention to the contractors. I am sure we have no better or more acceptable specimen of a contractor than Mr. Whiting, and I hope he has something to say on the subject.

Mr. Whiting.— Mr. President and gentlemen, I feel very much complimented in being invited here to-day. The subject under consideration is one in which I have been interested throughout my business life; and, as I was saying to Professor Sedgwick, many of the suggestions and recommendations made by your honorable board are very encouraging, as they are along the lines that we have always contended were of great importance to the milk business in general. For more than thirty years we have urged upon our farmers the importance of being more cleanly and more systematic in the care of their milk. We have urged that it could be done without any more trouble or expense, and, in short, that uncleanliness is only a bad habit.

I do not mean to insinuate that the farmers (many of them at least) are not willing to do what is right, when made to see it; but they are very much inclined to think that any invasion upon their old traditional customs is unnecessary and only an additional burden imposed upon them by their wicked contractors. In fact, as some of you know, they feel that we are responsible for about all of their woes; while we, on the other hand, try to show them that they are indebted to us for most of their blessings. Be that as it may, there is great opportunity for improvement without injuring or causing unreasonable expense to any one. There are so many good suggestions in your last report that I hardly know where to begin the discussion of them.

As Professor Sedgwick has said, there can be no hardship in cleaning up the cow stables; and the best farmers will not object to it, and those who do object should be compelled to do it.

I think the quality of the milk brought to Boston market is much better than it was ten or fifteen years ago; and, while we have many complaints from farmers that the standard is too high, yet I believe we are gradually working up to it, and every year it is being accomplished with less friction. Dr. Harrington, as you know, is doing good work in his department. We think he is pretty rigid sometimes, — possibly, a little unreasonable; but from personal experience we feel confident that he shows no partiality. I am a firm believer in the idea that whatever is really desirable for the promotion of any good cause or object can be accomplished if approached in a business-like and reasonable way.

The farmers feel that they are not receiving money enough for their milk, and I am inclined to agree with them.

And I will go a step farther, and say that I don't know of any one in the business who is getting enough or what he really ought. Now one way that the farmer is going to get more for his milk is by your assistance in getting better prices for it here, in convincing the consumers that, if they want a really good article of milk, they must be willing to pay for it. You cannot get something for nothing, which seems to be the desire of too many milk consumers in Boston.

One of the best suggestions that I have seen in your report — one which, I believe, if adopted, would result in the best good to the business generally — is the licensing of milk distributors. If the sanitary condition of milk is of so much importance to the health of a city or town, why should a man be allowed to engage in the delivery of it until he can show to the proper authorities that he has conveniences for doing the business in a decent and sanitary manner? In the first place, a man to engage in the business should be a man; and the absence of this condition would prevent many applicants. He should have facilities for doing his business, such as suitable cans, a respectable-looking team, and all the conveniences for caring for his milk while in his possession. In addition to this, let him pay a good license, — say a hundred dollars, — that will keep out a low class of milk dealers, who go into the business only for what they can make by cheating and defrauding honest dealers.

Men who intend to be square will not object to such a license; and it would materially help Dr. Harrington in paying the expenses of his office, and possibly save some poor innocent from suffering. In order to give a farmer more for his milk and encourage him to raise better milk, all the waste places must be stopped; and we, as contractors, feel that we are partly entitled to all the influence of a healthful public sentiment and reasonable laws.

We want your assistance in enforcing proper sanitary conditions among the farmers. We can work together in accomplishing this much needed improvement, for it is the fountain-head of the whole milk problem. Good milk can never be made from poor milk.

To my mind, the ideal way of carrying on the milk business in Boston — and one which, I think, may come in use, to some extent, before long — would be to have the milk brought to the city in large cans. the cans to be owned by the contractors. I would then filter the milk, — a process which, I am sure, would make it more cleanly, — and by cold-air process cool down to forty degrees, then put it up in cans or bottles, as required by the trade, after which I would replace in cold-air storage instead of the innumerable ice-chests used at present, some of which, I fear, are not any too clean. This plan would necessitate large storing and cooling capacity. But it would have the advantage of making the milk of uniform quality; and the cleansing and thorough cooling would, I am sure, improve the flavor and keeping qualities of the milk. It would also insure a prompt return of the cans to the farmers, as they would never go beyond the milk depot; and, by using this sized can, the number would be so much reduced that I think they could be hastily rinsed, and thus do away with much of the complaint of washing dirty cans. Another advantage would be that it could be made an attractive place for consumers to visit, and see for themselves where and how their milk is cared for. It would be imitating somewhat the plan adopted by Mr. Ellis, which, I am happy to say, is the best I have ever seen: he seems to accomplish everything in the care of his milk in a perfectly simple and natural way.

I should like to make a little addition to some of your rules which you have recommended. I think it would be of material assistance to the business. I have drawn up the following in connection with Section 1. I only added a few words. The section reads like this : —

"All cans, bottles, or vessels of any sort used in the sale, delivery, or distribution of milk to the consumer, must be plainly marked with the name of the owner of the milk route from which said milk is delivered, and must be cleaned or sterilized by the milk dealer before they are again used for the same purpose."

It seems important to me that each person handling milk should be held responsible for the part that he takes in it. If a man leaves milk at the door of a house, his name should be on the can, so that, if there is anything wrong about it, the trouble can be located. It would also assist in ferreting out complaints of constant thieving, not only of cans that are empty, but of cans that are full ; for, while a man is not obliged to have his own name on the can, if he can use anybody's can, it is a very easy thing for him to go to a door where these cans are set out at three or four o'clock in the morning, and take them.   This expense alone is a very serious one.

I am happy to pledge the support of the contractors in assisting you in any scheme that will promote the general interest of the milk business.

THE PRESIDENT.— The last word will never be spoken upon this subject — here, at any rate — until we hear from perhaps the most competent representative of the other side of the question, to whom this community owes a very great debt, and to whom this Association will listen with the greatest attention.   That is Dr. Harrington, of Boston.

DR. CHARLES HARRINGTON.— Mr. President and gentlemen, the ground has been so well and thoroughly covered that I feel that there is very little left for me to say.   I do not propose to say anything about the tuberculin test.   There have been enough hearings at the State House to show that it is not advisable to do anything further about that at the present time, but I want to say that I am heartily in sympathy in the movement for obtaining a supply of clean milk.   I think it may fairly be said that our supply of milk is pure enough, so far as adulteration goes; but I think it is very necessary that we should obtain a cleaner supply.   Now much can be done, it seems to me, by the rules and regulations suggested and by legislation, and a great deal can be done by educating the public sentiment a little more in the line of clean milk.   I think the consumers are very much to blame for the fact that our milk supply is not cleaner.   They do not insist on having a cleaner supply.   I believe in having the milk clean when it is milked, and kept clean until it is put on the consumer's table.   Our milk supply is subjected to more or less uncleanliness at its point of origin.   It is subject to more or less while it is in transit.   It is then subjected to a considerable source of contamination while it is in storage, and it is this last source which the public could very easily avoid if it only knew enough to insist upon it.   Our milk supply in Boston gets in here early in the morning and during the forenoon.   If the milk could then be distributed to the consumer, it would be in a great deal better condition than when it is distributed. The milk is carried from the railroad, where it is received, to the various stables of the delivering milkmen. Now I have taken the trouble to go around and examine all the stables in Boston where milk is kept and handled prior to its delivery to the customer; and, as a rule, the conditions in Boston are very good. I also examined the stables in the outlying towns, the stables of milkmen delivering milk within the city; and with some exceptions their condition was very good, or at least fair, and some of them were in a disgraceful condition of filth. Now there is no necessity of having this milk stored in any of these places, whether they are clean or filthy. The milk may just as well be delivered when it gets in Boston, but the public won't have it. If a milkman should address a circular letter to his customers, stating that on and after that date he was going to deliver milk at eleven o'clock in the morning, he would lose all his customers, because they would say: "We don't want it delivered so late as that. We want milk delivered early. We want it fresh." And so the milkman is obliged to send this milk, which they want fresh, which comes in by the railroad at eleven o'clock, and store it in his stable in his refrigerator, which, as Mr. Whiting has said, is never strictly clean ; and then the next morning at six o'clock it is delivered right fresh from the cow [laughter], and during this time it has had every opportunity to acquire new filth, and also to form a considerable multiplication of the bacteria that are already in the milk when it is sent down.

Mr. Gleason has touched on a point where I think I can cordially indorse him ; that is, on the power that the contractor has in assisting in this movement for pure and clean milk. Whether there are or are not regulations, the contractor has the right, and would undoubtedly exercise it, of shutting off the milk supply from any dairy where the cows and surroundings are not kept in a good sanitary condition ; and it would be only necessary, it seems to me, in some cases, if the contractor should insist upon that, that they would not receive milk unless it was clean.

As to whether the contractors and farmers get all they ought to for their milk, I do not know. It has always seemed to me that the contractors did fairly well.　They seem to be in a reasonable state of prosperity, and it always seemed to me that the farmers did not get quite all they ought to have.　I do not want to precipitate a discussion on that point; but I think, if the farmers knew the power that they might have if they should go out on a strike, they would get more money for it.

A MEMBER.— Do you keep cows, doctor?

DR. HARRINGTON.— Two.

THE PRESIDENT.— With regard to the last suggestions of Dr. Harrington as to cleanliness of the milk supply, Mr. Walker has, as I understand it, an improved milk-pail which we would be glad to hear about.　I do not know but Mr. Walker would be glad to say something about it in a word or two.

MR. F. H. WALKER.— Mr. President and gentlemen, I am pleased to be accorded the privilege of attending this meeting as a guest,

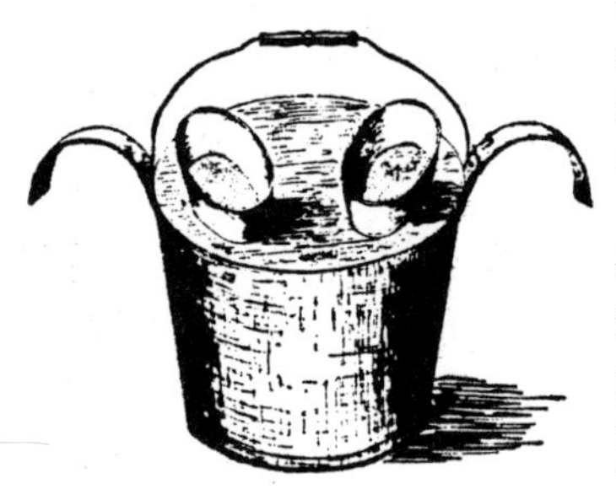

and to have the additional privilege of stating a few facts regarding the Climax Milk Pail, and results obtained from its use.

This device is a pail equipped with cover, funnels, and strainers in such a way that the milk, in its passage from the cow into the pail must go through these strainers. The pail is also supplied with hooks, which support it on the milker's knees.

I agree with Mr. Whiting and Dr. Harrington that more care should be exercised at the very beginning.　In fact, I believe, like the young lady school-teacher who took a refractory urchin over her knee, in going to the bottom of things.

I am positive, after careful investigation and trial, that the use of the Climax Milk Pail will accomplish certain results along the lines of convenience and cleanliness.　It will not change milk drawn from a diseased cow into a first-class, pure article.　It has nothing to do with the after condition of milk, caused by pouring or repouring into dirty cans or those requiring sterilization.　It will not prevent the spread of contagious diseases, such as typhoid and scarlet fever, when the milker is afflicted with one of these diseases. It is not offered as a solution of the milk problem in its entirety, nor as a cure-all. It does, however, accomplish more than the practice of grooming the cows, and in much less time. Careful grooming is a splendid thing, but very few people are disposed to take upon themselves this extra work. Yet, with the utmost precaution taken, hairs and other articles will drop into the open pail. The Climax Milk Pail cover keeps out of the milk, during the process of milking, dirt, hairs, and pieces of cow manure, which latter sometimes give a peculiar flavor to the milk.

In accomplishing what it does, the pail supplies a long-felt want; and it is perfectly amazing to me, gentlemen, that a device of this kind has not before been put on the market. If puddings, pies, and other foods, prepared in our homes, were exposed to contact with foreign matter, as is milk in the open pail, many of us, I fear, would be loath to partake of them. The continued use of the open pail is of course largely a matter of habit. To quote from Lord Lytton, with but little change, "Use and habit are powers far greater than the dictates of common sense in this world of ours."

At the Boston Food Fair last October, where the pail was first shown and where several hundred were sold, it attracted not only the attention of the every-day farmer, but was also personally shown to many in all walks of life, business and professional. Ninety-nine out of every hundred, I am certain, were favorably impressed with the device. Knowing, therefore, that public opinion — that average opinion of the people in which President Lincoln reposed the utmost confidence — indorses it, I hope to see it generally adopted. The pail is retailed at a reasonable figure, and the price is not a fancy combination one.

Upon investigation I find that devices of the general nature of the Climax Milk Pail are not unknown to the Patent Office; but on account of complex and complicated parts, and various silly notions embodied in their construction, these articles could not be produced at a reasonable price, and were, therefore, not put on the market. Some of the devices were as complicated as a Corliss engine, and decidedly impractical.

I am heartily in favor of rigid inspections, and of keeping clean and sweet all places of storage and all cans used for the reception of milk, also of Pasteurization of milk, if this is found beneficial and necessary. I believe that those practical, educated, and thinking men who are contributing so much time, study, and discussion to the better care and inspection of milk are doing a grand work. But inspection, however rigid it may be, will not accomplish everything. It ought to, and I hope will in the future, compel a more proper care of milk, stable, and surroundings. It is a fact, however, that inspection and experience born of inspection have done but little to prevent foreign substances from entering milk in the open pail. The idea has been to strain them out afterward. An ounce of prevention is certainly worth more than a pound of cure.

THE PRESIDENT.— Is there any gentleman here who wishes to say anything further about Section 4? We shall be very glad to hear from anybody, whether a member of this Association or not.

A MEMBER.— Mr. President, we have a gentleman here from Pittsburg who has been very active in the Farmers' Association, Mr. Harrington; and I should like to hear from him.

THE PRESIDENT.— We shall be glad to hear from Mr. Harrington.

MR. HARRINGTON.— Mr. President, I am a common farmer, a born hayseed. So you must not expect from me any words of wisdom. I have been for some years secretary of the Farmers' and Cattle Owners' Association, and I am certainly glad to see this movement in the line of cleanliness in milk production. I would say that our Association, as has been said by our president, Mr. Gleason,— that, in all reasonable matters bearing upon the production of clean, wholesome milk, the Cattle Owners' Association of Massachusetts is with the boards of health. There are some things which enter into this matter from a producer's standpoint which perhaps, as boards of health, we are apt to forget. In the first place, it must be realized that farmers at the present time are producing milk for the Boston market at next to nothing, if anything, above the cost. In fact, I firmly believe that just now milk for the Boston market is being produced by the farmers at less than cost.

The vast majority of the farmers of Massachusetts are holding on, hoping for better times and better prices, and are producing milk now at an actual loss, with a hope that in time they may better their condition. At a Farmers' Institute, only last week, it was demonstrated without a shadow of doubt that the cost of production was above the price received at the railroad station. Now we all wish to produce better milk; and, while we are willing to put forth every effort possible, the boards of health, I hope, realize — I believe they realize — that the condition imposed upon the farmers must imply very little added cost at the present time. Perhaps more can be done in the line of education than in the line of legislation. I believe the farmers are willing to come up to a better standard just as fast as they can or as fast as they realize the absolute necessity of it; but it must also be remembered that the vast majority of people,— as has been said, I think, by Dr. Harrington, of Boston,— a vast majority of people look at the cost rather than the quality. I sell my milk in the Pittsburg market, and I know that nine-tenths of the people in the city will look at a cent a quart before they will at the better quality of the milk.

Mr. Whiting.— The question under discussion, I believe, is whether this Association shall leave the tuberculin test optional with boards of health or whether they shall plainly state their position. Now the Farmers' and Cattle Owners' Association was organized primarily to oppose compulsory tuberculin. They oppose it. Compulsory tuberculin is a thing of the past. I am sure it will never again be required by the State of Massachusetts. I believe, if the Association here will pass the resolution that has been offered by Professor Sedgwick, just as it has been offered by him, that the Farmers' and Cattle Owners' Association, if there is legislation needed,— and there doubtless is,— is willing to go before the legislature and help in passing just such a bill. Last year there was passed also a bill which gave to the boards of health just the power which is in this resolution, minus the tuberculin provision. Our society added a proviso practically like the suggestion presented by Professor Sedgwick. That suggestion was not accepted by those who promoted the bill, and we defeated the bill. So, I think, it is safe to say that we defeated the bill. I know that to be a fact. Our Association went before the Committee on Agriculture. We looked up the members of the legislature, and a bill was reported. The promoters were given leave to withdraw. Now, if this Association will declare itself one way or another on this matter, the Farmers' and Cattle Owners' Association are ready to work with the boards of health in any way which will promote health, which will promote wholesome food, and which will promote clean milk. We stand unutterably committed on the question of tuberculin.

THE PRESIDENT.— Is there anything further to be said on this subject?

DR. SMITH.— I think that this Association should not leave the subject here without taking some position upon the subject of tuberculin. I do not mean to say that tuberculin should be compulsory throughout the State; but I think, as a scientific organization, we at least should not turn our backs completely upon a diagnostic agent which is just now beginning to increase in its use in the medical profession, on account of the delicacy of this diagnostic subject in proving tuberculosis. It seems to me that putting in a clause that tuberculin should not be used would imply that the Local Boards of Health of Massachusetts are doubting the value of tuberculin; and I think this is a serious mistake. At the present time I believe that there are men in the State who have their cattle tested, and who try from time to time to rid themselves of tuberculous cattle. However, that is done at present at the expense of the State; and, therefore, it is difficult to see how there is any difference between those men and the men who do not have their cattle tested. It seems to me that, if there are men in this State who will take upon themselves the personal expense of having their cattle tested, and having the affected cattle weeded out, this Association ought to give those men its heartiest support, and recommend its policy voluntarily. I mean that this body, as a scientific organization, should not consider tuberculin as a useless agent, when it is making progress throughout the world. To-day in Germany, for instance, it is used more than it was two or three years ago, and it will continue to be used; but I am not at all so sure that ten years from now it will not be used in Massachusetts. I am not at all sure that it will not be asked for by prominent men who are handling cattle. I think that time is coming; but I think it must come, of course, through co-operation of those who have charge of those animals.

DR. MILLER.— Mr. President, it seems to me that we can do no better than to adopt that article as just read by the chairman of the committee. It is impossible for every one here to-day to study it exactly, and I therefore move that the article be adopted as read by the chairman of the committee.

THE PRESIDENT.— Mr. Ellis has previously moved, if I understand him, that this article be amended. What is your pleasure with regard to the amendment proposed by Mr. Ellis?

PROFESSOR SEDGWICK.— Mr. President, if I may say one word in further explanation, I should like to say that I do not believe that this clause commits the Association pro or con. It simply sets this thing aside. It says certain things as printed already, and adds, "this shall not be construed as forbidding the sale or use of milk from cows not tested with tuberculin." It does not say that it is not a good thing to test cows with tuberculin. It simply says, if a man brings milk to the city, and is asked, "Have your cows been tested?" that the milk shall not be excluded because the cows have not been tested. It does not say that the Association does not believe in tuberculin or anything of that sort, and it has been very carefully arranged with that in view. I grant, as Mr. Ellis holds, that it seems, or might seem to any one reading it, to minimize somewhat the value of tuberculin. Personally, I am quite willing to take that stand. I do not feel that tuberculin is to-day in such a state that this body as a scientific Association, as Dr. Smith has said, needs to take any positive stand one way or the other on that matter; and I cannot see how this phrase, that "this shall not be construed as forbidding the sale or use of milk from cows not tested," throws any more than a very slight doubt on tuberculin. I think that it does throw such a very slight doubt; and I think that doubt is justified by the present state of the tuberculin question, so that I do not think that this organization will be facing backward if it takes this stand. It simply sets the thing aside : it says, for our present purpose, we shall not exclude milk from untested cows. I dare say, if this Association should take a vote, it would say, on the whole, it thought it well to test cows; but, in the present state of the question, it sets the whole thing aside, and throws only that very slight shadow which I have spoken of upon the use of tuberculin. I hope the resolution will be carried as it stands, because I believe greater good will be done by adopting it than by defeating it. As I understand the matter, it is not that these gentlemen, representing the Milk Producers' Union, Cattle Owners' Association, and so on, make any threats. It is not that. Nor are we afraid of any threats, if made; but simply forgetting the greater good we are willing to set aside, for the time being, and put out of consideration, the question of tuberculin-tested cows as milk producers.

MR. ELLIS.— Mr. President, it seems to me that is just exactly what is done. I am still obtuse enough not to see that question as the chairman of the committee does. It seems to me that without it, if you leave the whole matter in the hands of the local boards, you leave it exactly where a stand can be made without this Association expressing its opinion. If the Cattle Owners' Association care to, they can go before the legislature, and have some special act with reference to the tuberculin test. That has nothing to do with this. That does not affect this question at all, but this is putting this Association on record against the tuberculin test or it has no effect.

THE PRESIDENT.— Is anything more to be said upon Mr. Ellis's amendment? If not, all those in favor of the amendment proposed by Mr. Ellis will signify it by saying ay. [The vote was taken.] The chair believes it to be a vote: it is a vote. The section that "this shall not be construed as forbidding the sale or use of milk from cows not tested with tuberculin" is stricken out.

PROFESSOR SEDGWICK.—Mr. President, I voted under a misapprehension. It is possible others may have done the same. Dr. Durgin was talking to me, and by mistake I voted for Mr. Ellis's amendment.

THE PRESIDENT.— I am afraid one vote would hardly make any difference. The vote was not doubted.

A MEMBER.— I beg to doubt the vote.

DR. MILLER.—Mr. President, I think if you would read it, we could all understand it better.

THE PRESIDENT.— The question is upon Mr. Ellis's motion to strike out the words, "but this shall not be construed as forbidding the sale or use of milk from cows not tested with tuberculin." The question is now whether those words shall be struck out. All those in favor will please rise and stand until they are counted. [The vote was taken.] It is not a vote. The question now is upon the adoption of the article as reported by the committee. All those in favor of adopting the article as reported by the committee will say ay. [The vote was taken.] It seems to be carried by a unanimous vote. The next article with regard to which there is any amendment is Section 2; and, as I understand it, that was adopted at the last meeting, but it is now proposed by the committee to add to it a few words, which, I understand, are simply in the way of definition.

PROFESSOR SEDGWICK.— Section 2. This was adopted, as the President says; but it is proposed by the committee, voluntarily proposed on their part, to give a loop-hole for the men who cannot possibly afford a really good room, and to insert after the word "cleansing" "or in some room approved by the said Board of Health."

THE PRESIDENT.— Is it your pleasure to amend this article by adding these words, which do not change the sense of it? If you are so minded, will you please signify by saying ay? [The vote was taken.] It is adopted.

The next section amended or, in fact, not accepted at the last meeting of this Association is Section 4, which originally read, "All milk directly after it is drawn from the cow shall be at once taken to, and be at once filtered, cooled, and stored in, a room such as is described in Article II., Sections 1 and 2." The committee now propose that it shall read, "All milk directly after it is drawn from the cow shall be at once taken to, filtered, cooled, and stored in, some room other than the stable, and not containing any urinal or privy, nor used for sleeping or other domestic purposes."

DR. DAVENPORT.— Mr. President, if the chair will allow me a question, I did not quite hear back here just what that means. I would like to know whether it means that cans can be in the barn and milk poured into the cans after it is drawn from the cow and then removed, or that the milk-pail filled up full must be taken immediately to the barn or some adjacent room. Now that would make quite a difference in the expense and work of the farmer, as I understand by that clause. If it means every pail full of milk shall be carried from the stable before it is deposited in the cans, why, it means quite a heavy burden upon the farmer. If it means that it may be placed in the cans and the cans removed, why, that is quite a different thing. I should like an interpretation on that.

THE PRESIDENT.— I will ask the chairman of the committee to inform him.

PROFESSOR SEDGWICK.— This was the suggestion of only one member of the committee. As I understand it, the idea was that it was a bad thing to have cans standing near the tails of the cows, perhaps with open mouth, and it would contribute to general cleanliness if the man, after filling the pails, were to go into the next room and empty the milk there. Of course, if that involves very serious hardship, the committee might be willing to reconsider the matter; but it does not seem the proper thing to have the can behind cows, as it often is in the stable, and it does make more space needed. But, if the room were provided, as it should be, and then separated a few feet from the barn or from the stable, I do not know that it would be very serious, hardly more than to walk across from the yard to the place where the cans were set.

DR. DAVENPORT.— Mr. President, I should like further to know from you, not to invite trouble here, how that is to be done in a room. Would it not be well that it be done out of doors, to add to the word "room" "space"?

PROFESSOR SEDGWICK.— There is a qualifying clause,—" or some place approved by the Board of Health." If a man can show it is better to do it out of doors, I do not think there would be any trouble on that.

THE PRESIDENT.— It is moved and seconded that the section as originally read stand as the opinion of this Association. What is your pleasure thereon? All those in favor will signify by saying ay. [The vote was taken, and the motion was declared carried.] The only other section referred to the committee, on which I understand that no action has been thus far taken, is Section 2 of Article V.

Professor Sedgwick.— Mr. Chairman, in regard to Article IV., I think the suggestion of Mr. Whiting is very good. His suggestion is this : " All cans, bottles, or vessels of any sort used in the sale, delivery, or distribution of milk to the consumer, must be plainly marked with the name of the owner of the milk route from which said milk is delivered, and must be cleaned and sterilized by the milk dealer before they are again used for the same purpose." In other words, he introduces this to facilitate keeping cans clean. One of the greatest abuses is dirty cans, which arises under this system of trading cans and stealing cans, and all that sort of thing. It seems to me that would be a very good suggestion,— to change Article IV. He also suggests on this type-written sheet, " It shall be deemed a sufficient reason for forfeiture of license for any milk dealer to fill or use in any way a milk vessel for any other purpose than milk." I am sure it would be a good thing if it was understood to be a sufficient reason for the forfeiture of a license if the vessels were used for any other purpose than for milk. I think these are very valuable suggestions from Mr. Whiting, and I move that both of them be incorporated in Article IV.

The President.— Is it your pleasure that Article IV. be amended by introducing the words and sentences read to you by Professor Sedgwick ?

A Member.— Mr. President, I would like to amend that by changing one word,— " must be cleaned *or* sterilized."

Professor Sedgwick.— Well, Mr. President, in this case it is the milk dealer who is concerned; and he ought always to have a place where he can do the work properly. I do not think there would be a great deal of trouble arising in the city between the contractor and consumer ; and it would not be felt to be a hardship there to keep the word " and," while in the case of the farmer who had not reasonable apparatus it might be a real hardship. I do not care to insist on it, however, because I suppose practically he never will really get it thoroughly sterilized ; but I do not think it is too high an ideal for the man who sets up milk in his stable, near the tails of his horses, to try to rise to. I think that is where a great deal of trouble comes in, as Dr. Harrington has intimated also. These fellows who get milk from the contractor take it home, work it over, and set it by in

ways that are not at all desirable. Their cans might well be sterilized. I do not think it will be any great hardship for them to do it.
I hope the time will come when that work will be done, and that
milk will be kept where the horses' tails are not within ten or twelve
feet of the setting-up process.

A MEMBER.— What is meant by sterilizing in this case?

PROFESSOR SEDGWICK.— It means the destruction of all germs.

A MEMBER.— That is, what is the method?

PROFESSOR SEDGWICK.— Whatever means may be necessary to
accomplish it.

A MEMBER.— I think still it would be a hardship for the small
country dealer in a small country town.

PROFESSOR SEDGWICK.— That is a point I am ready to admit. If
that is true, I withdraw my objection. I think this Association is
too apt to think of the Boston system. I grant the value of that
suggestion, and am quite ready to make it " or " in the case of
smaller towns.

DR. BURR.— I think the most of these bottles may have come
from some house where there has been diphtheria or scarlet fever.
I think that was why it was insisted on that the dealer should sterilize his cans which had gone to the consumer.

THE PRESIDENT.— Will you amend this section as suggested by
Professor Sedgwick?

PROFESSOR SEDGWICK.— In regard to Dr. Burr's remark, he refers
to what is really a serious matter, especially in the bottle trade,
which has come in more and more. Bottles are left now in the
Boston system, bottles are left at the houses of the consumer; and
they may have been taken right into the room where people are
sick with diphtheria or scarlet fever, just because they are attractive
and instead of some other dish. They are then delivered to the
milkman the next morning; and, as Dr. Burr has said, the committee felt that they ought to be sterilized largely on that account.
That is undoubtedly a coming way for the spread of disease; but, if
it is true, as the gentleman says, that it would be too great a hardship in the smaller towns to have the bottles sterilized, I do not care
to insist upon it, but it seems to me that in time it ought to be done.

THE PRESIDENT.— The question, then, is upon the amendment

substituting the word "or" for "and." Is it your pleasure that the substitution be made? If so, you will signify by saying ay. [The vote was taken, and the amendment was declared adopted.] That finishes the general consideration of the portions of the articles and sections that were referred to your committee. Is it your pleasure now to adopt them as a whole, and instruct some proper committee to procure the necessary legislation to see that they go into effect?

PROFESSOR SEDGWICK.— Mr. President, I move that the Committee on Legislation be instructed to secure such modification of the existing law as shall be necessary to carry these recommendations and suggestions into effect.

The motion was seconded by Dr. Miller. The vote was then taken, and the motion was declared carried.

RULES SUGGESTED BY A COMMITTEE OF, AND RECOMMENDED BY, THE MASSA-CHUSETTS ASSOCIATION OF BOARDS OF HEALTH FOR ADOPTION BY THE BOARDS OF HEALTH OF THE STATE FOR THE PROTECTION OF MILK SUPPLIES FROM POLLUTION.

ARTICLE I.

SECTION 1. All persons engaged in the production of milk for sale, or in the sale, delivery, or distribution of milk, in the city or town of ——, shall annually, on or before May 1, make written application, on forms prescribed by the Board of Health of said city or town, for a permit or license.

SECT. 2. No person shall engage in the business of producing milk for sale, or in the sale or distribution of milk, in the city or town of —— after ————— without a permit or license to do so signed by said Board of Health, and under such conditions as said Board of Health may impose, revokable at the pleasure of said board.

SECT. 3. The conditions under which every cow is kept, whose milk is brought into any city or town, or kept, delivered, distributed, sold, or offered for sale, in such city or town, shall be made known to the local board of health of said city or town in such detail as the board may require, and shall be approved thereby; and no milk except that derived from such cows shall be so brought, kept, delivered, distributed, sold, or offered for sale.

SECT. 4. No milk shall be sold, offered for sale, or distributed in any city or town, unless the cows from which it is derived have within one year been examined by a competent authority, and shown, to the satisfaction of the Board of Health of said city or town, to be free from diseases dangerous to public health;

but this shall not be construed as forbidding the sale or use of milk from cows not treated with tuberculin.

SECT. 5. All persons having a permit or license to sell, deliver, or distribute, milk in any city or town, shall keep a copy of the same constantly posted in a conspicuous place on premises and vehicles from which milk is sold or distributed or in which milk is kept or delivered.

ARTICLE II.

SECTION 1. No milk shall be kept for sale or distribution, or handled, transferred from can to can, or stored, in any stable or similar place or in any room used in whole or in part for domestic or sleeping purposes.

SECT. 2. Milk shall be stored or regularly mixed, cooled, or poured from can to can only in a room not directly connected with a stable or stables, provided with a tight floor, and kept constantly neat and clean, the walls of the room being of such a nature as to allow easy and thorough cleansing; or in some room approved by the Board of Health of the city or town in which the milk is to be sold or distributed. The room aforesaid shall contain proper appliances for washing and sterilizing all utensils actually employed in the storage, sale, and distribution of milk in said building, and all such apparatus and utensils shall be washed with boiling water or sterilized by steam regularly after having been so used.

SECT. 3. No urinal, water-closet, or privy, shall be in the aforesaid room or any room directly connected therewith.

SECT. 4. All milk directly after it is drawn from the cow shall be at once taken to, and be at once filtered, cooled, and stored in, some such room as is described in Article II., Sections 1 and 2.

ARTICLE III.

SECTION 1. Milk kept for sale in any store, shop, market, bakery, or other establishment, shall be always kept in a covered cooler, box, or refrigerator, properly drained and cared for; and while therein shall be kept tightly corked or closed, and only in such location and under such conditions as shall be approved by the local board of health. .

ARTICLE IV.

SECTION 1. All cans, bottles, or vessels of any sort used in the sale, delivery, or distribution of milk to the consumer, must be plainly marked with the name of the owner of the milk route from which said milk is delivered, and must be cleaned or sterilized by the milk dealer before they are again used for the same purpose; and it shall be deemed a sufficient reason for forfeiture of license for any milk dealer to fill or use in any way a milk vessel for any other substance than milk.

ARTICLE V.

SECTION 1. Every person engaged in the production, storage, transportation, sale, delivery, or distribution of milk, shall immediately, on the occurrence of any case or cases of infectious disease, such as typhoid, scarlet fever, or diphtheria, either in himself or in his family, or amongst his employees or within the building or premises where milk is stored, produced, sold, or distributed, take care that the local board of health is notified of such case or cases, and at the same time suspend the sale or distribution of milk until authorized to resume the same by the local board of health.

SECT. 2. It shall be unlawful for any person suffering from a contagious or infectious disease, such as typhoid fever, scarlet fever, or diphtheria, to handle, transport, deliver, mix, taste, work over, or distribute milk, or to be in or about places where milk is stored, sold, or distributed, or to serve as a milker or milkman. No vessels which have been handled by persons suffering from such diseases shall be used to hold or convey milk.

THE PRESIDENT.— The next business upon the programme is " Remarks on the Use of Formaldehyde by Dr. Parks of New York, Dr. Brough of Boston, and others." Dr. Parks, of New York, is not here; and I understand some one will read his paper.

Mr. Charles E. Davis, clerk of the Boston Board of Health, then read Dr. Parks's paper, as follows : —

[*THE PREPARATION AND FREE DISTRIBUTION*
TO BOARDS OF HEALTH OF ANTITOXINE

REPORTING OF CHICKEN-POX

and

PROVISION FOR THE CARE AND ISOLATION
IN HOSPITALS OF PATIENTS ILL WITH
MEASLES]

THE PRESIDENT.—In accordance with the announcement upon your programme various questions have been suggested for discussion at this meeting, and I will read them in the order in which they have been received : —

1. What is to be the policy of the State Board of Health with regard to the preparation and free distribution to boards of health throughout the State of antitoxine, in view of the recent action of the legislature ?

2. How far away from a diphtheria and scarlet fever hospital is it suitable for a small-pox hospital to be located ?

3. Should boards of health require the reporting of cases of chicken-pox?

4. Should boards of health make provision for the care and isolation in hospitals, when requested, of patients ill with measles?

Those are the only four questions which have been submitted for discussion at this meeting. In what order will you discuss these questions, gentlemen?

DR. DURGIN.— I move, Mr. Chairman, that the first question raised, being of most vital importance, be discussed first; and I hope that we may have that question answered by the President of the Association.

MR. COFFEY.— I second the motion.

DR. DURGIN.— It is moved and seconded that this question be answered by Dr. Walcott. [The motion was adopted.] It is so voted, and the President has the floor. [Applause.]

THE PRESIDENT.— The question is, "What is to be the policy of the State Board of Health with regard to the preparation and free distribution to boards of health of antitoxine, in view of the recent action of the legislature?" The statement must be partly historical; and I shall endeavor to make it, of course, as little personal as possible.

I may call to the attention of the Association that there has been more or less discussion of this matter in the public press,— a discussion which has been limited entirely to the representatives of the Druggists' Association, so far as I am aware; for I assume that a recent communication by Mr. Canning in the *Transcript* is an official communication. I understand that he makes no question about his association with the Druggists' Association for the promotion of legislation in the interests of the druggists. In that paper there were various statements which do not seem to me correct; but there was one statement which I should like to meet, in the first place, and this is the statement that, after the general question of vaccination had been discussed before the Public Health Committee of the legislature and settled, some interested parties then introduced a bill for the making of vaccine lymph by the State Board of Health. As a matter of fact, those two measures were introduced simultaneously. One measure did not depend upon the success or failure of the other. The measure for the production of vaccine lymph, which I hold in my hand, Senate Document No. 179, was referred to the Committee on Public Health on Feb. 3, 1902, long before the close of the hearing upon the subject introduced by the anti-vaccinationists; and it reads as follows:—

SENATE No. 179.

(To accompany the petition of Samuel H. Durgin that the State Board of Health be authorized to produce antitoxine and vaccine lymph. Public Health.)

AN ACT

Relative to the Production of Antitoxine and Vaccine Lymph, etc.
Be it enacted, etc.
SECTION 1. Section four of chapter seventy-five, of the Revised Laws is amended by inserting after the word "institution," in the eleventh line thereof the words:—and may, for the free use of the people of the Commonwealth, produce and dispose of antitoxine and vaccine lymph.
SECT. 2. This act shall take effect upon its passage.

That proposed legislation was referred to the Committee upon Public Health, which, after a hearing or two and due consideration, reported that legislation was inexpedient.

At a later date, Mr. Adams, of Melrose, the chairman of the Committee on Appropriations, having had his attention called to the fact that a tuberculous cow, which had evidently been recently used for the purpose of producing vaccine lymph, had been found in one of the slaughter-houses of the Commonwealth, and had been found to be so grossly diseased that the inspector ordered it to be thrown at once into the rendering vat, again called the attention of the legislature to the necessity of some action. The matter was referred again to the Committee on Public Health, which at that time and for the first time during the session asked the opinion of the State Board of Health. A hearing was held, at which I personally, as representing the State Board of Health, went before the committee, and stated that this matter of producing vaccine lymph had been settled in almost all the civilized countries of the world in favor of a government supervision of it, for the reason that it was an article absolutely impossible of chemical analysis, that no examination extended beyond the individual specimen that might be submitted for examination, and that under those conditions it appeared to be essential that the whole process should be supervised by some authority from the beginning to the end, that that was practically the only protection which would be given to the public. Upon that statement, and some statements made by parties interested in the manufacture of vaccine lymph, the committee again took the matter under consideration. This was toward the end of the session. Three or four days before the final adjournment of the legislature the Public Health Committee recommended that the subject of producing vaccine be referred to the State Board of Agriculture, and the matter so stands.

Now to go back a few years, in 1894 or 1895, I am not quite certain which, the State Board of Health began an examination of the antitoxine products then for sale in the Boston market. They were found to be of such untrustworthy character that it seemed essential to the Board of Health in the exercise of its principal function, the protection of the health of the people of the Commonwealth, to see what could be done in the matter. We were dealing with an article which at that time had only recently been brought into general use. There were a great many questions with regard to its preparation which had not been answered anywhere. There was a great deal of question among intelligent men as to the value of the product. For every reason, then, it seemed to the Board of Health a sufficient justification for some intelligent investigation into the matter,—an investigation which was rendered very easy for us at that time because Dr. Theobald Smith had lately come to this part of the country to accept an appointment in Harvard College, and his services were available for the State Board of Health. With Dr. Smith's assistance an investigation was made of the whole matter of the production of antitoxine, which for thoroughness has not been surpassed anywhere; and I venture to say that the product which has been elaborated under Dr. Smith's superintendence has a character that is second to none produced anywhere in the world. At any rate, you gentlemen are familiar with what the product has accomplished; and in that direction it is not necessary for me to say anything more about it.

That preparation was begun under the general powers given to the board to protect the health of the people of this Commonwealth. We did not ask the permission of the legislature of Massachusetts to do it. We have never asked the permission of the legislature of Massachusetts to save human life : we have assumed there would be no question upon that subject. From time to time a statement has been made by the Board to the Committee on Appropriation of the manner in which the money appropriated for the use of the Board of Health should be spent. As you all know, at the beginning of the year the various State departments go before the Committee on Appropriations and explain the appropriations which they ask for. Beyond that committee there has never been any discussion in the legislature as to whether antitoxine was to be prepared or not. I would say that the Committee on Appropriations has always accepted without hesitation, as far as I know, the recommendations of the board, and has made the proper appropriation. The amount of money spent has averaged probably some five or six thousand dollars a year. In this last year, when the product of antitoxine and the use of antitoxine was somewhat less than in the preceding year, the board prepared and distributed 58,000 doses. That represents, as you see, a very small expense. The market value of that preparation, assuming the lowest price at which we find that it is sold in the city of Boston, would have been $87,000.

Now I think we probably should all agree that neither this community nor any community has a right to demand that the State should pay for the product which the public can get as easily, as promptly, and as safely at an establishment which makes an occupation of preparing and selling that drug. It should be remembered, however, that the Commonwealth has taken a very different position, with regard to a certain number of contagious diseases, from that which it has occupied with regard to disease in general. It has made it possible in the case of small-pox for anybody to go to the public authority and be vaccinated free of charge : no question has been asked about it ; and yet the vaccine quill is sold in the druggist's shop, and the doctor stands ready for a reasonable compensation to apply it. In diphtheria you are dealing with a product which commands a price beyond the possibilities of purchase by the ordinary laboring

man.   If you assume the presence of a case of diphtheria, in which
you are going to use such doses as have been used by the best practitioners in this Commonwealth, 40,000 to 70,000 units, you have got
entirely beyond the probability of any laboring man's purchasing this
agent of immunity from disease.   He has got to procure it free of
charge from some one, and it is for the benefit of the whole community that he should procure it as soon as possible.   By the lives
so saved the whole of us are benefited and protected.   For that reason the Board of Health has never had any question that it was per-
forming a very simple part of its duty in manufacturing this article
and distributing it as widely as possible through the agencies of the
boards of health throughout this Commonwealth.

When, however, the question was brought up as to the production
of vaccine lymph, I asked Dr. Durgin when he consulted me about
this matter, long before the legislature came together and long before
the question of the anti-vaccinationists had been considered by any
committee in the legislature, to insert in his bill a provision for the
manufacture of antitoxine.   It seemed to me the time had come
when it was well that the Commonwealth should take a position one
way or the other in this matter.   It had ceased to be a question of
experiment.   There is no question now that there are — I am very
certain that Dr. Smith would agree with me — establishments in this
country that can produce antitoxine, and can produce antitoxine of
a sufficiently good quality.   It is also true that antitoxine can be
examined so as to determine, in rather large quantities, whether it is
good antitoxine or bad antitoxine.   Of course, behind all that would
remain the question whether, if you depended entirely upon the sale in
the open market, the poor man would get it as he ought to get it;
but, at any rate, the time certainly had come when antitoxine and
vaccine lymph should be put upon the same footing, and, therefore,
the legislation before mentioned was asked for.   Now the action of
the legislature upon the face of it leaves the question in this position :
They were expressly asked to authorize the manufacture of anti-
toxine; and they, with great deliberation, declined to authorize it.
On the one hand, it is apparent to me that the withholding of that
permission, when it comes to the expenditure of money at the State
House, is generally construed to be a forbidding of the expenditure

of money. On the other hand, some members of the legislature say, "We didn't interfere with the practice, and therefore go on with your practice, even if it does mean the expenditure of money." In order to dispose of that part of the question, I will say that the Board of Health have determined to go on with the manufacture and distribution of antitoxine [applause] until they are restrained by some competent authority from so doing; and I should like to say that this unpaid board with great unanimity voted at their last meeting that they would personally contribute the money necessary to carry on this work if need be. [Applause.]

The production of vaccine lymph is, it seems to me, a far greater question than the production of the antitoxine of diphtheria simply for the reason, as I have already said, that there are absolutely no means of testing more than the individual specimen that is submitted to you; and that test would be a long one. There is no possibility of settling that question in an hour or a day or a week even: you can only settle it when the question ceases to be of any interest to the community. I think we may in that direction turn our attention for a moment to what is done in foreign countries. In Germany, where government is disposed to interfere to a far greater extent than we are supposed to on this side of the Atlantic, antitoxine is in the hands of a great commercial establishment. The government exercises a very rigorous supervision of all the methods of that manufacture, but it still leaves the business in private hands. On the other hand, the production of vaccine lymph is absolutely in the control of the government. They never have allowed that to go out of their control for the reason that every step of the process has got to be watched. In the first place, you have got to get a healthy calf; in the next place, you have got to get a set of clean men to do your work; and in the next place, the last place, you have got to remove it absolutely from the temptations of commerce. There must be no temptation whatever to keep a product that is inert or a product that has been improperly prepared. So long as you cannot correct the steps of that progress by any chemical or microscopical examination, you have got to depend upon authority, and you have got to depend upon authority exercised at every moment. There is no step of the process that can be safely left without constant and accurate supervision.

The expense which the State Board of Health estimated would attend this business was an appropriation of some $20,000 for the erection of a building sufficient, in the first place, to stable the animals; in the next place, to include all the biological laboratories which had got to be built with all the precaution that a biological laboratory for any purpose has got to be built; and, finally, the rooms for the storing and the housing of the people who are concerned in the distribution of this product. The Commonwealth has had the advantage thus far of a location upon the untaxed lands of Harvard College, at the Bussey Institute; and that location is still open to the Commonwealth without compensation, so that there is no sum of money included in this for the purpose of purchasing a lot of land. But it will be seen that the question was not of a place to house a certain number of calves or anything of that sort. It was a laboratory built according to modern methods, and with the expenditure of money, large expenditure of money, necessary for that purpose. It was also proposed, as our antitoxine establishment had outgrown its quarters, that that should be united with the vaccine establishment; that is, that we should give the antitoxine business a proper and convenient housing, which it has not hitherto had, and at the same time provide for the preparation of vaccine lymph. It was also estimated that the running expenses of that establishment would be about $6,000 a year. Now an original investment of $20,000 and an expense for maintenance of $6,000, when one of the products produced by that establishment in the last year had a market value of $87,000, would not seem a disadvantageous investment, even for the Commonwealth of Massachusetts.

That, gentlemen, is where the question stands at present. While the Board of Health is quite willing to take the position which it has taken for the present year with regard to the manufacture of antitoxine, with another legislature, and with a fuller discussion of this whole question, it must be remembered that the uncertainty cannot continue into another year, and that it really rests, I think, with this Association, with the local boards of health of this Commonwealth, as to what shall be done. It seems to me the opinion of this Association means more — it certainly does to me — than that of any other body of men in the Commonwealth; and, whatever the decision of this Association is, I, personally, shall stand by it. [Applause.]

Mr. Coffey.— I move the adoption of the following resolution : —

Resolved, That this Association fully indorses the decision of the State Board of Health to continue the production of antitoxine.

Dr. Durgin.— I second the motion.

The President.— You have heard the motion of Mr. Coffey. Is there anything to be said upon the subject?

Dr. Magee.— Mr. Chairman, I think we have touched on a very important subject this afternoon, one that ought not to be hastily gone over. Antitoxine is certainly important. Every man who is a practitioner of medicine knows what the State Board has done to save the lives of thousands of children. I should like to hear more discussion on the subject before it is passed. I should like to hear some other gentlemen.

Mr. Coffey.— Mr. President, in offering that resolution, I supposed, as the gentleman who has just sat down has said, that every man here who is connected with a board of health is fully aware of how much this antitoxine has done toward the diminution of diphtheria and the saving of life in this community. As I say, I supposed, as he has said, that every man knew that, that it was not necessary that it should be discussed or debated, that we were all aware of it, that it was a question that would pass without any discussion or debate, and that we simply put upon record our approval of the action of the State Board of Health in continuing the production of this antitoxine, that they may know that this Association, representing, as it does, the boards of health in the entire State, is fully in accord with and approves its action in continuing this work. I know in my own city we are indebted to the State Board of Health for antitoxine in practically unlimited quantities. We have a hospital for the care of diphtheria and scarlet fever, which is known as the isolation hospital; and there we take care of two hundred, three hundred, four hundred cases in the year, probably half of which are diphtheria. I know that our record there since the introduction of antitoxine has been marvellous: I think I may use that word with safety. We have reduced the rate of mortality in diphtheria to about 7 per cent., and that a few years ago would have been considered marvellous. When it is considered that we don't force anybody to enter that hospital, that the applications and admissions are all voluntary, no person is forced to send his child there against his will, it will be seen that, as a result, a large proportion of the cases that we get are the very worst type of the disease. In fact, we get a great many cases in which the doctor tells the people, the parents, the friends, that "there is no hope for this child unless you send it to the isolation hospital, and possibly they may be able to pull it through." We get about all of the intubation cases, I think, almost without exception: once in a while one stays at home; but, as a rule, all the intubations go there. And so our rate, as I said before, I think is marvellous, considering that fact, that we do get those very worst cases, and get a very large proportion of them—in fact, nearly all. That is largely due to the unlimited use — that the Board of Health have made possible by their free gift — of antitoxine. We have used there as high as 50,000 and 60,000 units for a patient, with splendid results, too. A great many cases that have hovered between life and death for a week have finally pulled through. As I said before, when I introduced that resolution, I did not suppose that it was necessary to make any argument in support of it. The feeling that I had was that we might strengthen the hands of the State Board of Health, and make them feel that behind them was this organization, representing, as I said before, the entire boards of health of the State. [Applause.]

Dr. A. E. Miller.— Mr. President, it seems to me that as physicians here we are all of one mind. We are all in favor of this resolution. We might do a great deal as a body of medical men to impress the next legislature. It is not long before we are going to vote; and I think we can wake up the masses of the people, so that we can elect a legislature who will favor this next winter, and will give the State Board of Health an appropriation sufficiently large, not only to enable them to manufacture antitoxine, but to manufacture a sufficient amount of vaccine virus. Both of those articles should be furnished by the State and given to every practitioner free of charge. We have a law that compels — at least, that is being tested somewhat now — people to be vaccinated; and these people, if they are compelled to be vaccinated, ought to know that they are to be vaccinated with something that is furnished by the State Board, and is the purest article that can possibly be had. We should all wake up on this point, and see if we can't get a body of men as a legislature next winter that will vote just right. [Applause.]

DR. MAGEE.— Mr. Chairman, that was my object in getting up, to have the matter discussed. I think it is a very important matter to have the representatives to the General Court men whom we know, and to go to them and insist upon those men voting for what we ask. Not only that, but — I see there are very few members here to-day — the medical societies, the district societies, should be interested in this one subject. It is an important one. Every member here who belongs to a district society should bring the matter up. We should go to our representatives, ask them to do as we wish, and show them the reasons why this should be done. That was the reason why I wanted a little discussion on the matter.

DR. HILL.— Mr. Chairman, we are all agreed that antitoxine is the thing. It may not be out of place to say that, being in charge of the laboratory of the Boston Board of Health, Boston physicians often come in and discuss with me whatever subjects may come up; and of course much of such discussion is on diphtheria. It is the universal impression that antitoxine is the thing to use. There cannot be any question in anybody's mind of its value in that direction. I would suggest as an amendment to the resolution, or an addition to it, if such is proper, a clause stating that the resolution shall be forwarded to the proper legislative authorities as the direct expression of the belief of this Association in the matter.

THE PRESIDENT.— The legislature that it ought to be addressed to is not in existence.

DR. HILL.— True, but it would be kept until the next session.

MR. COFFEY.— Mr. President, Dr. Durgin and myself discussed this somewhat while you were talking; and we thought that perhaps it would be wise to have this resolution adopted now, and then, at the January meeting or at the October meeting, probably at the January meeting, just about the time the legislature convened, a resolution might be introduced and passed that would embody not only antitoxine for diphtheria, but also vaccine lymph, and that the legislative committee of this Association might be instructed to go before the Committee on Public Health, or whatever committee would have charge of the matter, and urge the appropriating of a certain amount of money, in order that the State Board might carry out those ideas. But we thought that perhaps just now it would not be amiss to have a resolution indorsing the stand of the Board of Health in determining to keep on with the manufacture of antitoxine, while the question of vaccine lymph we might allow to remain in abeyance until January, when the thing would be ripe for action.

DR. DURGIN.— I want to indorse what has been said by our President in regard to the letter to the *Transcript* by Mr. Canning and the action of the legislature on the production of vaccine lymph. I was greatly surprised on reading the letter of Mr. Canning night before last. I had supposed Mr. Canning to be better posted on the facts than appears from his letter. It is stated in this letter that "a bill for compulsory vaccination was asked for, and that, after the bill making vaccination compulsory had been signed, the views of the Board of Health representatives seemed to undergo a change, and it was pretended that it was necessary, in the interests of the public health, that the State Board of Health should be given the power to manufacture and give away vaccine virus." It would have been easy for Mr. Canning to learn that no compulsory vaccination bill was asked for, and that this law was already on the statute book and had been there for the last forty years. It would also have been easy for Mr. Canning to learn that, instead of one of these petitions following the other, they were both prepared and introduced in the legislature at the same time, so that no " change of mind " on the part of the boards of health mentioned happened or was thought of except by Mr. Canning and possibly some other disinterested druggists.

Mr. Canning states that a proposition for the State's " supplying milk, running milk farms, manufacturing ice, constructing ice factories, the establishment of a great laboratory for the production of pure bread, the production of pure flour, the production of drugs and medicines, quinine, and every other drug or medicine which the people need, would be no whit different from the manufacture and distribution of vaccine lymph." I think it might be fair to say that Mr. Canning knows that the State does not command the use of milk, ice, bread, flour, or quinine, and that she has never considered that the public health required any legislation upon the subject. Mr. Canning ought to know that the State of Massachusetts, and almost the civilized world, has legislated upon the use of vaccine lymph as a public health measure and necessity, and has ordered its use. It ought not to be difficult for Mr. Canning to see a moral obligation on the part of the State to supply pure and active vaccine lymph the moment she issues her command for its use by her people. Would Mr. Canning or the other druggists question the right or obligation of the government's supplying the school-house and teacher, when it commands the education of the people as a safeguard of order and liberty, or do they see a whit's difference between the supplying of these and that of vaccine lymph, when the same government orders the use of vaccine lymph for the preservation of the public health? I think one of the most interesting things, however, in Mr. Canning's letter is the statement that "any opposition that was made by the druggists was made on principle, and not from interested motives." I would only say that this disinterested devotion to the public welfare, attended with so much expense and time on the part of the druggists, is a trifle phenomenal, and, if true, deserves more public recognition than has yet been given to it.

I hope the members of this Association will carefully consider, not only the clear obligation of the State in this matter, but the immense advantage in quieting the fears of our people as to the safety and activity of vaccine lymph by securing its preparation by our State Board of Health.

Dr. H. E. Marion.— Mr. Chairman, do I understand that this Canning who wrote the article in the *Advertiser* is of the firm of Canning & Patch, the druggists?

The President.— I think so.

Dr. H. E. Marion.— I thought that it would be well for every member of the Association to know the animus of that writer.

Dr. Chase.— Mr. President, may I inquire through you how many members of the Public Health Committee of the legislature are druggists? I understand that a number of the members are druggists. I should like to know how many.

Dr. Durgin.— I am told four or five.

Dr. Chase.— How large is that committee?

DR. DURGIN.— It has eleven members.

DR. STEVENS.— If it is in order, I should like to state my personal experience with vaccine. The last few weeks, as you know, we have had something of an epidemic of small-pox. In June, and up to the 15th of July, I procured 110 points, and used them in vaccinating people among my own patients. A very large proportion of these were revaccinations: some 12 were primary vaccinations. In not one instance have I had a successful vaccination from these 110 points,— not one instance, primary or secondary. I have procured since the 16th of July, from the same producer, points, and have vaccinated some of the people I tried before,— some of them I tried three times,— and in about 20 per cent. of them I have succeeded. The virus that I used first was dated good until August 5. The virus that I have been using lately was dated good until August 15. That that was marked good until August 5 absolutely failed. That that was marked good until August 15, an entirely new lot, seems to be succeeding. I don't know whether that is the general experience; but one of my neighbors, who has vaccinated very many more people than I have, told me that his experience had been exactly the same as mine, that he had only had one success with the virus marked good until August 5. It seems to me that it is pretty important, if you are going to vaccinate people, that we should have something that we can use as vaccine virus, and not a lymph that is inert,— and I believe that the vaccine to which I first referred was absolutely inert,— particularly in a town where small-pox is prevailing to a considerable extent.

DR. DAVENPORT.— The question has been asked how many of the Committee on Public Health were druggists. I should like to ask how many were practising physicians, if any.

DR. ABBOTT.— None.

DR. DAVENPORT.— The statement has been made that Mr. Henry Canning was of the firm of Canning & Patch. There was formerly such a firm, but it no longer exists. Mr. Canning is now in business by himself.

DR. H. E. MARION.— Drug business?

DR. DAVENPORT.— Yes. He is the Mr. Henry Canning of the former firm of Canning & Patch, who continues the drug business, corner of Green and Chambers Streets. He is the same person who reports to the Secretary of the Commonwealth, under the so-called Lobby Act, that he has paid to Benjamin N. Johnson, Esq., $1,685.25 for services and expenses in opposing the bill authorizing the State Board of Health to manufacture antitoxine and vaccine virus under Senate Bill 179.

DR. DURGIN.— I was in New York a few days ago, and the health officer there told me that 144 immigrants had recently been vaccinated, with success in only 6. He revaccinated with virus which was produced by the New York Board of Health, and there was over 50 per cent. of success on these same individuals.

MR. COFFEY.— I want to add to that, Mr. Chairman, the fact that at Worcester we do a wholesale vaccinating business every year. We vaccinate from 2,500 to 3,000 children every year before they enter the public schools. We begin vaccinating the last of August, and keep it up every Monday morning during the year until the school year ends. We vaccinate, as I say, from 2,500 to 3,000 children every year; and the number is constantly increasing. We have tried a number of various vaccine lymphs on the market; and something over a year ago we began to use the vaccine lymph produced by the New York City Board of Health, with the best results that we have ever had from any vaccine that we have tried. Last summer, when we had a little outbreak of small-pox at the city hospital in Worcester, we vaccinated some 8,000 or 10,000 people with that lymph. Dr. Clark, who does the vaccinating and has done it for seven or eight years, says that the percentage of successful vaccination is very much greater than with any other lymph that he had previously used; and we have never had any bad arms or bad effects whatever from it. We have had, as I say, splendid results. They sell it to us cheaper than we bought some of the lymph that was put on the market by commercial firms. We paid formerly $7\frac{1}{2}$ cents a point, and they furnish it to us for $6\frac{1}{2}$ cents a point.

A MEMBER.— Do you buy it direct from the board?

MR. COFFEY.— Buy it direct from the board. It is sent direct, and we get it usually twenty-four hours or surely forty-eight hours afterward. We have used in a year something like 12,000 or 15,000 tubes, and the physicians of Worcester now are using that largely.

We find that that gives better results. The physicians come to me very often and ask for that, when they have one or two private patients that they are anxious to have take.

A MEMBER.— Is that on the market?

MR. COFFEY.— Well, they sell it from the New York City Board of Health. They sell it to anybody who wants it. They make this, of course, for their own use in the city of New York; but they make more than they use, and they are ready to dispose of it. In an account in one of the magazines I happened to run on to it something over a year ago. I saw a description of the methods that they used in producing the lymph, and they struck me as being very painstaking. I suggested to Dr. Clark that we try it, as we were having trouble with some of the lymph that we were using at the time, having people who had been vaccinated come back for revaccination. He said, "All right," and sent for it with the result, as I say, that we have had splendid results from it. We have two nurses come down from the City Hospital and prepare the arms of the children by washing with a liquid soap and then subsequently with alcohol. We have done that for about a year or two years with, as I say, no evil results in the way of sore arms at all. No shields are used. A great many people who can well afford to pay for vaccination, I presume, come there; but we don't ask any questions. They come there, and we vaccinate them. We make them return, and look their arms over before we issue the school certificate. I don't know that we can ascribe to any other means the fact of Worcester's freedom from small-pox. Since last July we have had only three cases of small-pox in the city of Worcester, although it is, next to Boston, the largest city in the State, and all around us in the surrounding towns they have had a great deal of it,— towns that are connected with Worcester by trolley lines that are running in every half-hour or hour. We have only had, as I say, three cases of small-pox in about a year in the city of Worcester. I don't know what else to attribute it to except the thorough vaccination that is going on there. This began some years ago by starting with the vaccination of school-children in a small way; and it kept growing and growing until to-day, practically, I suppose, two-thirds or three-fourths of all the children that enter the public schools every fall are vaccinated at our office before they enter. The school department works in harmony with us, because no child is admitted to the public schools without a certificate. They don't give them the billet in the office of the superintendent of schools without first sending them to the health office to see if they have been successfully vaccinated or not. I must say that children who have moved from some other cities and towns of the State to Worcester come in with certificates in their hands, signed by physicians, that they have been successfully vaccinated; and on investigation, making them strip and letting us see whether they have been or not, we fail to find any evidence whatever of successful vaccination, or of any vaccination, in a great many instances. I cannot account for that in any other way than that perhaps a physician will vaccinate a child, and then later the mother or father will come in and say it took all right; and he will sit down and write a certificate, and give it to the mother or father without seeing the child. But I want to say that no child is admitted to the schools of Worcester in that way. We must ourselves see every child, and every one comes into the office. They strip, and we see whether they are successfully vaccinated or not; and, unless they are, we don't issue the certificate, and the school department refuses to give a billet until the certificate has been issued.

Dr. Davenport.— Mr. Chairman, I should like to say a word in regard to the examination and vaccination of school-children. The board of health started in the town of Watertown last year to have the school inspectors make a personal examination of the arms of all the children in the schools, and prepare a card catalogue of the number and character of the vaccination scars found, primary or revaccinations, whether satisfactory, indifferent, or what they were, and to urge the revaccination of all such children as were found not to have been properly vaccinated. We had three inspectors in the schools. One of these inspectors co-operated heartily with the chairman of the board of health, who happened to be myself; and there was a good deal of vaccination and revaccination done in one of the three districts. The other two inspectors did not co-operate heartily. Although I had acted as chairman of the board of health for ten years, I am not now on the board. It was said that there was too much interference and too much zeal, although it was, of course, without any personal interest, as I was not in practice in the town. We have had several cases of small-pox in the town. Some of them have been among school-children, but not in the well-vaccinated district. It has happened in some of the other districts. This card catalogue of the vaccination was to be kept on file in the office of the master or of the superintendent of schools, for convenient reference.

THE PRESIDENT.— The question before you is the vote offered by Mr. Coffey. I don't understand Dr. Hill insists upon his amendment.

DR. HILL.— No, I will withdraw it.

The vote offered by Mr. Coffey was adopted.

DR. MAGEE.— Now, Mr. Chairman, with your permission, I would like to make a motion that the Secretary of this Association be instructed to communicate with the secretaries of the district medical societies of this State, asking them to take some action, and recommending the antitoxine of the State and also the matter of the free distribution of virus. I think in that way you will bring the discussion before the medical men of the State, who are very much interested in the matter; and in that way you will get good results. There might also be communications with the various boards of health.

DR. A. E. MILLER.— Mr. President, I desire to second that motion.

THE PRESIDENT.—It is moved and seconded that there be an official communication from this Association to the respective district medical societies of the State upon the subject of the production of antitoxine and vaccine lymph. If that be your pleasure, signify it by saying aye.

The motion was adopted.

THE PRESIDENT.— It is so voted. The next question before you is the answer to the question,—

How far away from a diphtheria and scarlet fever hospital is it necessary for a small-pox hospital to be located?

I know of no one better able to answer that question than Dr. Abbott.

DR. ABBOTT.— This question came in on Tuesday; and I have looked up the subject somewhat, Mr. Chairman, since that time. In considering this question, the proper location of a small-pox hospital, we may be guided by the experience of those communities where the violation of the natural laws governing the spread of infectious diseases has been productive of serious harm.

The principal information upon this point comes, not from Germany, since Germany has neither small-pox nor small-pox hospitals, but from England, where both are abundant, and instances of faulty locations are often reported.

Several years ago the small-pox hospitals of London were established in districts of the city which were becoming every year more and more populous and densely settled. In the midst of several moderate epidemics of small-pox which occurred between 1877 and 1881, it was observed that the prevalence of the disease appeared to bear a direct relation to the distance of certain infected localities from one of these hospitals (the Fulham Hospital). Similar observations were also made at Sheffield, Warrington, and Hastings in later epidemics. In consequence of these observations the old small-pox hospitals of London have been abandoned, and a new location has been established several miles down the river, where some hospital ships are moored in the river, to which all patients are now taken for treatment. And what is the result of this change? According to a statement in the London *Lancet* of Feb. 22, 1902, during the present epidemic of small-pox in London, and while these hospital ships have been crowded with patients, the disease has broken out at Purfleet, a village just north of the Thames and about a mile from the ships : —

Dr. Thresh,* the medical officer of health of Essex, attributes the excessive prevalence of small-pox at Purfleet to the proximity of these

* "Hospital Ships and the Dissemination of Small-pox," by Dr. J. C. Thresh, the *Lancet*, Feb. 22, 1902, p. 495.

hospitals of the Metropolitan Asylums Board of London. Cases have followed one another in rapid succession since September last, until about one-tenth of the population has been attacked, and it has spread to adjoining parishes.

Vaccination has been much neglected in Purfleet: " The prevailing wind has been from the south-west; and in the cottages nearest, and exposed to the prevailing wind, out of every eight persons, one has been attacked. If such an epidemic prevalence had occurred in London, there would have been over a half-million cases in the past seven months. My impression is that the infection may be carried two or possibly three miles in the direction of the wind."

In an editorial in the same issue of the *Lancet* the same view receives substantial support in the following word : " These revelations are extremely inconvenient,"— that term " inconvenient " no doubt relates to the conclusions that had been already made, that had induced them to carry these ships down to that point — " and another result should be the recognition of the fact that *we cannot, by isolation, hope to get rid of small-pox*. The remedy is ready at hand, and consists in placing revaccination on the same basis as primary vaccination. With the German method we shall avoid small-pox outbreaks, but with primary vaccination alone we can never hope to do so."

Hence we find that the local government board of England has arrived at quite definite conclusions upon this subject. The following statement is quoted from their memorandum, or circular, of January, 1895 :—

Small-pox hospitals have again and again served to disseminate that disease to neighboring communities, and this, to use the words of the Royal Commission, " in spite of precautions almost in excess of any that would have been anticipated " (L. G. B. Memorandum, 1895).

It is not certain, what distance they are dangerous to surrounding populations, but it may be accepted that it is *not safe* to erect a small-pox hospital :—

(1) On a site within $\frac{1}{4}$ mile of a hospital, either general or for infectious diseases, or of a workhouse or similar institution, or of any aggregation of 150 to 200 persons.

(2) On a site where it would have within $\frac{1}{2}$ mile a population of 500 to 600, whether in one institution or in dwelling-houses.

These distances are not to be taken as absolutely fixed, and the case of a considerable population resident just outside such limit would call for serious consideration.*

* "Himes's Practical Guide to the Public Health Acts," p. 639. See also Copnall's " Infectious Diseases and Hospitals," p. 232.

The exceedingly contagious nature of small-pox is one of its peculiar characteristics. In this respect it surpasses all other diseases. Whooping-cough may be communicated from one person to another at a short interval of space, and so may scarlet fever and diphtheria, especially when the two parties, the sick and the well, are in a small closed apartment. With small-pox, however, the case is otherwise; and, according to the observations of Dr. Thresh, the infection may be carried two or possibly three miles in the direction of the wind.

I think this might be modified, perhaps, by other statements that have been made; that is, that large aggregations of cases several cases in one house or one building, would constitute a greater danger to the community than a single case.

This peculiar tendency of the infection of small-pox to be transmitted through the air for considerable distances is illustrated in Dr. Powers's report of 1882, from which the following figures and conclusions are quoted: —

ADMISSIONS OF ACUTE SMALL-POX TO FULHAM HOSPITAL, AND INCIDENCE OF SMALL-POX UPON HOUSES IN SEVERAL DIVISIONS OF THE SPECIAL AREA DURING FIVE EPIDEMIC PERIODS.

CASES OF ACUTE SMALL-POX ADMITTED.	IN EPIDEMIC PERIODS SINCE OPENING OF HOSPITAL.	INCIDENCE ON EVERY HUNDRED HOUSES WITHIN THE SPECIAL AREA AND ITS DIVISIONS.				
		On Total Special Area.	On Small Circle 0–¼ Mile.	On First Ring ¼–½ Mile.	On Second Ring ½–¾ Mile.	On Third Ring ¾–1 Mile.
327 . .	Mar., 1877–end of 1877,	1.10	3.47	1.37	1.27	.36
714 . .	Jan., 1878–Sept., 1878 .	1.80	4.62	2.55	1.84	.67
679 . .	Sept., 1878–Oct., 1879 .	1.68	4.40	2.63	1.49	.64
292 . .	Oct., 1879–Dec., 1880 .	.58	1.85	1.06	.30	.28
515 . .	Dec., 1880–Apr., 1881 .	1.21	3.00	1.54	1.25	.61
2,527 . .	Five periods	6.37	17.35	9.20	6.16	2.57.

Conclusions Relative to the Spread of Small-pox in the Neighborhood of Hospitals.

1. There has been in each epidemic period an excessive incidence of small-pox in houses in the neighborhood of the hospital as compared with more distant houses in Chelsea, Fulham, and Kensington.

2. The percentage of houses invaded in the neighborhood of the hospital has become gradually smaller as the distance of the houses from the hospital has increased.

This gradation has been very exact and very constant.

3. Houses upon the chief lines of human intercourse with the hospital have not suffered more than houses lying in other directions from the hospital.

4. In point of time there has been a very marked relation between the varying use of the hospital and the manifestations of excessive small-pox in the neighborhood.

This relation has not shown itself, while the use of the hospital has been for convalescents only.

5. The appearance of excessive small-pox in houses around the hospital has never been delayed until the hospital has become full, or nearly full. It has been always most remarkable at the time when admissions to the hospital were beginning to increase rapidly.

In the succeeding months of active operations, though the use of the hospital may have gone on increasing, the excess of small-pox upon the neighborhood has habitually become less marked.

6. On comparison of different epidemics an almost constant ratio is observed between the amount of the hospital operations and the degree of excess of small-pox in the neighborhood.

7. The machinery of the hospital administration, with inclusion of defects in that machinery, does not account for the peculiarity of small-pox incidence within the three parishes of Chelsea, Fulham, and Kensington since the establishment of the hospital.

8. There must have been some condition or conditions operating to produce the observed distribution of small-pox around the hospital that have pertained to the hospital as such, and that have been in excess of the condition of small-pox extension as usually recognized.

9. During the present epidemic period, and most probably during former similar periods, there has arisen in the atmospheric circumstances of the time peculiar facility for the dissemination in an undamaged state of any matter that may have been given off from the hospital.

A similar occurrence has recently taken place in the city of Everett on a smaller scale. Everett is a city of peculiar conditions. It has had an exceptionally rapid growth, having increased its population more than tenfold in the past thirty years (population in 1870, 2,220; and in 1900, 24,336), while at the same time it is one of the smallest cities in point of area, having less than three square miles of territory.

Early in the present epidemic a case of small-pox was found in a house opposite a railway station and in a quite densely settled district. The case was quarantined at this house; and as soon as other cases occurred they were taken to this house for treatment, the house being made a temporary hospital. As a natural result, several other cases occurred within the next six months in the neighborhood of this house.

I have here Dr. Thresh's more recent statement, published in June in the *Medical Magazine.* There is hardly time to read any further conclusions from it, but I think what I have stated sufficiently covers the subject.

DR. A. E. MILLER.— I would like to ask Dr. Abbott the distance where there was 2½ per cent. I did not get that.

DR. ABBOTT.— One mile; that is, between the three-quarter mile and one mile, the outer ring of the circle.

DR. CHASE.— I would like to ask Dr. Abbott what the capacity of the small-pox hospital was. It makes a great difference, I understand.

DR. ABBOTT.— The Fulham Hospital?

DR. CHASE.— Yes.

DR. ABBOTT.— It must have been pretty large, I think. It probably held, I should judge, three or four hundred patients, though I don't know. But I know the new one down the river is already holding to-day, or held during the last two or three months, about thirteen or fourteen hundred at a time.

DR. CHASE.— The minimum distance, then, should be, did I understand, a quarter of a mile or a mile?

DR. ABBOTT.— A quarter of a mile.

DR. CHASE.— Then, if the hospital is such as we ordinarily have in our towns for small-pox patients, one to accommodate, say, a dozen patients, a shorter distance than a quarter of a mile would suffice would it not?

Dr. Abbott.— I should think it might. I think the general rule would be to put it as far away as you can.

Dr. Hill.— Mr. Chairman, as far as I am aware, the Massachusetts experience in the matter of carriage of small-pox to a distance hardly agrees with the English experience; and I should like very much to hear some of those who have had experience in Massachusetts with small-pox talk on that point. I think there are a number of other men that feel the same way.

Dr. Field.— I think that in Lowell the small-pox hospital must be between a quarter of a mile and half a mile from the poor-farm. I doubt if it is much over a quarter of a mile. I do not know of a case of small-pox ever arising in the poor-farm. They are both on the same land; and it is about five minutes' walk, four minutes' walk, from one to the other.

Dr. Magee.— I have had a little experience this year in small-pox. I had three cases of small-pox in a house on Oak Street. The area between the houses was about 4 feet, and we have had no contagion from that. I also had three cases on Cross Street, where the area was 15 feet on one side and 20 on the other: no contagion from that. We have had in the town of Andover some twelve cases, and the area between the houses there was somewhere about, I should judge, 150 feet: no contagion from that. But we had a little field surrounding the poor-house, and we have had small-pox from that. So far as contagion is concerned, I think it is something that is pretty hard to define. That has been my experience the last few years with small-pox. We have had no contagion outside from those houses, and the windows have been open at times no doubt; and neighbors have been within 15 feet on one side and 20 on the other, within four feet in one case. The windows not only had screens in, but I guess the screens were raised once in a while.

Dr. A. E. Miller.— Mr. President, I should like to ask the gentleman who relates this experience if one reason why they have not had contagion has not been because they have had thorough vaccination of the individuals around, and that vaccination prevented the contagion.

Dr. Magee.— In my cases I can't say that they have been vaccination, for I don't know.

Dr. A. E. Miller.— I should be inclined to think there had been thorough vaccination.

The President.— Dr. Swarts, haven't you some Rhode Island experiences that might be interesting?

Dr. Swarts.— Well, as to the location of hospitals in connection with the spread of the disease, I think most of us in Rhode Island do not have that fear of the spread from isolation spoken of; that is, if the isolation is what it should be, there should not be any spread. One instance occurred where I was called upon to decide whether a patient should be removed from a house which was 20 feet distant from a school of about 200 children, and the question was whether the school should be closed or not. I told them to continue the school. I thought they were safer within bounds than without. Of course, the equations of every individual case and of every hospital must be taken into consideration. If your isolation is absolute, you may have 1 or 50 patients; and if the possibilities of spreading the disease are good, as undoubtedly they may be in the London hospitals, where they have so many cases, and where the neighborhood possibly is a negligent one, I should think the spread might be considerable. I think that it is a question of all conditions present which you must take into consideration, not simply the area, the location of the hospital, and having any number of cases surrounding it, but who the people are who have the cases in charge, the methods of isolation, the care which is taken of the patients to prevent desquamation from being carried through windows or by the attendants. I think so many factors come into the question that I personally, and I think most of the officers in Rhode Island, would have very little fear to locate a hospital within the inhabited area of the city, the only objection being public prejudice; that is, we feel that, if we have a hospital, it should be under proper control and proper conditions, and that the spread of the disease will depend, not upon the location of the house, but the care of the individual.

Dr. Palmer.— Mr. Chairman, I am one of the victims of popular prejudice in the care of small-pox; and I think there is a great deal yet to be learned about its contagiousness. If I relate the experience in Framingham, it may possibly be instructive. There were two cases during the past winter. One was in a private house, isolated there; and there was no further trouble from it. The second case came down in a hotel; and the man went to the dining-room, and to the dining-room table, after he was thoroughly broken out. He was isolated, as Dr. Abbott says, the best that could be done,— and this was the cause of my undoing,— in a private house, at least 150 feet away from any other one; and there was no other case from it. The only point that I want to make is that I think we don't know absolutely yet where small-pox comes from or how far it may be carried. We know only in a measure. If any people were exposed in the second case to which I referred, it was the people round and about that hotel from which the case was taken.

DR. OTIS H. MARION.— How many were vaccinated?

DR. PALMER.— The precaution was take to revaccinate those who were exposed in the hotel; and the hotel was quarantined, and no one allowed to go in or out until we thought they were safe.

DR. HILL.— Mr. Chairman, since no one else will ask the question, I shall have to ask Dr. Shea about the Northampton Street hospital.

THE PRESIDENT.— Dr. Shea, we shall be glad to hear your experience.

DR. SHEA.— Mr. President, before we establish a hospital for small-pox, we always see that the neighborhood is well vaccinated; and, as a result, we have no cases near our hospital. That has been our experience. At the beginning of this last epidemic we sent a squad of physicians, and we vaccinated the neighborhood for a mile each side of the hospital; and the district shows that we have not had many cases round the hospital there. I think it would be prudent for any town or city, before it establishes a small-pox hospital, to see that in the immediate neighborhood, within a radius probably of a quarter of a mile, all the families were well vaccinated.

DR. ABBOTT.— Mr. Chairman, I should like to add one or two words upon this. These cases are mostly, you might say, negative evidence of isolated cases, perhaps, that have been brought up; but these conclusions of the Fulham Hospital were made from 2,527 admissions in one building, and the aggregation of that number of course adds to the value of the conclusions. In regard to this particular point of vaccination, Dr. Thresh's more recent article brings up this very point, because the London anti-vaccinationist is a pretty busy person, and picks up every point in the argument that he possibly can against vaccination. He says :—

It has been urged that the fact that no cases have occurred amongst the garrison at West Purfleet [that is, a government institution] or amongst the lads on board the training ship, "Cornwall," [near by this, at West Purfleet, a little distance from that village], both within three-quarters of a mile radius of the ships, prove that the infection is not air-borne. Certainly, at first sight, it does appear singular that these should have escaped. But the reason is very simple. The barracks lie to the extreme north of Purfleet, in the portion where only two cases of small-pox have occurred ; but the immunity of the garrison is due not so much to the position of the barracks as to the fact that every inmate has been *revaccinated*, save a few who had had small-pox previous to the present outbreak.

So this vaccination of the people in the surrounding neighborhood is a pretty important one, after all.

Dr. Palmer.— Mr. Chairman, if I may be allowed, I should like to ask a question. If it is out of order in this discussion, you will rule it out. I should like to ask the opinion of those present as to the temperature that will affect the activity of vaccine virus. That question has been brought to my mind recently. I find a great many physicians keep their vaccine, very conveniently, right on their desk beside them, to use when it is necessary, while I have been told by the agents of the mercantile houses that it is necessary that it be kept constantly in a cool place. If any one can give light on that, I should like to have it.

The President.—Dr. Smith, cannot you help us to an answer?

Dr. Smith.— Mr. President, vaccine virus maintains its efficiency at a variety of temperatures. The best temperature is that of the ice-chest, about 55 degrees Fahrenheit; but it will remain efficient at a higher temperature, provided it is in the form of glycerinized lymph. If it is dried on the end of points, the more rapidly will the vaccine organisms be destroyed. It depends largely upon the manner in which the virus is put up for use. I should like to ask whether the question was asked concerning the dried virus or the virus that is mixed with glycerine.

DR. PALMER.—What I refer to is the tubes of the glycerinized lymph.

DR. SMITH.—It seems to me that the ice-chest temperature would be the better temperature. Within the period within which virus is usually used I think the ordinary temperature probably would not destroy it, though it might destroy it a trifle faster than a lower temperature.

THE PRESIDENT.—If there is nothing more to be said upon this subject, we will proceed to the consideration of the third question :—

Should boards of health require the reporting of cases of chicken-pox?

Perhaps you can say something about that, Dr. Chase.

DR. CHASE.—I don't know exactly why I should be called upon to speak upon that subject. We have authorities here on small-pox, and I don't pose as one. But I know how closely chicken-pox simulates small-pox; and I am called on frequently to settle the diagnosis, and a difficult one. I will admit that I was the one that asked that question, but not the one that proposes to answer it. In some places, chicken-pox is obliged to be reported because of its frequent simulation of small-pox. In the town in which I live our board does not require the reporting of cases of chicken-pox; and I am here to learn, if I can, what we ought to do, require it or not require it.

DR. MAGEE.—Mr. Chairman, I may have something interesting to say on that subject. Two months ago or more in my city there was reported a case of chicken-pox by one of our physicians, who is quite a bright man; and the agent of the board of health went to see it. He doubted the diagnosis of the physician. He came to me about it. I told him that something should be done. He doubted the diagnosis. The physician objected to any local doctor going in to see the case. Finally, we sent for our friend Dr. Morse; and, after the man had supposed chicken-pox for two weeks, it turned out to be a case of small-pox. We have had similar cases of that kind. I think myself that it is the duty of physicians and boards of health to insist on the report of so-called cases of chicken-pox or all cases of eruptive disease, especially at a time when small-pox is quite prevalent. There are a great number of physicians who have not seen cases of small-pox. In the town of Andover, I have had twelve cases of small-pox; and Dr. Morse can bear me out in my statement. A gentleman contracted small-pox in the city of Boston, or we think he contracted it there. His was a very light case. He attended to his business, with the exception of two or three days. He had a headache and a backache and chills and a little vomiting, and the doctor who was attending him thought he had chicken-pox. He went along; and his wife contracted chicken-pox, so called. His four children, from the ages of two to seven or eight, contracted chicken-pox, so called. But they were all cases of small-pox,— six in that family. His book-keeper contracted small-pox, his brother-in-law and his sister-in-law contracted small-pox; and they were all reported chicken-pox.

A MEMBER.— And his father-in-law.

DR. MAGEE.— And his father-in-law, yes.

A MEMBER.— The mother-in-law escaped.

DR. MAGEE.— But I had those cases. This was in a town where the board of health, to say the least, is not very particular. This went along, and we have had twelve cases of small-pox in the town of Andover, and were very fortunate to get rid of it with only twelve cases. We have had one death. I have given you the source of contagion. I think myself, if that case had been reported in proper time, probably eight out of the twelve would have been vaccinated in proper time, and would not have had small-pox. I certainly think it is important to report cases of chicken-pox to the boards of health; and they should send a physician immediately or call on the proper authorities to go and examine those cases, especially where chicken-pox is reported in an adult. Many people believe that you cannot get chicken-pox in an adult; but there are cases of chicken-pox in the adult, there is no doubt of that. When you get chicken-pox in persons of — well, above eight years of age, I certainly think they ought to be reported, if not under; but my idea is that all such cases should be reported.

Dr. Durgin.— From the experience we have had in the city of Boston in the last thirty years it is safe to say that you are much better off in calling for the report of cases of chicken-pox, and looking them up. If you don't, you will occasionally have some undiscovered cases of small-pox spreading the disease.

Dr. Magee.— Our board of health in the city of Lawrence insists on the reporting of chicken-pox cases.

Dr. Durgin.—We have called for the report of cases of chicken-pox in Boston for quite a good many years. We look them up, and find some cases of small-pox among them.

Dr. Magee.— In the children there?

Dr. Durgin.—Both children and adults. I am glad the preceding speaker has mentioned the fact that it is not safe to conclude that you don't get chicken-pox among the adults.

The President.— Are you satisfied, Dr. Chase?

Dr. Chase.— Perfectly satisfied. Thank you, doctor.

The President.— The next question is, Should boards of health make provision for the care and isolation in hospitals, when so requested, of patients ill with measles?

I have to ask for some volunteer upon that matter. I don't know who is an authority upon the subject.

Dr. Chase.— Mr. Chairman, as Dr. Currier, the acting superintendent of the south department of the Boston City Hospital, is present, perhaps he will tell us a little about the experience there.

The President.— We shall be glad to hear from Dr. Currier on the subject.

Dr. Currier.— It seems very important to me that measles should be isolated at the very first sign of any symptom. The cough especially, and the coryza, and the koplik spots inside the cheeks have been proved to be preliminary symptoms. Every case is followed by the measles eruption. The measles eruption with these symptoms, if not isolated, will certainly cause an epidemic in any hospital or elsewhere, whether the exposure is direct or indirect.

Dr. Chase.— Mr. President, I should like to know what the practice is in Worcester about admitting measles patients to the contagious hospital.

Mr. Coffey.— Mr. Chairman, there is no provision made in Worcester for caring for cases of measles in the isolation hospital there, although we have felt a great many times since we have erected the hospital that we ought to have made provision for it. At the outset, while we considered it, the extra expense involved made us fearful that, if we asked for the amount necessary to care for measles with diphtheria and scarlet fever, we might not get anything, so that we did not ask to include measles in the amount asked for. Since we have been operating our hospital, now about six years, we have in a great many instances felt the need of accommodations for cases of measles. There has been a number of times persons taken sick at hospitals and boarding-houses and at some of the schools. There are a large number of preparatory schools in Worcester, from which we get quite a number of patients with diphtheria and scarlet fever. We have also had applications to care for measles, but have been obliged to refuse because no provision was made for the care of measles. But we have asked for an appropriation to make an addition to our hospital there; and it is our intention, if we obtain that appropriation, to make provision for the care of a number of cases of measles,— perhaps not to attempt to take care of them in any general way, but those isolated cases that arise,— servants in private families, patients in hotels, boarding-houses, and at those schools that I speak of. In every community there must be a large number, of course, varying with the size of the community, of cases of that kind, where it is extremely difficult, if not impossible, to properly treat and isolate a case of measles without putting the family to a great deal of inconvenience; and I think that, when the communities, as they are now doing throughout the State, make provision for the care and treatment of contagious disease, some arrangement ought to be made to treat measles, those isolated cases that I speak of. I know that in a large community it would be very difficult, perhaps, to build a hospital large enough to care for measles when it becomes epidemic in the thickly settled section; but, as I said, some provision ought to be made, in my judgment, for those cases that occur, as they frequently do, in houses and institutions and hotels, where it is almost impossible to properly treat and care for them.

DR. PERRY.— Mr. Chairman, there is one other point along that line which has not been touched upon; namely, the cases of measles which are complicated with pneumonia. Among the very poor these cases not infrequently occur, and, I venture to say, vex the physician and tax his powers more than almost any cases he is called to attend. Then, again, an empyæma demanding surgical interference may be a sequel of a pneumonia starting from measles. Still, if the patient has measles, in many cities he cannot be taken to a hospital; and, if the patient is very poor,— for instance, a city physician's patient,— you can see that the nursing and the general care of the patient would be very inadequate, perhaps, with our present lack of special arrangements, for the treatment of such patients. Since measles complicated with pneumonia must be attended to as cases of measles, it would seem that especial provision in our contagious hospitals should be made at least for such cases as have a coexisting pneumonia or require surgical attention.

DR. FIELD.— What has been said seems to show that boards of health popularly consider measles a milder disease than scarlet fever or diphtheria, and I imagine that Dr. Abbott would tell us that in some epidemics that is far from being the truth. I remember that in Lowell fourteen or fifteen years ago we had an epidemic of measles, in which more persons died than died from scarlet fever and diphtheria together for several years. We lost 108 people, I think, from measles, when Lowell was a much smaller town than it is now.

DR. MAGEE.— Wasn't it complicated with something, doctor?

DR. FIELD. — I presume there were complications, as there very often are with measles; but it was measles.

DR. MAGEE.— Do you remember that epidemic, doctor, at all?

DR. ABBOTT.— No.

DR. MAGEE.— It is very rare that you lose a case of measles without some complication.

DR. ABBOTT.— The fatality is inside of 4 or 5 per cent. usually.

The PRESIDENT.— Is there anything more to be said upon this subject? If not, there is one other question that has been submitted; and that is,—

Is it advisable that any municipality of 50,000 or more population shall discontinue its bacteriological laboratory, and depend again upon such assistance as the State Board of Health can render it?

I should like to say, before asking general discussion upon the subject, that, so far as the State Board of Health goes, our resources are taxed to the utmost; and it is not possible to do any more with the present appropriations or with the present room than is already done. No one is better aware than myself that what the State Board does is a very insufficient protection for the Commonwealth in this direction. It does seem to me that there is absolutely no question that a municipality of 50,000 people ought to provide a bacteriological laboratory of its own. There are so many questions that modern civilization demands of such a laboratory that every municipality fifty or forty or thirty miles, even, away from Boston, should be in condition, when called upon, to answer them.

DR. MAGEE.— Is there any law pertaining to that?

THE PRESIDENT.— No. Perhaps Dr. Davenport has given some consideration to such a question as that. He is a scientific man with a laboratory.

DR. DAVENPORT.— Mr. Chairman, I have not had much experience in that regard. My municipality was only of 10 to 11,000; and, as I said in my previous remarks, I am no longer chairman or even a member of the board of health, for the reason of alleged undue activity. [Laughter.] The institution of a bacteriological laboratory in charge of one of the school inspectors was one of the forms of activity which was displayed. Curiously enough, my fellow-practitioners did not support me in the manner I had anticipated. Some of them even privately told me I was interfering with private professional business in carrying out the school inspection in the thorough manner I was having it done.

THE PRESIDENT.— Dr. Spencer, you have had charge of a bacteriological laboratory in Cambridge. Cannot you tell us something upon this subject?

Dr. SPENCER.— Mr. President, we could not dispense with it, — could not dispense with it, never should consider it for a moment.

Mr. COFFEY.— I want to say that in Worcester we have had a bacteriological laboratory for seven or eight years. I think we were the first east of New York to establish one; and we certainly would not think of dispensing with ours, because very frequently we are able to get a diagnosis from our bacteriologist within five or six hours after the culture comes in. That would be impossible if we were obliged to send it to Boston, to the State Board of Health. We have cultures brought in sometimes in the forenoon; and at three or four o'clock in the afternoon the bacteriologist is able to make a diagnosis, and does frequently, and the patient is removed to the hospital within five or six hours after the case is first reported. That, of course, would be impossible if we were obliged to send the culture to Boston. It is such an advantage that we would not want to dispense with our laboratory.

DR. MAGEE.— We have none in our city.

DR. PALMER.— It might be of interest, Mr. Chairman, if I were to state that in connection with the little cottage hospital in Framingham, we are doing something of that work ourselves.

THE PRESIDENT.— Your population is how much, doctor?

DR. PALMER.— Only 11,000.

Dr. PERRY.— Mr. Chairman, there is a municipality of even 65,000 inhabitants that has had a bacteriological laboratory established — this is now the third year. I have just received intimation that the discontinuance of that laboratory was being considered. It was established by the local board of health late in 1900, in compliance with a demand registered in the unanimous vote of the local medical society. It seems to me most inexpedient that a department which despite its niggardly appropriations has been so efficient and successful from its very beginning, as a recent statement signed by sixty-nine physicians who have used the laboratory and now demand its continuance vouches that department to have been, should now be discontinued on account of an expense of a few hundred dollars a year.   Thus to imperil the lives of thousands of the residents of that municipality seems to me an outrage against sanitary progress little less than criminal.   Far from any discontinuing or crippling of this department, it would seem that the confidence which the laboratory has already won among the medical men of that municipality warrants an increased appropriation commensurate with its present necessities and its constantly growing importance and usefulness.

I should like to hear from our State Inspector upon this subject.

THE PRESIDENT.— Dr. Morse, we shall be glad to hear what you have got to say.

DR. MORSE.— Mr. President, that is something that I have not given very much attention to; but I think it would be a serious reflection upon the city of Somerville to withdraw its bacteriological laboratory.   I think more could be done with it if the board of health would make certain regulations which they do not now require, insisting upon patients ill with diphtheria having two negative reports from their throats before releasing them from quarantine.   It seems to me that the bacteriological laboratory at Somerville should be equal in efficiency to any other in the State.

DR. ABBOTT.— Mr. Chairman, this opens up quite an important phase of this question, which in a general way is, I think, one that may be made useful by large cities to the surrounding neighborhood. I refer particularly to the city of Springfield, which maintains a bacteriological laboratory in which work is done for quite a large territory, extending, perhaps, thirty or forty miles in any direction from Springfield, even over into Connecticut, I believe; but that is, perhaps, outside the question.   It is a very convenient thing for that neighborhood to have one so located that material can be sent there from those towns and a reply can be had very soon, compared with the time which would be consumed in getting material down to Boston and getting the reply back again.

DR. LOWELL.— Mr. Chairman, as the bacteriologist of the city of Somerville, I should like to state how things have worked there.   For the year 1900, that was the year before the laboratory was established, the work was practically all done by the State Board of Health laboratory. To be exact, the laboratory was established late in the year 1900. During that year there were 520 cases of diphtheria reported. During that year the State Board of Health laboratory examined 322 cultures for diphtheria. During the year 1901, the first part of the year, the city physician, Dr. Perry, examined the cultures (for three months). I was appointed in April, and examined them for the rest of the year, and am examining them now. In the year 1901 there were 340 cases of diphtheria reported, and there were 801 cultures examined. For the year 1902, for the first six months or up to date, there have been some 96 cases of diphtheria reported. Up to the first of July I have examined 500 cultures for diphtheria. That is about four cultures and a half or five cultures for each case of diphtheria reported. There have been 96 cases reported; and I have had over 90 of those come through the laboratory for examination, for diagnosis, or for release or negative for release. I think those figures alone show pretty conclusively to what extent the physicians of Somerville have appreciated a local laboratory.

Dr. DURGIN.— I want to apologize for forgetting one question which was sent to me instead of to Dr. Walcott. It was from Dr. Fiske, of Fitchburg, and was concerning the collection of the expenses for caring for patients with infectious diseases.

DR. FISKE.— I included all other contagious diseases, any case of quarantine. In cases of quarantine for contagious disease, whether cities and towns where the cases occurred supported the families during quarantine, and, if so, to what extent, and what proportion of the families ever paid back a rebate to the city or town for the quarantine as under the Public Statutes ?

DR. DURGIN.— We don't quarantine families for small-pox in Boston. We take the patient to the hospital, clean up the house and what is left in it, vaccinate all exposed persons and watch them for two weeks. Cases which go to the hospital, if their legal settlement is in the city, we take care of, and say nothing about it. If their legal settlement is in any town within the Commonwealth, that town must by law pay the reasonable expense of taking care of the patient. If they have no legal settlement in any place within the State, then the State itself pays the bill for reasonable expenses.

DR. FISKE.— Mr. Chairman, in towns or cities that have not an isolation hospital for scarlet fever or diphtheria, for instance, I presume the families are quarantined with the case; and in that case there would not be any expense to that city or town during the quarantine.

DR. DURGIN.— In Boston we pursue this course with regard to scarlet fever and diphtheria. A case is reported. The house is visited at once by an officer of the board of health, to see if isolation is satisfactory. If it is, the patient is isolated there by order of the board of health. A card is at once put up, indicating that the board has assigned those quarters for the isolation of that case. No bills are incurred by the board of health. The patient is left under the care of the attending physician and the family. If, however, that case is not isolated to the satisfaction of the board of health, it is at once removed to the hospital. As to paying the bills there, I am not certain whether any of the expense is collected from the patient or from the State.

THE PRESIDENT.— Perhaps Mr. Coffey can answer those questions.

MR. BODWELL.— Mr. Chairman, if you will allow me, I hope there will be a general expression on this question. I am speaking for myself and of small-pox. In Salem, when we have a case of small-pox, we take the patient to the hospital. We have this winter quarantined the house afterwards, and it has been very expensive. For instance, within two weeks we have had a house quarantined where there are eighty in the house, of course we paying all expenses; and that is very expensive. I thought I should like to have an idea of how many places were doing that sort of business.

MR. COFFEY.— At the meeting in Boston — either the last meeting or the annual meeting, I have forgotten which now — this matter was discussed under the head of small-pox; and I stated then that at Worcester, since 1894, we have not quarantined any house in small-pox. We do as they do in Boston. The patient is removed to the small-pox hospital; and immediately our inspectors go in and disinfect the house, and everybody in the house that has been exposed is vaccinated. A visit is made every day to that house for two weeks, to ascertain if any person who was exposed is ailing. Otherwise, we don't in any way interfere with the family. We have had two or three outbreaks of small-pox since 1894. That year was the first year we began to do that. We had some 20 cases that year, and we did that all through that epidemic. We had no trouble in suppressing it. And we have not had any trouble in suppressing the disease through these other outbreaks that we have had. We have had no spread from the place of outbreak to other places, have had no difficulty whatever. There is no expense attached to it; and, consequently, there are no bills to be paid. Now, in diphtheria and scarlet fever, we don't force anybody to go to the isolation hospital. The hospital, to begin with, is too small to accommodate all of them. We have gone on the theory that we would allow people to voluntarily decide whether they should send their children to the hospital or not, and that has worked very satisfactorily. We don't quarantine. A card is put on the house, " Scarlet Fever " or " Diphtheria." The schools are notified, and the libraries and some of the public institutions are notified of every case. In certain trades and occupations we refuse to allow the members of the family to go to their work. For instance, men engaged in the grocery and provision trade, who are handling food, or who are driving the delivery wagons of grocers and butchers, and visiting houses,— those people we do not allow to pursue their usual avocations. They must either send the child to the hospital or must cease work. Sales-girls in dry-goods stores, girls who work in the large corset factories, who are handling goods that might act as fomites to spread the disease,— in those cases we say to the people: " This child must go to the hospital, or you must cease work. You can take your choice." In most cases they allow the child to go to the hospital. We don't consider that we are responsible in any way for the loss of that person's services, and no bills have ever been rendered to us; and consequently we have never paid any bills for that.

Now I would like to ask a question; and I think the doctor, perhaps, had it in mind. A new law has been passed recently, which is a change from the law that has been in force for a great many years in relation to the payment of settlement cases. Under the old law those bills were paid, without any question, by the overseers of the poor. The bills were rendered to the overseers of the poor. Under the new law, when a case of contagious disease is taken charge of by any city or town, and expense entailed, the board of health of the city or town in which that case may have a settlement is notified. Until within a year that notice was always sent to the overseers of the poor. This new law makes a change, and necessitates the sending of the notice to the board of health, who are obliged, under the law, to turn it over to the overseers of the poor to ascertain settlement. If the settlement is in the city or town to which the notice is sent, then they acknowledge the settlement. The question that I would like to have answered is this: Has any city or town that is represented here to-day by its city solicitor or by any case in court determined whether that settlement money is to be paid by the board of health, or, as in the past, by the overseers of the poor? This case has come up in Worcester, because the overseers of the poor have notified me that these notices that we have received from other cities and towns, that they were caring for persons who have a settlement in Worcester, must be paid from the appropriation of the board of health. As a matter of fact, the board of health has no appropriation for any such purpose. This law went into effect, I think, this year, on March 26, and consequently we have no appropriatron for that purpose; and yet the overseers of the poor have notified us that under the law we shall be obliged to settle any claims that are made upon us by any other city or town of the Commonwealth.

Dr. Magee.—— Contagious diseases?

Mr. Coffey.—— For any contagious disease which is treated by that city or town. Any expense incurred in the treatment of cases of contagious disease by any city or town is now required, as I said, to be reported to the board of health of the town instead of, as formerly, to the overseers of the poor; and the overseers in Worcester contend that the payment must be made from the appropriation for the board of health. You know this is a new law that was passed, I think, by this last legislature, which changes the law which pauperized persons afflicted with contagious disease. The old law included them in the general pauperization of persons who are aided: the new law exempts those persons who are treated for contagious disease, and says they shall not be pauperized; and, consequently, the overseers of the poor have refused to pay. They say that under the general laws, and under some decisions that have been given, no money can be expended by the overseers of the poor that is not expended for the benefit of paupers, and that this new law exempts these people from being paupers, consequently that they cannot spend their money for that purpose. The fact is that the laws require that the notice shall be sent to the board of health instead of, as formerly, as I said before, to the overseers of the poor. What I wanted to know was, Has any city or town had it settled or determined by any opinion from a lawyer of standing, or by the courts, or even by the State Board of Lunacy and Charity, whether that money is to be paid from the appropriation of boards of health, or, as formerly, from the appropriation of the overseers of the poor.

DR. FISKE.— Mr. Chairman, Mr. Coffey has touched on a vital point of my question. It was on account of this new law that I put the question, because the board of health of the city of Fitchburg has had that very trouble. We had a case of diphtheria occurring in a neighboring town, in a poor family who had a settlement in our city; and, after the case was entirely recovered, the bill was sent to our overseers of the poor. They repudiated the bill, sent it back to the town where the case occurred, and then various correspondence occurred between the town and city. It finally came into our office, and we declined to pay the bill; and it went back again to the town. But, in looking the matter up, we found that under the new law the board of health had the jurisdiction in the matter rather than the overseers of the poor. We had no appropriation to pay that expense, and our board of health referred it to our mayor. That bill was put in simply as a bill or claim from that town against our city; and that bill as a claim bill went through our city government, was referred to the Committee on Claims, was acted upon, and our city government voted to pay it out of the incidentals on the approval of our board. It was not paid out of the appropriation of our board. But I should like to know how we should act in the next instance.

THE PRESIDENT.— I am afraid this discussion will have to be continued, as it is time for the boat.

Adjourned.

JOURNAL OF THE
MASSACHUSETTS ASSOCIATION OF BOARDS OF HEALTH.

ORGANIZED 1890.

[The Association as a body is not responsible for statements or opinions of any of its members.]

| VOL. XIV. | May, 1904. | NO. 2. |

THE MASSACHUSETTS ASSOCIATION OF BOARDS OF HEALTH was organized in Boston, March, 1890, with the following objects: the advancement of sanitary science; the promotion of better organization and co-operation among local boards of health, and the uniform enforcement of sanitary laws and regulations.

THE JOURNAL OF THIS ASSOCIATION has for fourteen years faithfully reflected the views of the public hygienists of Massachusetts. As the only one of its kind in Massachusetts, the Journal has had its own field, which, however, it has not yet fully occupied. With the October issue of the year 1903, a policy of expansion was adopted. The subscription list showed an immediate and most gratifying increase, so that this, the fourth issue has a total circulation of over 1,200 copies.

In order that the Journal may appear within the next month after each quarterly meeting of the Association, the dates of publication will be FEBRUARY, MAY, AUGUST and NOVEMBER of each year.

THE JOURNAL will contain the papers read at the meetings of the Association, verbatim reports of the discussions, editorials, abstracts, reviews and hygienic notes of professional interest. Subscription rates, $1.00 per year. Reprints furnished at cost price.

All communications concerning the ASSOCIATION should be addressed to the Secretary of the Association, JAMES C. COFFEY, CITY HALL, WORCESTER, MASS.

All bills not relating to the Journal, and MEMBERSHIP DUES ($2.00 per year), should be sent to the Treasurer of the Association, DR. JAMES B. FIELD, 329 WESTFORD ST., LOWELL, MASS.

All communications concerning the JOURNAL, copy, proof, subscriptions, advertisements, etc., should be addressed to the Managing Editor, DR. H. W. HILL, 607 SUDBURY BLDG., BOSTON, MASS.

EDITORIALS.

THE UNITED STATES SOCIETY FOR THE STUDY OF TUBERCULOSIS.

The appointment of a committee, composed of Drs. Trudeau, Biggs, Welch, Sternberg, Flick, Osler, and Jacobs, to draw up a Constitution and By-Laws for the new "United States Society for the Study of Tuberculosis," by a meeting of those interested in the tuberculosis problem, held in Philadelphia on March 28th, is the final outcome of a struggle which has been going on for over a year between the various interests in that field of endeavor.

At the meeting of the American Congress Tuberculosis held in New York city in the spring of 1902, the President of the Congress, Dr. Henry Holton, and some of his prominent associates, became deeply impressed with the fact that the interests of the crusade against tuberculosis would best be served by an entire reorganization of the Congress. This they attempted to bring about by the election of an entirely new list of officers, which was accomplished in a perfectly proper and legal manner. Dr. Daniel Lewis, Health Commissioner, was induced to accept the presidency of the Congress and Dr. George Brown of Atlanta, Ga., was chosen Secretary. After the adjournment of the Congress the former Secretary, Mr. Clark Bell, refused to be governed by the action of the Congress in electing new officers, declining to recognize their appointment, and soon after claiming that the real officers were elected after the adjournment by a so-called "Executive Committee," the formation of which and the authority for which is shrouded in mystery.

The officers regularly elected by the Congress applied for and received articles of incorporation as officers of the American

Congress on Tuberculosis, and became thereby the only organization entitled to the use of that name. Notwithstanding this, however, the mysteriously created "Executive Committee" and its appointees continued to use that name, and in addition settled upon St. Louis in the summer of 1904 as the time of their meeting, which was the place, and practically the time decided upon by the regular officers of the incorporated Congress for the holding of its meeting.

Not wishing to enter into an open conflict with the organization so mysteriously created, the officers of the incorporated Congress decided at a meeting held on May 7th, 1903, to eliminate one element of confusion by postponing the time and changing the place of meeting to April, 1905, and Washington, D. C. They were also influenced in making this decision by the fact that the International Congress on Tuberculosis was planning to meet in Paris in 1904, and they did not desire their meeting to conflict with it. At the same meeting the officers appointed a committee of some of the leading scientific workers in the profession to direct the more scientific work of the Congress, and they further decided to invite all the medical organizations whose members were eligible for membership in the American Medical Association to send delegates to the Congress.

At the Washington meeting of the American Public Health Association in October of last year, members of the staff of the Henry Phipps Institute endeavored to enlist support for the organization of a new national tuberculosis society for the express purpose of inviting the International Congress on Tuberculosis to hold a meeting in this country in 1905, it being stated that acceptance of the invitation was already assured. The supporters of this movement were entirely opposed to union or affiliation with any existing American anti-tuberculosis organization. Much to their surprise it was soon announced that the Paris meeting of the International Congress had been postponed until 1905 on the plea of not desiring to conflict with the meeting of the so-called "Clark Bell Congress" in St. Louis.

To the difficult task of endeavoring to bring order out of this chaos, a physician, Dr. Knopf, whose name has for several years been a prominent one in anti-tuberculosis literature, directed his efforts by sending an open letter to some of the weekly medical journals in which he outlined the situation, and commented freely on what he considered to be the deficiencies in the lists of prominent supporters of some of the existing organizations. He also issued a call for "all interested" to meet in Baltimore on January 29th. While "all interested" may not have been present, there were indications that, had circumstances permitted, several distinct national organizations would have been projected before the end of the meeting.

The most decided effort to produce harmony was the submission of an offer of the American Congress on Tuberculosis through its President, Dr. Daniel Lewis, to permit a committee, of some of the persons present at this meeting, to assume charge of the affairs of their organization and do with it what seemed best for the general interests involved. Towards this end Dr. Lewis stated that the Congress had changed its corporate name to American Anti-Tuberculosis League at the suggestion of one of the prominent supporters of the Phipps Institute plan.

From the tone of the discussion it became apparent to all that nothing could be settled at that meeting, and under the masterful direction of Dr. Welch the meeting finally voted to submit the whole question to a Committee to be appointed by the Chairman, and to be bound by its decision.

The members of this Committee, which included Drs. Biggs, Osler, Trudeau, Theobald Smith, Bowditch, Knopf, Jacobs, Bracken, Flick, and Ravenel, met subsequently in New York, and after some discussion it was generally understood that a large majority of the Committee were favorable to the plan of accepting the offer of the President of the Anti-Tuberculosis League made at the Baltimore meeting. It was considered wise, however, before settling the matter definitely, to enlarge the membership of the Committee, and to hold another meeting.

Advantage of this change was taken by those supporting the

Phipps Institute movement, who had from the first vigorously opposed affiliation with any existing organization, by inviting the Committee to hold their next meeting in Philadelphia on the date previously set for the presentation of a paper by Dr. Maragliano before the Phipps Institute.

The enlargement of the Committee naturally increased the Philadelphia representation upon it, and the holding of the meeting in that city insured the entire attendance of that representation while lessening the attendance from distant points, so that by actual count fifty per cent. of the persons present resided in Philadelphia or vicinity. With the assistance of a few ardent supporters from outside of their district, the Philadelphians were manifestly in control of the meeting, and it was seen beforehand that it would be useless to attempt to follow the plan of recommending affiliation with the Anti-Tuberculosis League, which had been deemed the wisest course by a majority of the Committee as originally constituted.

The struggle attending the birth of the Society, and the experience and results obtained from the Tuberculosis Exhibition and series of lectures held in Baltimore, have shown conclusively the need of an organization which will bring to the immediate attention of the profession as a whole and to the general public the essential truths concerning the nature, dissemination, prevention and treatment of the great plague.

That the United States Society for the Study of Tuberculosis will be a well conducted, thoroughly scientific and valuable organization no one questions for an instant. We hope that it will not confine itself to the scientific and more detailed clinical study of the tuberculosis problem, but will, as well, conduct a campaign of education for the benefit of the mass of the medical profession and the public, which was the aim and object of the American Anti-Tuberculosis League.

UNIFORM STANDARDS IN PUBLIC HEALTH ADMINISTRATION.

An excellent editorial on this subject in the *Journal of the American Medical Association* calls attention to the very varying practice in the large cities regarding the reporting of infectious diseases, the placarding of houses, and the extent of isolation required. The editorial urges that some understanding should be reached resulting in uniformity of procedure, and recommends that the American Medical Association should take up the consideration of the subject.

The ASSOCIATION which this JOURNAL represents was founded to promote uniformity of precedure amongst the local Boards of Health of this State, and it is therefore fully in sympathy with the general principles advocated by our contemporary. Of five or six different procedures only one can be the best. To find this best and to adopt it should be the aim of all interested in hygienic administration. The recommendation that this subject should be taken up by the American Medical Association involves, however, an unintentional but none the less poignant reflection, perhaps not altogether undeserved, on the hygienic associations of this country. It is reform from within, and not under compulsion from without, that is the best and most sincere, as well as the most creditable and encouraging. In hygienic matters the reforms should be initiated and carried out by the hygienists themselves. The American Public Health Association, the Conference of State Boards of Health and the local State hygienic societies constitute bodies not only the best informed on these subjects but the most likely to have weight with the public hygienists generally. The American Medical Association, representing the medical profession as a whole, is entitled to, and does, carry great weight, but the hygienic associations represent specialists in hygiene who have evolved, many of them from the medical profession, and it is no more proper that the American Medical Association should recommend procedures to the public hygienists than that the American Medical Association should recommend procedures to their own ophthalmological section or to their section of pathology and bacteriology.

The fact that official public hygienists have been slow in securing national or even State uniformity in many details furnishes, perhaps, some excuse for an appeal elsewhere. The fact that such an appeal has been made should be a sufficient spur to us in this at present rather neglected line.

MEDICAL INSPECTION OF SCHOOLS.

American Medicine, Feb. 27, '04, contains this item in the column on "Foreign News and Notes":

"MEDICAL SCHOOL INSPECTION ABROAD.—An exchange says: The foreign custom, universal in France and Germany, of insisting upon each child entering school, and at regular intervals thereafter submitting to a medical examination, is an example worthy of emulation in vaunted up-to-date communities. The question of vaccination and the control of contagious epidemic are the only occasions when medical intervention is usual in the schools in this country. Abroad it is customary to appoint school physicians, whose duty it is to examine twice a year all the pupils with reference to the senses, the spinal column, the development of the limbs, and to make recommendations for their special instruction on account of stuttering, etc. Not their least important work is the quarterly or in some cities semi-monthly sanitary inspection of school rooms and buildings. It is one of the duties of teachers to call the attention of the school physician to any pupils whose state of health during the interval since the previous visit creates suspicion. The physician can, however, in case of sick pupils, only notify the parents formally of the child's condition, their treatment being left entirely in the hands of the family physician. It is proposed by the French medical fraternity to have the school physician's duties extended to an inspection of the condition of the dwellings of sick school children, and also to give advice concerning the architecture of schools and the division of school hours."

The medical inspections thus vaunted are at most semi-monthly. It is interesting to compare this item, written recently, with the following paragraphs from a paper by Dr. E. M. Greene, Philadelphia Medical Journal, Feb. 16, 1901.

"The first city in this country, or abroad, to establish a system of daily medical inspection in all the public schools was Boston. Since then similar methods of inspection have been adopted in New York City, Chicago, and in most of the large cities, as well as in many of the smaller towns. Within a few years we may expect to see some method of medical inspection in general used throughout the country. The important questions are how comprehensive and searching an inspection is desirable, or practicable, and how to organize and conduct the work in the most efficient manner.

Medical inspection of schools, both public and parochial, was begun in Boston in the fall of 1894, and was secured only as the result of 4 years of persistent effort on the part of the efficient and progressive chairman of the Boston Board of Health, Dr. Samuel H. Durgin. The immediate occasion which made his appeals successful was the unusual prevalence of diphtheria in Boston during the year 1894.

The system of inspection is under the control of the Board of Health. The School Committee co-operates cordially in the work, by giving permission for inspectors to enter the school buildings and examine pupils, and by directing teachers to watch for cases of illness and to bring them to the notice of the inspectors."

TYPHOID FEVER EPIDEMIC AT COLUMBUS, O.

Mr. R. Winthrop Pratt, Engineer of the Ohio State Board of Health, has very kindly furnished us with the following notes of the recent epidemic in Columbus:

In the early part of the present year there occurred at Columbus a typhoid fever epidemic of considerable proportions. Out of the city's population of about 140,000, there were 1606 cases and 162 deaths during the months of January, February and March. The typhoid fever death rate previous to this time had never been as great as that of many other cities. This fact led many of the citizens, including several physicians, to believe that the water supply was quite safe, although sources of pollution were known to exist.

WATER SUPPLY.—Columbus is supplied with water from the following sources: 1st. The Scioto River; 2nd. Filter Gallery on the bank of the Scioto River. 3rd. Alum Creek, and 4th, wells driven along the bank of Alum Creek.

At the "West Side Pumping Station" water is pumped from the first two sources and supplied to the central or business part of the city as well as to the western and northern portions. About 11,000,000 gallons per day are supplied by this pumping station and the proportion drawn from the river direct depends upon the quantity available from the filter gallery. The latter is used when possible but is never able to furnish enough water for any considerable time so that the raw river water is almost always being pumped into the mains in greater or less amount.

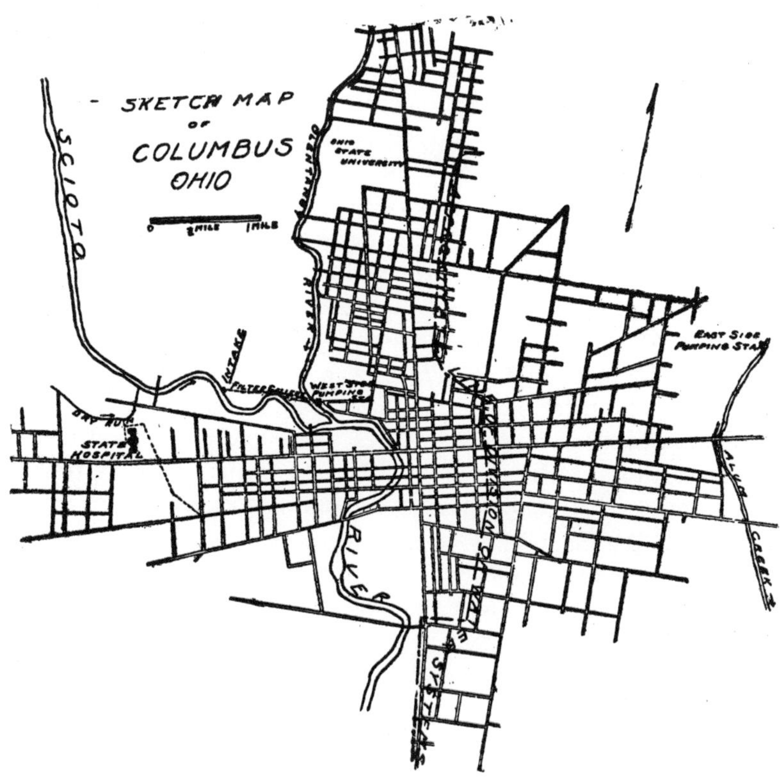

Just previous to the epidemic 3,000,000 to 4,000,000 gallons per day, out of the 11,000,000 pumped at the West Side Station, was raw river water.

At the "East Side Pumping Station" water from Alum Creek or from driven wells near by, depending upon the quantity available from the latter, is supplied to the eastern portion of the city. The quantity from this source is perhaps 75 per cent. of that furnished by the West Side Station.

The approximate dividing line betwen the districts supplied by the East Side and the West Side pumping stations is shown on the map.

DISTRIBUTION OF CASES. Almost without exception the typhoid fever cases occurred among the residents of the district supplied with Scioto River water or among the business men, who, though residing outside of this district, were supplied with Scioto River water at their offices. This fact proved that the water supply was the cause of the trouble and also showed that the Scioto River rather than Alum Creek was infected.

SOURCES OF POLLUTION OF THE SCIOTO RIVER. The watershed of the Scioto River above Columbus covers an area of 1070 square miles and consists principally of farm land, although several communities, acting as serious sources of pollution to the river water, are located upon it.

Within 65 miles of Columbus, 27 towns and four institutions exist upon the river or its tributaries, representing a population of about 43,000, while the sewers of six of the towns and three of the institutions discharge directly into the river or its tributaries, representing a population of about 30,000.

CAUSE. Although there are many places which might have infected the river water with typhoid bacilli, investigation has shown that by far the most probable cause of the epidemic was the State Hospital for Insane, one of the institutions mentioned, located within the city limits of Columbus.

The sewerage system at this hospital is rather unusual. The domestic sewage from the institution, which is occupied by some

1600 people, is collected in an 8-inch or 10-inch cast iron sewer laid within a 36-inch storm water sewer. A short distance away from the institution buildings the sanitary sewer leaves the storm sewer and connects with the city's sewerage system; but the storm sewer discharges into Dry Run, which is a small intermittent stream entering the Scioto River about a mile above the water works intake.

Shortly after the epidemic broke out an inspection showed that connections between the sanitary sewer and laterals, coming from various parts of the institution, were made in at least two cases by simply discharging the laterals into the big storm sewer and constructing a bulkhead immediately below the point of discharge, through which bulkhead the open end of the main sanitary sewer projected. Under these conditions, with every storm, the water collected by the storm sewer carried the accumulated filth from behind these bulkheads into Dry Run and thence to the river. Moreover one of the bulkheads was found to be broken, permitting some of the sewage to flow continuously into Dry Run. It was necessary to take twenty-two and a half tons of putrefying sludge out of the storm water sewer in order to clean it.

Twelve cases of typhoid fever had occurred at the institution one year previous to the epidemic, since which time there were no reported cases until January 3rd, 1904. The case reported on this date was soon followed by seven more, two of which died.

Typhoid fever had occurred to a greater or less extent at Kenton, the Girls Industrial Home, near Delaware, and at Arlington, all having sewers discharging into the river or its tributaries, and possibly at the Stone Quarries, a small settlement of unsanitary character 3 miles above the intake of the Columbus water works.

There is no doubt that the Insane Hospital discharged the greatest amount of sewage into the river with the exception of the cities of Kenton and Marion. Therefore, considering this as well as the proximity of the institution to the water works intake (one and one-half miles following Dry Run and the river), the extremely low stage of the river at this time, and the fact that there was typhoid fever at the institution at least ten days previous to the beginning of the rapid increase in the cases in Columbus, it seems fair to conclude that the principal factor in causing the epidemic, if not the sole cause, was the State Hospital.

MONTHLY RECORD OF CASES.

Month.	Cases Reported.	Deaths.	Annual Death Rate per 100,000
December, 1903	40	4	34
January, 1904	725	35	300
February, "	798	94	805
March, "	83	33	283

In April the reported number of cases and deaths were both much decreased.

DAILY RECORD OF CASES.

	Jan.	Feb.	Mar.		Jan.	Feb.	Mar.
1	1	138	9	17	2	19	2
2	0	52	4	18	24	25	2
3	0	29	1	19	48	22	1
4	1	28	4	20	24	27	0
5	8	26	5	21	44	4	4
6	3	48	3	22	35	21	0
7	3	16	7	23	41	8	0
8	7	74	2	24	16	15	0
9	4	34	1	25	43	19	2
10	1	26	3	26	25	14	4
11	5	19	5	27	48	5	0
12	9	15	2	28	35	2	2
13	26	36	1	29	47	4	2
14	34	12	2	30	81	.	2
15	43	36	2	31	23	.	1
16	47	13	4				

APRIL QUARTERLY MEETING

OF THE

Massachusetts Association of Boards of Health.

The quarterly meeting of the Association was held at the Brunswick Hotel, Boylston Street, Thursday, April 28th, 1904, the luncheon beginning at 1 P. M. Dr. H. P. Walcott presided.

THE CHAIRMAN: The Association will come to order. We will listen to the records of the last meeting.

(Records read by the Secretary, Mr. James B. Coffey.)

THE CHAIRMAN: Is there any change to be made in the record as read? If not, it will stand as the record of the last meeting of this Association. The Executive Committee, in accordance with your by-laws, report to the Association, with the recommendation that they be elected, the names of the following gentlemen:

George B. Robbins, Boston.
John A. Morgan, M. D., Hyde Park.
Stephen DeM. Gage, Lawrence.
William C. Doherty, Lowell.
Leonard Huntress, M. D., Lowell.
Joseph S. Hart, M. D., Lincoln.
Martin T. Field, Salem.
Caleb A. Page, Somerville.
Wesley R. Lee, M. D., Somerville.
Edward B. Hodskins, M. D., Springfield.
D. P. Cilley, M. D., Westboro.

THE CHAIRMAN: It is moved that these gentlemen be elected members of this Association. If that be your pleasure, you will signify it by saying aye.

THE CHAIRMAN: These gentlemen are duly elected members of the Association. Is there any incidental business to come before the Association at this time? If not, we will proceed to the regular programme of the afternoon. The first item is a paper on "Sanitary Dangers of Certain Occupations," by C. E. A. Winslow. I have the pleasure of presenting to the Association Mr. Winslow.

THE SANITARY DANGERS OF CERTAIN OCCUPATIONS.

BY C. E. A. WINSLOW, M. SC.
Mass. Inst. of Technology.

Sanitary authorities exist to protect the citizen against dangers which in his individual capacity he is unable to avoid. First, water supply, milk supply and food supply, must be safeguarded, since the life of every citizen depends upon these necessities. Second, the insidious spread of contagious diseases must be checked, since unrecognized cases of diphtheria or of small-pox menace the safety of all with whom they may come in contact. These two vehicles of disease, infected food and infected persons, threaten every individual in the community and rightly challenge the most ardent efforts of the sanitary engineer and the public hygienist. Of the less general dangers which affect only certain classes of individuals none can, I think, be more important than those connected with trades and occupations. The force of economic necessity too often makes it impossible for the factory operative to escape from the unsanitary conditions which surround him. He is helpless unless the State, or that matured public opinion of which the State is the expression, shall come to his aid. Therefore he has a special claim upon the consideration of such an association as our own.

Thanks to the admirable statistics collected by the Registrar-General of Great Britain, we have a pretty precise idea of the extent to which health may be affected by various trades and occupations. Dr. Tatham's figures, for example, show that the general death rate of Plumbers, Painters and Glaziers, and of Cotton and Linen manufacturers, is nearly twice, that of Potters, Earthenware manufacturers and File-makers is more than three times, that which obtains in the professional and agricultural classes. Unfortunately American vital statistics, both State and National, are so inaccurate and so incomplete that comparable data for this country are wanting. Such figures as we possess indicate the same startling discrepancies; and Dr. C. F. W. Doehring in the Bulletin of the U. S. Department of Labor for January, 1903, cites statistics for our own State according to which the average life of factory workers in Massachusetts is only 36.3 years against 65.3 for farmers.

The cause of excessive mortality varies widely in different occupations. Most prominent perhaps are those trades liable to accidents in the operation of machinery. English regulations class under four heads the mechanisms which prove most often dangerous, (a) Prime movers, (b) Mill-gearing and belts, (c) Machines for manufacturing purposes, (d) Hoists and other lifting tackle. Mules, looms, circular saws, planing machines and power presses all add their quota of victims. The manufacture of explosives should be placed under this head, with certain electrical processes in which the liberation of charges of high voltage may be the result of careless handling.

Of far greater importance, although less dramatically impressed upon the public mind, are the harmful effects of those occupations in which the worker is subjected to the breathing of excessive quantities of dust. The increase of tuberculosis and other pulmonary disorders due to this cause is unquestionably the gravest feature in the hygiene of occupations. Dust in various trades differs widely in character, but from the fine metallic particles produced in needle-making to the fragments of stone inhaled by quarrymen and the fine fibrous material which fills the air of a carding-room, all in varying degrees produce their bad effects. Dr. Doehring in the paper above cited gives a list of 38 injurious varieties of dust, and in Dr. Thomas Oliver's classic work on "Dangerous Trades," it is shown that in 19 different dusty industries the death rate from tuberculosis and other diseases of the respiratory system is more than twice that of the agricultural class. The rate among agriculturists being taken as 100, that of Potters and Earthenware manufacture is 453, that of Cutlers 407, that of File-makers 373, that of Glass-makers 335, etc. Less serious but yet appreciable is the danger from metallic dust to Miners, Iron and Steel workers, Gun-smiths and Needle-grinders—from stone dust to Masons, Stone-cutters and Cement-makers—from fibrous dust to Shoddy-makers, Rope-makers, Rag-pickers, Cotton and Woolen mill operatives, Carpet-makers, Flax and Hemp carders, and opera-tives in horsehair factories—from wood dust to Coopers and Carpenters—from flour dust to Millers, Bakers and Confec-tioners.

Next to dust, excessive temperature and moisture probably contribute most to make certain industries unhealthful. The effect of such conditions upon the general resistance of the or-ganism and particularly upon the vaso-motor system of heat regulation is well understood; and Laundry workers, Glass-blowers, Iron and Steel workers and the operatives in wet spin-ning rooms pay a heavy tribute of deaths from tuberculosis and other pulmonary disorders in which these form a predisposing cause.

Another important series of industrial disorders are the intox-ications due to the introduction into the system of certain metal-lic poisons. Plumbism is the familiar example of this class. If deaths from lead poisoning among all occupied males be taken **as one, the comparative mortality in England is, among** Lead workers, 211; among File-makers, 75; among Plumbers, 21; among Painters and Glaziers, 18; among Potters, 17; among Glass-makers, 12, while Copper-workers, Coach-makers, Gasfitters, Locksmiths, Calico printers, Enamellers, Solderers, Type founders and others suffer to a lesser degree. Mercury poisoning occurs among the makers of thermometers and other physical instruments, the makers of incandescent electric light bulbs and other electrical supplies, and in certain more restricted industries. Cases of arsenical poisoning, though becoming year-ly more and more rare, are not entirely abolished. Copper and zinc poisoning are not unknown; and chromium sometimes affects workmen in bichromate works and those who use dyes containing this metal.

Still another group of diseases are caused by the fumes of various non-metallic chemical substances. Carbon bisulphide as used in certain processes for treating india rubber and gutta-percha produces severe hysteria and exhaustion. Strong acids and alkalies sometimes overcome the workmen engaged in their manufacture. Benzine, as used in cleansing, and certain other commercial spirits, more rarely cause toxic effects. Here, too, we may mention the manufacture of fertilizer, rendering, bone-boiling, tanning and other industries accompanied by the production of noxious odors of decomposition which slowly undermine the general vitality.

Finally, as a last class of occupation diseases, there are certain bacterial maladies which under unusual conditions may be transmitted by trade materials. Cases of typhoid infection among laundry workers are so common as to warrant their inclusion under this head. Anthrax affecting wool-sorters and the handlers of hides is a typical case in point; and those vocations which bring men much in contact with the lower animals lead, though rarely, to infection with glanders, foot-and-mouth disease and other disorders.

In looking over this list of the dangers to operatives from accident, from dust, from heat and humidity, from metallic poisons, from noxious fumes and from infectious diseases, it seems obvious that most of them are preventable and thus legitimately within the field of sanitary science. The fencing of machinery, with proper regulations as to its operation—the removal of dust by special ventilation and the substitution of processes in which no excessive amount of it is formed—the regulation of humidity and temperature, the government of lead and other chemical factories by such rules as shall prevent the ingestion of poisonous substances, are all practical preventive measures. The problems, however, are various and complex, and each industry requires detailed study and specific treatment. So in England, the country which first took the lead in factory legislation, we find a maze of statutes under the general heading of Mines and Factory Acts, which have gradually grown up year by year to meet the exigencies of individual cases. Beginning in 1802 with an act for preserving the "health and morals" of apprentices in cotton mills, various statutes provided for general sanitary conditions, and in 1883 a bill for the government of white lead works recognized the principle of special regulations for particular trades, a principle extended by the Act of 1891, so that such rules can be drawn up by the Factory Inspectorate for any industry certified as dangerous by the Secretary of State. A similar development has taken place in Germany, where factories must receive authorization dependent on compliance with elaborate rules as to general ventilation, removal of dust and fumes, temperature, lighting, proper rooms for meals, lavatories and cloak rooms, water-supply, protection from accidents, and exclusion of women and children from dangerous and exhausting processes. The special trades for which regulations have been drawn up in England and Germany are shown in the appended table, taken from Oliver.

INDUSTRIES FOR WHICH SPECIAL RULES HAVE BEEN ENACTED.

ENGLAND.

1 Bichromate works
2 Bottling of aerated water
3 Brass and alloy mixing and casting
4 Bricks, glazing of, by lead
5 Chemical works
6 Earthenware and china
7 Enameling of iron plates
8 Electric accumulator works
9 Explosive works in which dinitro-benzole is used
10 Flax spinning and weaving
11 Lead (red and orange) works
12 Lead (white) works
13 Lead (yellow) works
14 Lead smelting works
15 Lead, yellow chromate of
16 Lucifer match factories
17 Paint and color works, and extraction of arsenic
18 Skins and hides, sorting
19 Tinning and enameling of metal ware
20 Tinning and enameling of iron hollow ware
21 Transfers (lithographic) for decoration of china, etc.
22 Vulcanizing of india rubber
23 Wool sorting
24 Wool combing

GERMANY.

1 Basic slag works
2 Bichromate works
3 Brick works
4 Brushmaking works and horsehair spinning
5 Cigar factories
6 Chicory works
7 Electric accumulator works
8 Glassworks
9 Hackling and preparing rooms in textile factories
10 Lead, color and acetate of lead works
11 Letterpress printing works
12 Lucifer match works
13 Sugar refineries
14 Vulcanizing of india rubber
15 Wire-drawing mills

Less elaborate systems of factory legislation are in force in France, Austria, Belgium, Holland, Sweden, Switzerland and other European countries. It is, however, significant to note that the two nations which have advanced farthest along this path are the two leading commercial powers of the Old World, and that one of them at least owes its ever increasing pre-eminence to the general application of the broad scientific principles of economy of force upon which such legislation is founded.

Turning to the United States we find the regulation of dangerous trades in a primitive and undeveloped state. We lack even statistical information as to the extent of occupation diseases; we wholly lack scientific study of existing factory conditions. In our State of Massachusetts there is indeed a Department of Inspection of Factories and Public Buildings under the Chief of the District Police, but the officials of this department, however able and efficient, cannot properly solve such complex problems as those of factory sanitation without special expert assistance. Chapters 104 and 106 of the Revised Laws, under which for the most part they work, contain several admirable general principles. It is provided, for example, in Section 51, Chapter 106, that "a factory in which five or more persons are employed shall, while work is carried on, be so ventilated that the air shall not become so impure as to be injurious to the health of the persons employed therein, and so that all gases, vapors, dust or other impurities injurious to health, which are generated in the course of the manufacturing process or handicraft carried on therein shall, so far as practicable, be rendered harmless." This is good so far as it goes. It does not apply, however, to small factories or to workshops where men only are employed. It gives no power to deal with such special evils as lead or arsenic poisoning. Even with respect to ventilation general provisions are useless unless applied in the form of such detailed and specific regulations as can be drawn up only by expert sanitary authorities.

The backwardness of factory legislation in this country is no doubt in part due to the fact that we have never had the gross evils which elsewhere become so patent as to demand drastic measures for their redress. Evils exist, however, and though less obvious than those which caused Sir John Simon to speak of "the canker of industrial disease" gnawing at the root of England's national strength, it is high time that we gave them some attention. From the figures in the Census of 1900 I find that there were 127,000 persons in Massachusetts engaged in trades shown by investigation in other countries to be more or less prejudicial to health, including 38,642 foundry and machine shop workers, 26,211 house and sign painters, 17,696 brick and stone masons, and 8112 plumbers and gas and steam fitters. In the more intensely dangerous trades we find 2395 cutlers, 289 emery wheel workers, 89 file makers, 264 grinders of kaolin and other earths, 270 operatives in needle and pin factories, 758 persons engaged in the making of pottery, terra cotta and fire-clay products, and 449 workers in shoddy mills. Judging from analogy it seems probable that the unregulated conduct of these industries and certain others is causing a constant drain upon the health of the community; and in spite of the absence of good vital statistics or scientific factory inspection specific instances every now and then attract our notice. The spread of the disease, Anthrax, in Lynn from a morocco worker who had handled infected hides, was noted in the newspapers only a few weeks ago. The death rate from consumption in Massachusetts according to the United States Census of 1900 was 2.5 among all males, 3.7 among marble and stone cutters and 4.1 among masons; and Dr. T. J. Dion of the Quincy Board of Health writes me that the excessive prevalence of tuberculosis among the stone cutters in that city is a well known fact. In Chester is a factory of which Dr. C. J. Shepardson, a leading local physician, says, "We have a mill in town where quartz or silex is reduced to sandpaper, etc., which has been responsible for a great many deaths. Not much work is done there, however, and I think the force of employees is kept so low that the law as it now exists is not applicable to the place."

At East Douglas is an axe factory, in relation to which Dr.

Titus P. Holbrook allows me to quote the following statement: "I have been in practice in East Douglas since 1863 with the exception of some thirteen years following 1872. I have seen quite a number of cases of so-called grinders' consumption. I have examined one case post mortem. I found the smaller bronchial tubes thoroughly filled with the grindstone grit; the lung in the lower part looked like and felt like the liver after cooking. The symptoms are excessive dyspnœa on slight exertion, dry cough and great prostration. The grinders are from the Polanders and Finns for the past dozen years. The disease takes hold of them more frequently, and is more rapidly fatal than among the grinders of former years and of other nationalities. When I came here 40 years ago I found the victims among the Yankees who had ground some 20 years before. Those would grind 18 or 20 years before having to give up work. The French Canadians were then grinding. They could work 12 to 16 years. They became frightened off, and the Swedes took up the work. They would get the disease in 8 or 10 years. Now the Finns and Polanders are at it, and they last only 3 to 5 years, and the disease is more common among them."

It is not surprising to find on an examination of Massachusetts Registration Reports that while the death rate from consumption for the period 1881-99 was 2.5 for the whole State, it was 3.4 for the town of Douglas.

Nearer home I visited within a month a twine mill not five miles from where we are gathered at this moment. I wish I could take you through that factory and show you the dry spinning room with its clear normal air, the carding room filled with clouds of fine choking dust and the wet spinning room with the hot damp deadly atmosphere of a tropical forest. In the first department you would see average healthy factory workers alert and cheerful; in the last two, the women and children, some of them palpably under age, with dull eyes and feverish cheeks, stand or sit listlessly by their machines, stolidly going through the mechanical routine which brings them daily nearer to the inevitable end. The factory inspector had made his visit a few days before mine; but being neither a medical man familiar with the symptoms of tuberculosis, nor a sanitary engineer, versed in the laws of ventilation, he found no fault except to suggest that the few insufficient ventilating fans which had been installed should be put in operation. When I went through the factory some of them were running and some were not; and as the superintendent told me of the admirable quality of twine he was turning out I could not but feel that the cost as paid in human lives was far too high.

These are isolated cases only. Granted. Yet I believe that in the discussion this afternoon the members of this Association may add many more from their own experience. We have already enough in my judgment to warrant us at least in looking further. We need exact knowledge of conditions here in Massachusetts. We want the State census of 1905 so planned as to furnish statistics of occupation mortality which shall be full and accurate. We want the Legislature to appropriate money for a special investigation of the risks and dangers of factory life by the State Board of Health, which, having solved the fundamental problems of water supply and sewage disposal, should be our pioneer in these new fields. With the facts once in hand, the members of this Association will not be slow to apply the needful remedies. It is the pride of sanitary science that it is founded on the unchanging rock of Nature's laws. Yet we study the world as it is only to make it better; and I believe that the informing motive of our profession, whether we are conscious of it or not, is a deep-rooted enthusiasm for the progress of that humanity which in such diverse individuals is so mysteriously one. These twin impulses, the love of truth and the love of man, are together irresistible, both should impel us to remove the cruel conditions which make it necessary for even one individual to barter the health of tomorrow for the livelihood of to-day.

The Chairman: Mr. Winslow's very interesting paper is before you for discussion. I hope it may give rise to questions and to additional information.

DR. BECKWITH: I would like to ask if the reader of the paper or any one else knows whether people working in celluloid factories have their health impaired. I have seen two or three cases in which there has been a great loss of strength and weight, and also some impairment of the kidney function. In fact, I have found two or three cases where there was a good deal of albumen in the urine, and it has seemed to me as though there was something in the process of making celluloid that perhaps caused this.

THE CHAIRMAN: Have you come across that, Mr. Winslow?

MR. WINSLOW: I have not.

THE CHAIRMAN: Dr. Abbott, I think you might say something to the point.

DR. ABBOTT: The reader of the paper has covered the ground so fully that I have but little to add to what he has said, except to amplify one or two points. I will answer the last speaker, in regard to celluloid, that I visited a celluloid factory in the village of Zylonite, part of the town of Adams, some years ago—I think it is not in existence now—and went through the whole factory, noting the different processes. It seemed to me that the principal danger there, aside from the tremendous danger of fire, was that of breathing the spirits of camphor. I understood the superintendent of the factory to say that occasional cases of headache and some irritation of the throat were about all that really were to be feared. The fact is, as the reader said, we do very little about this subject in this country in consequence of the want of information upon the subject. Any sanitary body has to have, of course, information first, and then it can go ahead with prevention afterwards. The information is almost all foreign. The laws in Massachusetts put this whole work in charge of the district police, but the district police— perhaps through want of funds—have not, as they have in other countries, any efficient and intelligent medical authority under their control to supervise the work; so that the laws which have been framed at their instance have been mostly laws in regard to ventilation, plumbing, etc., which, of course, are important, but there is not much of anything upon other points. The general term "sanitary" appears in those laws, but that term needs to be more specifically defined, in order to amount to anything. The occupations which the reader has spoken of as most dangerous to health are those which have to do with the metallic poisons, lead, arsenic and corrosive sublimate, also the poison of phosphorus which is involved in the trade of match making, and the dust producing occupations. Then another occupation which is a source of danger is that of persons who are exposed to alcoholic excess—that is, bartenders and saloon-keepers. Every life insurance man knows very well that a bartender or saloon-keeper will not be taken as a risk except under restricted limitations.

Some years ago I visited a paper mill in Maine, where I was surprised to see that the people were far better protected than in any mill I have ever seen in this State. That was Mr. Warren's mill, the Cumberland Mill.

THE CHAIRMAN: He was a Massachusetts man.

DR. ABBOTT: Yes, sir. The fact is, in the paper mills there are two classes of people, one class which is exposed to danger and one class which is not. The first class comprises persons who take the rags and dust them. The dusting men, perhaps, first of all, and then the women who sort the rags in the mill, are constantly exposed to danger from dust. Also, as Dr. Withington found in an inquiry made for our board some fifteen years ago, there is the exposure to small-pox, which is not so great as it used to be since greater precautions are taken in paper mills with reference to the vaccination of employees.

In the sorting room of Mr. Warren's mill where the women sort the rags, every person has in front of her a machine, or a part of a ventilating apparatus, which is connected with a general shaft running through the room by which all the dust is taken away from the mouths and faces of the operators and deposited in a shaft outside the building. The other class in the paper mills that handle the finished paper after it has been through the various processes are not exposed to any danger whatever. The clean paper has been thoroughly disinfected by the processes to which the rags have been subjected.

With regard to arsenic, I can say this. I visited some ten years ago a mill in this State where 200 pounds of paris green were then made annually. The complaint then had nothing to do with the operatives, but it came from the people outside who were afraid of the arsenic being distributed around the surrounding region for a quarter of a mile. One farmer allowed his whole crop of hay to rot on the ground for fear his cows would be poisoned by eating it. But the condition of the operatives in that mill surprised me. Almost every man in that establishment had sores upon the face, eyes, nose, ears, mouth, hands and other parts of the body, due to the neglect of the greatest of all laws, the law of cleanliness—absolute cleanliness—which has more to do with this subject than anything else. People handle these metallic poisons and then take their lunch without washing—that is where the trouble very largely comes from, handling poisons and then contributing those poisons to the food every day, right along, day after day. I have seen the same thing in other factories of similar nature.

The figures, it has been said, are unreliable in this country. There are no figures in this country upon this subject that really amount to anything except, perhaps, those of some of the great industrial insurance companies. One reason for this unreliability is this. In this State the statistics on this subject were begun in 1842, and were continued for nearly forty years. They were published in the registration reports for all that time, but they gave the average age at death, which does not amount to anything. It has no significance whatever upon the subject. Let me illustrate. A major general dies at seventy years of age, we will say, as a general rule, and a lieutenant dies at perhaps thirty or forty years of age. Is that of any value to show that the position of a major general is any more healthful than that of a lieutenant? Not one bit. It is a question of age. In an old ladies' home the average age at death is seventy; in an infants' asylum it is two. Is one for this reason to be considered any more healthful than the other? Not a bit. These figures were on a wrong basis. When we can get down to the proper basis of comparing the deaths in each industry at certain ages with the living at similar ages we shall have something to rely upon.

PROF. SEDGWICK: In view of the paper which has been read and the fact that members of this Association are stationed as sanitary pickets, as it were, all over the State, I hope that any one within whose knowledge there may come information regarding cases of damage to health due to special occupations will be kind enough to communicate with Mr. Winslow and inform him of the fact. And in view of the statements which have been made by the secretary of the State Board of Health that we lack authentic information even in this State, which is noted for its leadership in sanitary science, I would like to suggest the passage of a resolution requesting the Legislature to set in motion some machinery looking toward the gathering of accurate information. It so happens that this is a very good time to do this, inasmuch as there is a committee of the Legislature now considering just such questions, namely, the Committee on Relations of Employers to Employees. With this idea in mind I am going to submit for your consideration, and if possible for your adoption, the following resolutions which, if they should come with the authority of this Association, might, I believe, do a real good at the present juncture in bringing about legislation looking towards the end desired. I should like to move, Mr. President, that this Association adopt, and through its secretary forward to the proper persons, the following resolutions:

"Whereas, investigations in other countries have shown that certain trades and industries, when conducted without due sanitary supervision and regulation, are injurious to the health of the operatives employed; and

"Whereas, exact information is lacking with regard to the extent of such evils, if any, in Massachusetts, be it

"Resolved, That the Massachusetts Association of Boards of Health, in Boston assembled, April 28, 1904, respectfully urge the General Court to direct the State Board of Health, with such aid as it may require from the chief of the District Police and the Bureau of Statistics of Labor, to investigate and report upon the sanitary conditions of factories, workshops and other places of employment in the Commonwealth of Massachusetts, with respect to all conditions which may endanger the life and limbs or be prejudicial to the health of persons employed therein."

THE CHAIRMAN: You have heard the resolution introduced by Prof. Sedgwick. What is the pleasure of the Association with regard to them?

DR. SMITH: It seems to me better that this Association should not undertake to get information concerning the dangers to life and limb of employees. It seems to me we have got enough to do to give our attention to unsanitary conditions and to those conditions which lead to certain diseases, and I would move an amendment, that that particular phrase be stricken out.

PROF. SEDGWICK: I am willing to accept that amendment, Mr. President.

THE CHAIRMAN: Do I understand that it is the pleasure of the mover of the resolution to so amend it that it shall read, "all conditions which may endanger the life or be prejudicial to the health of persons employed therein?"

PROF. SEDGWICK: I think Dr. Smith wished to omit "life and limb" both.

THE CHAIRMAN: "With respect to all conditions which may be prejudicial to the health of persons employed therein." I understand that is the form you are now willing to leave it?

PROF. SEDGWICK: Yes.

THE CHAIRMAN: The essential part of the resolutions then will now read, "to investigate and report upon the sanitary conditions of factories, workshops and other places of employment in the Commonwealth of Massachusetts with respect to all conditions which may be prejudicial to the health of persons employed therein." It is moved and seconded that these resolutions be adopted.

DR. MILLER: I was going to suggest that we leave in that word "life." I think it is important to have it in there—"life and health."

DR. SMITH: I simply made the suggestion to narrow down the inquiry to matters of sanitation. If the Association intends to go into the question of accidents it seems to me that is somewhat beyond our scope. It belongs to an entirely different body —to a body of engineers—to determine the conditions that endanger the limbs of persons, and not an association of this kind. The two functions, it seems to me, are quite distinct. While I think that we should certainly support these resolutions, as being of very great importance, it seems to me that what I suggest is much simpler than the broader statement that is contained in the original draft. All conditions that militate against the health of individuals may in the long run affect life of individuals. It seems to me the two terms, health and life, are more or less synonymous.

THE CHAIRMAN: What is your pleasure with regard to these resolutions? It is moved that they be adopted. If that be your pleasure you will signify it by saying aye.

(The motion was carried.)

THE CHAIRMAN: It seems to be the unanimous sense of this Association. The next paper upon our programme is by Dr. S. J. Russell, city physician of Springfield, on "Trichinosis."

(EDITOR'S NOTE.—Dr. Russell's paper, describing certain cases of Trichinosis, was read, but was not submitted for publication in time for use in this issue.)

THE CHAIRMAN: Dr. Russell's paper is before you for discussion.

DR. CHAPIN: I should like to ask one or two questions. Was this animal fed on offal?

DR. RUSSELL: It was fed on offal from the city of Springfield.

DR. CHAPIN: Then I want to know whether all the pork was from one animal, and also how the pork was cooked that caused the trichinosis.

DR. RUSSELL: On the first examination I questioned the patients about the pork. They said they had eaten very little, and it was well cooked. I forgot to state that the blood examinations, made in every case, showed an increase of eosinophiles, ranging from sixteen to sixty per cent.

DR. CHAPIN: Did you find on further investigation that the pork they had eaten was cooked a long time in the ordinary manner, like roast pork or friend ham or boiled ham—just how was it cooked?

DR. RUSSELL: I found that some of the pork was in the form of sausages which were eaten raw, but they claimed that most of the pork was very well cooked. Some ate raw pork and others ate the sausages raw.

DR. CHAPIN: Was it your opinion that some of them ate only the well cooked pork, or do you think all of those that were affected ate pork which was practically raw?

DR. RUSSELL: I think most of the pork was under-done.

DR. CHAPIN: Was there more than one animal infected?

DR. RUSSELL: Just one.

DR. CHAPIN: Did any other people eat of that who were not taken sick?

DR. RUSSELL: There were a few who ate a very little of it and were not taken sick.

Dr. Smith: This disease, while it seems to be comparatively rare in our own country, is yet more prevalent than is generally supposed. It is probable that mild cases occur, which are diagnosed as something other than trichinosis, and the true facts in the case are not discovered unless the body of the person should reach the dissecting room, and there the trichinosis may be found. Dr. Williams of Buffalo has made a rather careful study of the prevalence of trichinosis in our country, and he found that not less than five per cent. of the bodies that were examined contained trichinæ. This would indicate that the infection is commoner than we suppose, but that the dose is also less than that which people consume who eat meat raw. In Europe, as probably most of you remember, the outbreaks were at one time very extensive. The manner of the meat distribution there is so different from that which subsists in this country that outbreaks are traced more easily to their source. In the smaller towns and villages the animals that are slaughtered are consumed on the spot, so that a single pig may reach a large number of consumers, and epidemics in which hundreds of people have been involved, and in which the mortality has been relatively very high have been traced to single pigs. With reference to the cooking of meat, it is probable that now and then large masses of meat, although apparently well cooked on the surface, still retain living trichinæ near the bones. A few years ago my attention was called to some cases of trichinosis in one of our charitable institutions in the State. So far as was known at that time, the meat was thoroughly cooked. All precautions were being taken, and yet unquestioned cases of trichinosis occurred in this institution. The hogs were examined by removing small bits of tissue with a harpoon, and I think in over half of the cases trichinæ were found. Hence it may occur that infection with trichinæ will take place in families where pork is usually very well prepared, but where certain portions of it have not been subjected to the heat necessary to kill the trichinæ, where in other words the pork is underdone. This may account for the five per cent. of cases which have been found in the dissecting room and at autopsies by Dr. Williams. Of course the remedy is in all cases to thoroughly cook the pork. In fact, that is probably the the only remedy, unless the industry of raising hogs should be completely changed, and that of course would greatly augment the price of this kind of meat. Trichinosis in this country was practically unknown until the habit of certain foreigners of eating meat underdone or raw was brought with them. In France the disease is practically unknown, because the people cook all their meat, though, so far as we know, the statistics of the examination of pork show that the pigs in France are no less infected than in other countries. Practically the only remedy we have is to instruct the people to cook the meat as thoroughly as possible.

The Chairman: If there is nothing else to be said upon this subject, we will proceed to the next paper on the programme, "The Transmission of Infection by means of Footwear," by Dr. Francis P. Denny and Mr. J. Albert C. Nyhen of Brookline.

THE TRANSMISSION OF INFECTION BY MEANS OF FOOTWEAR.

BY DR. FRANCIS P. DENNY AND MR. J. ALBERT C. NYHEN
Brookline Board of Health Laboratory.

The experiments which are here reported were carried out by the writers in the Brookline Board of Health Laboratory, with the object of determining in a general way how readily infectious material will adhere to shoes, and how long and how far it will be carried in that way.

These experiments, which have been of a very simple nature, have consisted chiefly in putting some growth of the Bacillus prodigiosus (a red-pigment-producing non-pathogenic organism) on various parts of our shoes before going out from the laboratory to attend to our regular duties. On returning to the laboratory after varying intervals of time, each part of the shoe which had been infected was thoroughly rubbed with a moist cotton swab, and then the swab was rinsed in a tube of melted gelatine, which was then plated. The bacilli, if recovered from the shoes, appeared in the plates as characteristic red liquefying colonies.

The parts of the shoes which were inoculated were the under surface of the sole and heel, the lower edge of the side of the sole, the instep, and a few tests were made by inoculating some of the small holes in the O'Sullivan rubber heels. When entering the laboratory on our return, care was taken to avoid having the parts of the shoe which we had inoculated come in contact with the floor, which might have become infected with B. prodigiosus from some of the earlier experiments. In a number of control plates made from the parts of the shoes which had not been inoculated, B. prodigiosus was never found.

The tests were made during all the different seasons and under very varying conditions of weather and temperature. The amount of walking that was done while the bacilli were on the shoes varied considerably, but was usually more than that of the average physician for the same length of time.

The total number of tests made was 126. The results are given in the following table:

Duration of Tests.	Sole +	Sole −	Heel +	Heel −	Instep +	Instep −	Side Sole +	Side Sole −	Rubber Heels +	Rubber Heels −	Rubber O'rshoes +	Rubber O'rshoes −
½ hour	1	1	1	.	.	.	.	.	.	.	.	.
1 "	5	13	5	7	.	1	2	.	.	.	2	2
1½ "	4	5	4	1	1	1	.	.	.	.	.	.
2 "	3	3	2	1	.	1	1	.	.	.	.	.
3 "	1	3	1	1	3	1	.	.	.	.	.	6
4 "	.	.	.	.	3	.	4	.	.	2	.	.
5 "	.	.	.	.	1	.	.	.	.	.	.	.
6–8 hours	.	2	.	.	.	2	.	.	.	.	.	.
8 to 12 "	.	2	.	1	2	.	2	.	4	1	.	.
24 "	.	1	.	.	2	1	2	1	.	.	.	.
48 "	.	.	.	.	1	1	.	1	.	.	.	.
72 "	.	.	.	.	1	1	.	2	.	.	.	.
5 days	.	.	.	.	.	1	.	.	.	.	.	.
8 "	.	.	.	.	1	.	.	.	.	.	.	.
9 "	.	.	.	.	.	1	.	.	.	.	.	.
	14	30	13	11	15	11	11	4	4	3	2	8

Some of these data may be summarized as follows:

In thirty-seven tests where the *soles* were inoculated and where plates were made after intervals varying from one to three hours, the bacilli were found in thirteen (35 per cent.)

In twenty-two tests with the bacilli on the *heels* for a similar length of time, the plates were positive in twelve (55 per cent.) This would seem to show that bacteria will remain longer on the heel than on the sole, although the number of tests made is rather small to justify that conclusion.

In twenty-six tests where the *instep* was inoculated and plates were made after intervals varying from one hour to nine days, the results were positive in fifteen (58 per cent.)

In fifteen tests with the bacilli on the lower edge of the *side of the sole*, eleven were positive after intervals varying from one to seventy-two hours (73 per cent.)

As was to be expected, we found that the bacilli remained on the side of the sole and the instep for a much longer time than on the sole or heel. In ordinary walking on the sidewalks there is very little friction on the instep and the side of the sole. In some of the tests we could actually see for several days the growth which we had put on the instep. On the contrary, cross-country walking will very quickly remove any material from the instep or the side of the sole.

In seven tests where the *holes in the rubber heels* were inoculated, four were positive after intervals of four to nine hours.

Ten tests were made with the bacilli on the soles and the heels of *rubber overshoes* which were worn when there was snow on the ground. Of four tests with a one hour interval, two were positive and two negative. Of six with a three hour interval, all were negative.

With the exceptions about to be mentioned, the bacilli used in these tests were from fresh blood serum cultures. Eight of the tests were made using bacilli, which had been dried and pulverized. The powdered bacilli were put on a sheet of paper on the floor, and the foot was pressed over them. Six of the eight tests were positive after intervals of one to one and one-half hours.

Six tests were made using mucus, in which some growth of B. prodigiosus had been mixed; three were positive and three negative.

It seems probable that the bacilli actually persisted on the shoes in a much larger proportion of cases than would appear from our results, for many conditions were present to prevent all the bacilli appearing in the plates. Thus, all the bacilli were not necessarily removed from the shoe by the cotton swab, and probably all the bacilli removed on the swab were not washed out by the melted gelatine. Furthermore, some of the bacilli were doubtless overgrown by other bacteria, especially by some very abundant forms which rapidly liquefied gelatine.

These experiments having shown that footwear experimentally infected with bacilli will carry the infection to a distance, it remains to consider: (1.) under what conditions are shoes likely to become infected; (2.) what is the danger of the transmission of disease by the feet; (3.) what precautions should be taken to prevent the transmission of disease in this way.

INFECTION OF THE FEET IN THE VICINITY OF CASES OF CONTAGIOUS DISEASE.

It is certain that the floor of a room occupied by a contagious case becomes infected. Flugge* and others have shown that fine bits of secretion are given off as a spray in the act of coughing, sneezing and loud talking. These droplets disperse themselves to varying distances from the patient, and then sink onto the floor and other surfaces. Fine particles of epidermis from persons desquamating also find their way to the floor. In unmodified smallpox some of the many thousand scabs given off from each patient during desquamation are sure to drop on the floor despite the watchfulness of the attendants. If one looks carefully, one can actually see these scabs on the floor about the bed of a smallpox patient who is at the height of desquamation. What is true of such gross particles will be equally true of the smaller particles of epidermis in scarlet fever and others of the exanthemata.

---

*Deutsch. med. Wochen. Oct. 14, 1897, p. 665.

From the results of our experiments, it is certain that a person walking over an infected floor may carry off some of the infectious material on his shoes. One of the writers found a scab clinging to the foot of a patient in a small-pox hospital, and also on the sole of a rubber overshoe, which he himself was wearing in visiting the hospital. Wright and Emerson* found diphtheria bacilli on the soles of the shoes of three nurses in the diphtheria ward of the Boston City Hospital.

It is often possible for a physician to visit a contagious case without coming in contact with any infected objects, except with his hands in examining the patient, and with the soles of the shoes on the floor. The hands are always disinfected on leaving the patient, but the feet are usually neglected.

Is it necessary or desirable that precautions should be taken by physicians and others visiting a contagious case, to guard against carrying away infection on the feet? In many instances we believe it is unnecessary, for the reason that while it is possible for pathogenic organisms to be carried from the room on the feet, there is comparatively small chance for the infection to pass from the floors to which it has been carried to the mucous membranes of susceptible persons.

Under the following conditions it seems to us important that precautions should be taken:

(1.) *In the more serious contagious diseases,* and those which from the point of view of the public health are especially important; for example, small-pox, plague and foot-and-mouth disease.

(2.) *Under any circumstances, where it is considered necessary to have a strict quarantine;* for example, if it is considered necessary to keep a sheet wet with a disinfectant at the door of the patient's room, then certainly care should be taken to prevent infection being carried out on the feet of those leaving the room.

(3.) In scarlet fever and diphtheria, where a physician or other person is going very directly from a contagious case to rooms or nurseries where there are small children who play on the floor.

---

*Centralblatt fuer Bakteriologie. 1894. XVI. p. 112.

(4.) *In contagious hospitals.* In a hospital where a large number of contagious cases are collected together, the floors must be very thoroughly infected, and if persons are passing back and forth from one part of the hospital to another, for example, from the scarlet fever to the diphtheria side, without taking any precautions with their feet, there is great opportunity for the transmission of the contagion. It is not necessary that persons should actually pass from one side of the hospital to another, in order to have the infection transmitted by the feet. This may take place if the attendants from different sides use any rooms or corridors in common. In some contagious hospitals, which are considered models of their kind, the nurses from different departments use dining rooms and other rooms in common. It seems to us very important that in the construction of a contagious hospital provision should be made for the complete separation of the nurses caring for the different diseases.

PRECAUTIONS TO GUARD AGAINST CARRYING INFECTION ON THE FEET FROM ROOMS OCCUPIED BY CONTAGIOUS CASES.

On leaving the room the soles of the shoes may be immersed in a disinfectant, or the sole may be thoroughly wiped with a towel or cloth wet with a disinfectant. Rubber overshoes afford a very convenient and satisfactory method of protecting the shoes from infection as they may be put on before entering the sick room or hospital and taken off on leaving. They are easily disinfected themselves by immersion in a disinfectant solution. The nurse who is taking care of a patient isolated at home may put on rubber overshoes in passing through the house on going out for her daily exercise.

INFECTION OF FOOTWEAR FROM SPUTUM.

The habit of spitting on the sidewalk and floors of public places is still very common. On almost every sidewalk which is much used one can see sputum at intervals of only a few yards.

Mucus adheres readily to the sole of the shoe, and if a person steps on fresh sputum it may cling to the edge of the sole or low instep, and so be carried for a long time. It is not necessary here to speak of the dangers from sputum. It is well to remember that besides tubercle bacilli, other pathogenic bacteria may be present, for example, the influenza bacilli, pneumococci, and the diphtheria bacilli.

It is certain that any bacteria which are on the sidewalks may be carried to the floors of our own houses. In this way persons of refinement are exposed to disease through the filthy habits of others. To protect the public, therefore, spitting on the sidewalk should be an offence punishable by law, and this law should be enforced. It is our belief that footwear plays an important part in the dissemination of the tubercle bacillus.

INFECTION OF THE FEET FROM FECAL MATTER AND URINE.

Shoes may become contaminated in fields and gardens with fecal matter used as fertilizer and also in alleys and other more or less secluded places. Fecal matter is very likely to become adherent to the instep where it will be carried for a long time. The chief danger of fecal contamination is from typhoid bacilli.

The work of Richardson* and others has shown that typhoid bacilli in large numbers are often present in the urine in typhoid fever, and that they persist for a long time—months and sometimes years after recovery. Persons urinate out of doors much more frequently than they defecate and often in places where persons walk. The soles of the shoes may become contaminated with urine, and especially with soil saturated with urine.

If typhoid bacilli are brought into houses in material on the shoes, they may then be carried to articles of food by means of flies.

In military camps the feet probably play an important part in the spread of typhoid fever. If from lack of discipline or the indifference of the commanding officers, the men do not always use the sinks, the excreta (urine and feces) may become thoroughly disseminated in the camp by the soldiers' feet.

---

*Journal of Experimental Medicine. Vol. iii. No. 3. 1898.

The report of the committee* appointed to investigate the prevalence of typhoid fever in the camps during the Spanish War calls attention to this means of spreading the disease. The conditions of camp life, and especially the exposure of food to flies, are very favorable for the transmission of typhoid in this way.

FOOTWEAR IN THE TRANSMISSION OF ANIMAL DISEASES.

Feet probably play an important part in the transmission of animal diseases. The floors of barns and stables are sure to become contaminated with excreta, which is carried about on the shoes of the men and on the feet of the animals. If pathogenic organisms are in the excreta or on the floor, the animals' fodder is likely to become contaminated, as hay and ensilage are often walked over and tossed about on the floors.

Veterinarians and other visiting barns infected with foot-and-mouth disease should take special precautions to avoid carrying the infection on their shoes to other herds.

The point which we wish to emphasize most is the importance of footwear in disseminating tubercle bacilli. There is a great deal of sputum on our sidewalks, much of it is tubercular. We are carrying it about on our shoes and into our homes. The prevention of spitting on surfaces where people walk should receive the attention of all who are engaged in public health work.

THE CHAIRMAN: Before proceeding to the discussion of this paper I should like to call the attention of the Association to the fact that at the time of our annual summer outing with the authorities of the city of Boston in Boston Harbor—I may say one of the most agreeable occasions of the year—the laboratory of the State Board of Health for the preparation of vaccine matter and anti-toxin will be in operation. The building is externally complete, and will be occupied probably in June, so that in July we shall be able to show the members of the Association the establishment in actual operation. The building is at Forest Hills,

---

*Vaughan ; Boston Medical and Surgical Journal. May 18, 1899. p. 480.

within 10 minutes of the South Station by the quick trains of the New York, New Haven & Hartford Railroad, and the building at Forest Hills is a distance of only two or three minutes walk from the railroad station. It would be very possible for the members of the Association, as they come to Boston, to spend an hour or two in the inspection of that establishment before taking the steamer for the island in Boston Harbor, and I hope the members of the Association will take advantage of the opportunity offered. The paper of Dr. Denny is now before you for discussion or question.

DR. HARRINGTON: Dr. Denny's very interesting results suggest to me the desirability of the extension of such an investigation so as to determine how much danger of carrying infection may reside in women's skirts, through the senseless custom of dragging them over dusty sidewalks and staircases, gathering up all manner of filth which must necessarily be carried into the household. I know that it is a common practice on getting home to shake the skirt, in order to detach as much as possible of the dirt that has adhered during the walk. I hope that Dr. Denny will look into this matter, for it seems to me that there may be even greater danger of transmission of infection by skirts than by footwear. Another suggestion occurs to me. In place of putting on rubbers in passing to and from a contagious case, why would it not be well to use some sort of sandal made of stout paper, which, after use, could be burned? When one wears rubbers they must afterwards be disinfected, whereas with a very cheap sort of paper sandal the necessity of disinfection would be done away with.

DR. CHASE: I would like to say a word about the practical carrying out of these suggestions of Dr. Denny as to shoes. At the Brookline Board of Health Hospital we have two or three pairs of rubbers in the robing room at the entrance of the diphtheria ward, and also of the scarlet fever ward, and I find it a very easy matter to slip on one of these pairs of rubbers; and if another physician is along he does the same; but if his feet do not fit the rubbers he wipes off the soles and heels of his shoes with a solution of corrosive sublimate on a towel after finishing the visit to the scarlet fever ward. In visiting private patients we do not always do this; but now that our patients with dangerous contagious diseases are more and more generally cared for in hospitals, it is worth while, and is more necessary than ever to take this precaution to prevent cross infection. We all know the comparative frequency with which physicians bring home scarlet fever to their younger children, the children going around on all-fours. Within a year I have had in my care the one-year old child of a physician, who is very sure he himself brought home scarlet fever to his baby. He was taking care of a number of scarlet fever patients at the time, and it is very possible he brought home the infection on his feet. It is so easy and simple a matter to adopt Dr. Denny's timely suggestion that I hope others will try it as we have in Brookline.

Mr. WINSLOW: In connection with this scheme it is worth while to recall the typhoid fever epidemic in Springfield in 1892. I think the experts believed that the infection was carried from a tobacco field, in which typhoid bacilli occurred in human excreta, to a well in which milk cans were sunk. In that case infection was carried on the feet of workingmen.

Dr. SWARTS: The reader of the paper might have mentioned one other opportunity of investigation, made possible by the introduction of water filtration by means of what is called the sand-bed filtration, where the surface of the bed must necessarily be scraped at intervals, and the employees who do the scraping must necessarily tread upon the cleansed surface of the bed as they remove the scum of the bed, and after passing over a field well fertilized with night-soil it would seem to be possible that the footwear might carry a considerable quantity of innoculating material by which the whole of the filtering bed might become infected in this way. That is one of the objections to the use of sand-bed filtration, as compared with mechanical filtration, where it is not necessary to tread upon the bed in order to cleanse it. I would like to ask of the representatives of the

State Board of Health having control of all water supplies in the State whether they extend their labors to the control of the changing of shoes by those operatives who are scraping the beds; if not, whether it would not be a good idea to control such a condition.

THE CHAIRMAN: I seem to be left as the representative of the Board to speak upon that matter. It does not seem to me a matter of any consequence, because we assume that the typhoid bacilli do get upon the surface of that bed in any case. It is exactly what the sand bed is there for—but they don't get through it.

DR. DURGIN: I would like to ask Dr. Chase if he recollects what stage of scarlet fever this child was in when the foot-wear of the doctor was supposed to take the infection away.

DR. CHASE: He had quite a number of scarlet fever patients at the time, and they were in various stages of the disease. He could not tell from which patient he brought the contagion home, but he was positive he himself brought it to his child.

DR. CHAPIN: Dr. Denny's paper is a very interesting one, and investigations of this kind cannot help being extremely suggestive and useful. But at the same time I cannot but feel that we should be very careful in making deductions from them. Of course, it must be admitted from what he has told us today that the infection of a number of diseases can be transmitted from one place to another on the feet; but, as Dr. Denny himself well said, what we want to know is what are the chances of that infection getting from the feet to other living beings. What we want to know in all these investigations—and in all our study of the infectious diseases—is the exact mode by which the virus passes from the sick person to the well. We want to know the path followed in the majority of cases. I wish we were sure of this, but it does not seem to me that at present we really know very much about it. It appears that most of our notions are guess work. Now, it is possible to guess that the shoes are an important factor in carrying the disease from one person to another. It is possible to guess that the clothing is an important factor—that money, library books and school books are important factors—that the disease germs may be blown in the air from one person to another, and the disease spread in that way. So far as actual knowledge is concerned we appear at present to be very much at sea. Now, instead of guessing that the disease may be spread in the way mentioned, we are at liberty to guess that it is very rarely spread in any such way. We are at liberty to guess that, as a rule, the transmission of infection is pretty direct; that the disease poisons, the bacilli in diphtheria, for instance, are almost invariably transmitted in a pretty direct manner from the sick person to the well. Thus a person who is infected with diphtheria bacilli drinks out of a tumbler and some one else drinks out of the same tumbler shortly after before it is dry. A person who is infected with diphtheria puts a pencil in his mouth, and some one else puts that same pencil in his mouth within a few minutes and becomes infected. Those are direct means by which the bacilli are carried from one person to another. Now, one may guess that this is almost the sole manner in which disease is spread from the sick to the well. That guess has a good deal back of it. There is much to make us think that this guess is correct. Thus we find that it is not very easy for a person who has scarlet fever or diphtheria to infect others. All of you have noted plenty of instances where persons with scarlet fever or diphtheria have mingled freely with susceptible persons for days and weeks, and perhaps only one or two have become infected from them. Furthermore, we know that in diphtheria there are a large number of unrecognized cases of the disease, a very large number of persons who are not sick at all, but who are yet infected, and who are mingling freely with people in every walk of life and on all occasions, and it seems to me that opportunities for direct infection are very great indeed. So when we see that very often when there is close communication between sick and well, infection does not take place, that the infection appears to be somewhat difficult, and is not readily carried from one to another, we should be very chary of attributing very much importance to the carrying of the poison of diphtheria and probably of scarlet fever and the other diseases, on clothing or books or shoes or anything of the kind. Of course, we must admit that such a thing is possible. There is no doubt but that it occasionally occurs. But if we place so much stress upon the carrying of disease in fomites, as is usually done, are we not straining at a gnat? It seems to me that we are, and that we are drawing away public attention from the real source of the trouble, the real source of the extension of the contagious disease, namely, the existence of a very large number of unrecognized cases which are not sick at all, but are yet infected with the bacilli or other organism causing the disease. We know that this is the case in diphtheria. We have every reason to believe that it is so in other diseases, and I think we should hesitate very much before we unduly alarm people about any danger which may come from carrying the disease germs on the feet or on dresses or clothing or books or money or things of that kind, where there are a number of changes between the sick and the well and where considerable time elapses.

Of course, it is very much easier to blame inanimate objects, like books and shoes and clothing, for carrying disease than to blame a person who is perfectly well. No one who is perfectly well, who has had no sign of sore throat or eruption, likes to think that he can be the bearer of disease; but we know that can happen in diphtheria, and we believe that it can in other diseases. It is these persons themselves, it seems to me, that do the harm, and not the clothing or other material things carried by them.

Where a doctor brings home diphtheria to his children—which by the way, it seems to me, is a very rare thing, for I have almost never known of a physician carrying contagion in my experience of twenty years, and I have been on the lookout—is it not infinitely more likely that the physician has the diphtheria bacilli growing in his throat, that he has been infected himself from some one of his patients and has carried it home to his children in that way than that he has carried it home on his overcoat or his whiskers or his shoes? As regards scarlet fever we do not know that it is a bacterial disease, and we do not know with certainty the seat of infection, but we have reason to believe that the mucous secretions are infectious as they are in diphtheria, and also that well persons may have an infected throat or nose. In the case mentioned by Dr. Chase is it not more likely that the physician carried the disease home on his mucous membranes than on his clothing? It seems to me that in most instances it is the living person rather than inanimate objects that carry contagion, and that this is what we ought to teach.

THE CHAIRMAN: Is there anything else to be said on the subject of this very interesting paper?

DR. DENNY: I would like to say that I agree wholly with what Dr. Chapin has said—that infection is usually transmitted very directly from person to person, and usually from mild and unrecognized cases, and I don't think that the public should be stirred up about things of this sort. I should not think of bringing such a subject to the attention of the public. But it seems to me worth while to call to the attention of men who are engaged in preventing the spread of contagious disease the possibility of such a transmission, and especially the possibility of the transmission of tuberculosis. We don't know certainly how much danger there is from the sputum, which is around on the sidewalks or on the floors of our houses. Possibly we get infected more directly from other cases, but still, at the present time, when so much is being said and done to prevent the spread of tuberculosis from sputum, it seems to me as though we ought to consider the possibility of tuberculosis sputum being carried about in this way.

THE CHAIRMAN: If there is nothing more to be said upon this subject? Is there any other business to be brought before the Association at this time?

THE SECRETARY: I move we adjourn.

THE CHAIRMAN: If that be your pleasure, I will declare the Association adjourned.

ABSTRACTS, REVIEWS, NOTES AND NEWS.

Boards of Health are asked to send the Managing Editor notes of not more than one hundred and fifty words relating to new regulations passed, legal cases prosecuted, outbreaks of infection, unusual problems encountered, or other matters the publication of which may further the attainment of the objects of the Association.

References are indicated by numbers.   See list at end of column.

ANTI-VIVISECTION BILL AGAIN DEFEATED.—House Bill No. 174 of this year, which forbade any animal experimentation whatever to Municipal Board of Health or Hospital laboratories throughout the State, and permitted to the State Board of Health only inoculation tests, was reported "leave to withdraw" by the Committee on Probate and Chancery, May 4th, 1904. Substitution of the bill for this report was rejected in the House by a vote of 90 to 35, or 72 per cent. against the bill.

This bill required the appointment of a Commission of three to supervise animal experimentation, "one of whom and only one" should be a physician. Ex-Governor Brackett, who supported the bill at the hearings, sat beside the Speaker during the debate. Dr. Wheatley of Abington, a member of the Massachusetts Association of Boards of Health, Mr. Grady of Boston, the leader of the Democrats in the House, Mr. Cox of Boston and Mr. James Clark of Medford all spoke against the bill. Dr. H. L. Plummer and Mr. A. L. Gavin, both of Boston, also opposed the bill. Mr. McManus of Natick supported the bill, and so did Mr. Woodhead of North Adams, notwithstanding that the Board of Health of North Adams signed the protest against it.

Thereafter, in the Senate, substitution of the bill for the adverse report was urged, May 11th, by Senator Callender. The bill was again defeated, 16 to 7, or about 70 per cent. against it.

At the hearings, Dr. Harold C. Ernst appeared against the bill as the representative of the various Massachusetts Colleges and Universities, Hospitals and Boards of Health, presenting for the latter the official protests of Boards of Health from 31 of the 33 cities of the Commonwealth, and from 50 of its towns. The Boards of the remaining two cities also signified their opposition to the bill, but failed to sign the protest.

AGAINST THE TOY PISTOL.—At a meeting of the Berkshire District Medical Society, Feb. 26, 1904, it was voted that;

"*Whereas,* 406 deaths from tetanus were reported as occurring in the United States in July, 1903, as a result of fourth of July celebrations, 363 of these deaths having been caused by toy pistols loaded with blank cartridges, and 17 by cannon crackers,

"*Resolved,* That the Berkshire District Medical Society is in favor of any legislation and municipal ordinances which will effectively stop the sale and use of toy pistols, blank cartridges and cannon crackers.   *L. C. SWIFT, Secretary."*

IMPORTANT HEARING RELATIVE TO THE PROTECTION OF WATER SUPPLIES.—By a recent statute the State Board of Health of Massachusetts was authorized to "make rules and regulations to prevent the pollution and to secure the sanitary protection of all such waters as are used as sources of water supply." Acting under the provisions of this Statute (Revised Laws, Chapter 75, Section 113), the State Board of Health has made rules and regulations for several of the public water supplies of cities and towns, including Salem, Cambridge, Marlboro, Haverhill, Taunton, Pittsfield, Fitchburg, the Metropolitan Water District and several other places.

The density of the population in Massachusetts has increased to such a degree that it has become necessary to provide every possible safeguard for the many sources of water supply in order to protect them from the inevitable pollution which the collection of human beings in the neighborhood of such sources is bound to produce.

The city of Taunton acquired the right to take the waters of some of the great ponds in Lakeville, the largest fresh water areas in the State. But the natural beauty of these lakes had already induced a considerable number of summer cottagers to acquire land and erect buildings upon the immediate borders of these lakes, and for this reason an application was made to the State Board of Health to make such regulations as would protect these waters from pollution. Hence an attempt is being made by these property owners, among whom are several Indians, who claim direct descent from Massasoit, through seven or eight generations, to repeal the statute already mentioned. As the general tendency of legislation since 1878 has been to give greater, rather than less protection, to public water supplies, it can hardly be expected that this attempt will prove successful. The experience of Pennsylvania towns, in which the most serious epidemics have occurred in consequence of water pollution, was due largely to the absence of such statutes as Massachusetts fortunately possesses.

A hearing was held at the State House on Monday, May 2, at which the petitioners were heard, asking for the enactment of a new statute, the effect of which would seriously impair the value of such regulations. At the time of going to press the result of the hearing was not known. *S. W. ABBOTT, M. D.*

UNDERTAKING AND EMBALMING.—By a resolve of the Legislature, March 28, 1904, the Massachusetts State Board of Health was directed to investigate the necessity for a desirability of legislation to regulate undertaking and embalming. The Board reported May 4, 1904. We give below the paragraphs from the report bearing most explicity on the matter.

"As a result of this investigation (of the existing laws and conditions relating to undertaking and embalming) it is apparent that there is already vested in local Boards of Health a power in such matters exceeding that conferred upon the State Board of Health, and entirely adequate to ensure that the undertaking business will continue to be carried on, as at present, in a manner generally satisfactory to the community." * * *

"In regard to the question of embalming, the Board is distinctly of the opinion that, whatever value this practice may have in other respects, it cannot be regarded as necessary for, or contributing to, the protection of the public health. In the absence, then, of any necessity for new legislation to ensure the safe conduct into or through other States, of dead bodies shipped from this State in accordance with the requirements of existing statutes, and in the freedom from menace to the public health under existing conditions, the Board respectfully suggests that if for any reason new regulations to control the business of undertaking and embalming appear to be desirable, it must depend upon issues foreign to those upon which the Board feels itself competent to report."

AERIAL INFECTION FROM SMALLPOX HOSPITALS.—In the course of a suit, the Attorney-General and Others vs. the Mayor, Aldermen and City of Nottingham, England, recently heard before Mr. Justice Farwell, (Feb., 1904), much evidence concerning the extent and manner of distribution of infection from smallpox hospitals was considered. The Medical Officers of Health of the Essex County Council, of Basford, of Glasgow, of Bradford, and of Lambeth, testified that in their opinions aerial convection of the infective agent of smallpox is a serious source of danger in the neighborhood of such hospitals. The M. O. H.'s of Nottingham, Liverpool, Brighton, Staffordshire and others, did not agree with this, but believed that the spread of smallpox from a smallpox hospital is almost always to be ascribed to mal-administration in permitting intercourse with the people of the neighborhood to continue to a greater or less extent.

In summing up, Mr. Justice Farwell gave a long and closely reasoned opinion, and dismissed the case with costs, on the ground that the aerial convection of smallpox was not established by the evidence.

This case is interesting on account of the conflicting testimony given, but also because of the evidence that some smallpox hosvitals at least so not spread infection.

FEDERAL REGULATIONS CONCERNING VACCINES AND ANTITOXINS.—Rosenau, in a letter to *American Medicine,* calls attention to the act, signed July 1, 1902, "to regulate the sale of viruses, serums, toxins and analogous products in the District of Columbia, to regulate interstate traffic in said articles, and for other purposes."

This law requires that all establishments, native and foreign, engaged in such work, shall hold an unsuspended and unrevoked Government license, and prohibits interstate commerce in any product made in an illicit or unauthorized manner. It requires that every package of any such product shall bear the name, address and license number of the manufacturer, together with the name of the product, and the date beyond which it may become inert. False labelling is punishable by $500 fine, or imprisonment up to one year, or by both.

The U. S. Pub. Health and Marine Hosp. Service must detail an officer to inspect establishments having interstate commerce, and the Surgeon-General of this service, together with the Surgeon-Generals of the Army and Navy, constitute a board which may make rules, etc., controlling the licenses. The Director of the laboratory of this Service must examine the products, and licenses may be revoked for faulty methods of manufacture, faulty construction, faulty administration, impurities or weakness of products; already during a little over a year of operation of this law, four licenses have been revoked, and others have been refused, pending the making of indicated reformatory changes.

A STANDARD ANTITOXIN UNIT FROM AMERICAN SOURCES.—In the letter of Rosenau, just quoted, it is stated that his laboratory is engaged in the preparation of a standard toxin, after the character of Ehrlich's standard toxin, and that this standard toxin will be distributed to all interested in testing antitoxins. At the present time American laboratories depend principally on Ehrlich's laboratory for their supplies of such standard toxin. The ready determination of antitoxic strength in terms of a standard unit having general acceptance will be of considerable advantage to the whole country.

DIPHTHERIA MORTALITY WITH ANTITOXIN.— The Chicago Board of Health has recently published statistics concerning 7435 cases of diphtheria, which received antitoxin. Amongst these the death rate was 6.5 per cent., while in the remaining, non-antitoxin cases, the death rate was 35 per cent., or more than five times as great. In other words, eight deaths out of ten in the latter group occurred simply from neglect of a simple and readily obtainable form of treatment, available to the poor as well as to the rich.

THE TWENTY-NINTH ANNUAL MEETING OF THE NEW JERSEY SANITARY ASSOCIATION was held Dec. 4, 1903. The proceedings have been published and are all excellent. We cannot forbear quoting a few paragraphs from the brief address of the President, Dr. John S. Leal, Health Officer of Paterson, N. J., although all interested in scientific hygiene should read the article itself. "We must teach that the great sanitary bugbear of the past—filth, filthy water and filthy air— are in themselves of little sanitary importance, and that measures directed against them alone, however commendable they may be, are not demanded by sanitary science.

"True sanitary science wars against infection whether it chances to be in filth or in purity, in filthy air or water or in that which is pure. It is just as dangerous, if not more so, in what is pure as in what is filthy. The measures used against it may incidentally aid in accomplishing other good things, but their prime and true object is the destruction of the infection.

"The converse is also true that measures which properly belong to public decency, public comfort and public policy may also incidentally aid in the fight against infection."

THE STATE LABORATORY OF HYGIENE OF NEW JERSEY, now under the directorship of R. B. Fitz-Randolph, late Associate-Director of the Hoagland Laboratory, Brooklyn, has reached a high standard of efficiency, but while enjoying the confidence of the State Board of Health and of public hygienists throughout this country, it has received scant financial support from the Legislature of the current year. The same Legislature was prevented only by the Governor's veto from wrecking the excellent Sanitary Inspector law, emanating from the New Jersey Sanitary Association and approved by the well-known sanitarian, Dr. Henry Mitchell, secretary of the State Board of Health, passed one year ago, and received with general acclaim by the leading hygienists of New Jersey.

We would assure such legislators that they need not fear prosecution for adulteration should they mix brains with their legislation, notwithstanding the fact that, strictly speaking, such a compound might often properly come within the scope of the clause forbidding the addition of "substances foreign to the well-known article under whose name they are offered for consumption."

A CHANGE IN THE BOSTON BOARD OF HEALTH.—The Hon. Edwin L. Pilsbury, whose term of office expired May 1, 1904, failed of reappointment. Mr. Pilsbury, whose capacity and courtesy all members of this Association will remember with admiration and pleasure, has been a member of the Board for about twelve years, and has proved an excellent and efficient public servant. Political pressure at the last moment was alone responsible for his non-appointment. We cannot but regret the reason as well as the fact.

His successor, Dr. T. B. Shea, chief medical inspector, was selected by the Mayor independently of the political movement referred to, and his appointment illustrates two excellent principles—promotion of an officer who has proved his efficiency in a subordinate position and the choosing for a responsible technical and professional position one with training and experience for its important duties.

THE MAYOR OF SAN FRANCISCO has made it his business to deny the existence of plague in that city, and to obstruct all efforts against its spread. He has recently removed the whole City Board of Health, in whom the people had confidence, and has replaced them by men in sympathy with his policy. Six cases of plague were reported by the U. S. P. H. and M. H. S. as present in the city during February, 1904. (8.)

We cannot but regret that the distinguished visitor from the East should so far forget the courtesy due to the chief executive of the only American city which has yet shown him extended hospitality as to overstay his welcome, especially when that chief executive takes pains to state that the distinguished visitor has never been present at all. We suggest that the plague—or the Mayor—should align himself with the real facts as soon as possible.

DR. PETER H. BRYCE, for many years the Secretary of the Provincial Board of Health of Ontario, has recently been appointed Medical Inspector of Immigration, under the Dominion Government. He has established a detention hospital in Quebec, and is building also a hospital for the treatment of emigrants. He is in charge of the Medical Service to the Indians throughout the Dominion. His successor in the Secretaryship is Dr. Charles H. Hodgetts, of whom we hope a conduct of affairs reaching the high standard set by Dr. Bryce. The reports of the Board contain much of interest, particularly the recent one describing the work of Dr. John A. Amyot, Bacteriologist to the Board, on sewage purification at Berlin. If Dr. Hodgetts will inaugurate his term of office by an appeal to the Government to print his reports on paper, and with type, not quite so wholly disreputable as Dr. Bryce has been compelled to use, he will confer a great favor on those at a distance, whose chief acquaintance with the Provincial Board of Health work must necessarily be had from their pages.

DR. U. O. B. WINGATE, whose name has long been a household word in hygienic circles, a well-known member of the

American Public Health Association, and a thoroughly sound and efficient public health officer, was recently removed from his position as Secretary of the Wisconsin State Board of Health because, as one of the members of the Board put it, "the plum should be passed around." To Dr. Wingate this "reason" involves a tribute, since no one can imagine that it would have been offered had a better one been available. To Wisconsin and to its State Board the "reason" is a disgrace not easily to be forgotten or forgiven by the hygienic world.

DR. E. A. DE SCHWEINITZ died in Washington, Feb. 15th, 1904, of uræmia. He was chief of the Bio-chemic Division, Bureau of Animal Industries, U. S. Department of Agriculture, and was known everywhere for the high character of his work, particularly in the bacteriology and chemistry of tuberculosis.

MR. GEORGE C. WHIPPLE, at one time Biologist to the Boston Water Board, and for the last six years Biologist and Director of Mount Prospect Laboratory, Brooklyn Water Department, has recently resigned to go into private practice as a Sanitary Expert in New York City.

CHEMICAL DETECTION OF RAW MILK.—Raw milk, treated with a solution of orthomethylaminophenol sulphate, followed by hydrogen peroxide, develops a brilliant deep red color. If heated at a temperature of 75 C. for half an hour, the milk will no longer react. Higher temperatures destroy the reaction more rapidly, but a temperature of 70 C. for an hour does not prevent the reaction. Raw milk, masquerading as scalded or Pasteurized, can be recognized by this method. So delicate is it that one per cent. of raw milk added to scalded milk can be detected. (5.)

AN INDIAN SNAKE-STONE.—The well known stories concerning stones capable, when applied to snake bites, sometimes to mad-dog bites, of adhering to the wound and absorbing the poisons, have been put to the test by H. Watkins-Pitchford, Government Bacteriologist in Pietermaritzburg, Natal. The stone tested came from India, accompanied by a statement from the (white) owner that he had obtained it from a native whose life the stone had saved in his (the owner's) presence.

Careful tests on rabbits, using the venoms of various poisonous snakes, and following in the application of the stone the ceremonies described, exactly in the native fashion, showed, as might have been expected, that the stone had absolutely no effect whatever upon the symptoms or fatality caused by the snake poison. (7.)

A NEW METHOD OF GROWING ANAEROBES.—B. R. Rickards, 1st Asst. Bacteriologist, Boston Board of Health Laboratory, devised the simple plan of inverting ordinary tubes of solid media, inoculated in the ordinary way, in the ordinary solution of pyrogallol and alkali, contained in a tumbler or other convenient receptacle. For liquid media, a U-tube, with one end sealed, and this half filled with the inoculated medium, is similarly inverted with the unsealed end in the pyrogallol. For plates, the liquefied nutrient jelly is poured into a sterile erlenmeyer, and after solidification of the jelly, the flask is likewise inverted. In all cases, the pyrogallol solution rises in the medium container as the oxygen is absorbed. A fuller account is to be found in the Centrablatt fuer Bakteriologie.

SEWAGE PURIFICATION TESTS IN COLUMBUS, O.—About $50,000 have been appropriated for the testing of the various known methods of purification, the tests to run for a year from about July 1, 1904. The object is to determine the best conditions for Columbus, but the broad views shown in the planning of this work, and the character of the men who will conduct it, ensure that much will be added to the general stock of knowledge on this subject.

Mr. George A. Johnson, who was a member of the laboratory force which conducted the well-known water-filtration experiments in Louisville in 1895-96, under Mr. George W. Fuller, and who has since been engaged in similar work in Cincinnati, Washington, St. Louis and other cities, will be in charge. Mr. A. E. Kimberly of the Lawrence Experiment Station of this State will be First Asst. Chemist. The First Asst. Bacteriologist has been selected, we believe, but his name has not yet been made public.

DISEASE, OTHER THAN TYPHOID FEVER, FROM MILK.—During an outbreak of acute sore throat in England, traced by Vincent to one of two dairies, from which the infection had been distributed, a death occurred also from acute septic colitis, and Vincent convinced himself that this also was due to the use by the patient of the infected milk. (6.)

PNEUMONIA HAS BEEN PLACED ON THE REPORT-ABLE LIST in New York City, for the first time, it is said, in any city of this country. This is a marked recognition of the infectious nature of the disease, and of its increased ravages in late years.

The impression seems to be growing that even the ordinary colds are infectious, but these, as well as pneumonia, require a lowered condition of vitality in some form in the recipient before simple transmission of the infective agents becomes significant. We suggest that those Boards of Health which feel inclined to place pneumonia on the reportable list should be prepared to support their views by statistics, showing the average number of cases which can be traced to a single original case, amongst members of the same household and others closely associated with the patient, as has been done in tuberculosis.

TUBERCLE BACILLI IN OLD LIBRARY BOOKS.— Those who are in the habit of separating stuck-together leaves in public library books with finger-tips moistened with their own saliva, may, if well, become infected with tubercle bacilli, or if consumptives themselves, place their bacilli where others, following the same practices, may remove them to their own mouths.

Mitelescu, examining the books of a public library, chiefly from the fiction department, found that one-third of those over two years in use yielded tubercle bacilli from the leaves, when these were washed, and the washings centrifugalized and injected into guinea-pigs.

On clean paper the bacilli die out readily, from drying, but when dirty leaves stick together, evaporation is impeded, and the bacilli live longer. They were not found in books less than two years old (although we do not understand why), nor on the covers of any of the books. (10.)

It must not be forgotten that consumptives may infect books in the mere act of coughing, or even laughing and talking, when the book is open before them, and that such infection is more likely to remain active, shielded as it is from the action of sunlight and air when the book is closed, than similar infection of ordinary exposed surfaces. While it is unlikely that any large number of people become infected from this source, the handling of library books with moistened hands, a bad habit at best, receives additional condemnation from these results.

REGISTRATION OF TUBERCULOSIS.—Lecturing for the Phipps Institute, Dr. Herman M. Biggs of the New York Health Dept. points out that the objections to this can be met easily by providing that no action will be taken in the cases reported, unless the circumstances are such that administrative interference is necessary or desirable.

This is the principle on which the Boston Board of Health has proceeded since registration was made compulsory and comparatively little difficulty has been found in securing registration under this understanding.

FREE HOSPITALS FOR CONSUMPTIVES IN TORONTO.—This hospital, situated about ten miles outside of Toronto, is to be opened as soon as the necessary funds for furnishings, etc., are secured. A site near the new buildings of the University of Toronto Medical Faculty has been decided upon for a free dispensary for consumptives. So far about $400,000 has been expended in anti-tuberculosis work in Ontario by the National Sanitarium Association.

A PUBLIC TUBERCULOSIS CLINIC has been opened by the New York Health Department, near its headquarters, 55th Street and 6th Avenue. Diagnosis, circulars of information, treatment, sputum cups, etc., are offered free to indigents. A special corps of trained nurses is provided to care for poor patients at their homes. The co-operation of charitable organizations for the supply of fuel, ice, etc., has been secured. Suitable cases are sent to hospitals or sanitaria. Special attention is paid to preventing the spread of the disease, particularly amongst the children of the infected families. (9.).

ARE ALL SPECIES OF ANOPHELES HARMFUL?— Hirschberg throws doubt on *Anopheles punctipennis* as a transmitter of malaria, while confirming the capacity of *Anopheles maculipennis* in this direction. His method was to permit the mosquitoes to bite patients suffering from malaria in favorable stages, and then after waiting the proper interval, to section the mosquitoes and search for the parasites within them. In 58 tests with *A. punctipennis* he did not succeed in finding parasites at all, while in 48 tests with *A. maculipennis,* 8 positive results were obtained. (2.)

DENGUE, OR BREAK BONE FEVER, a hitherto mysterious affection of the Far East, is now ascribed by Dr. Graham of Beirut to a parasite transmitted by mosquitoes after the manner of malaria.

MEDICAL INSPECTORS APPOINTED.—Forty medical inspectors have been recently appointed by the Health Department of Philadelphia, pursuant to a recent act passed by the City Council. These medical inspectors are to give their entire time to the city, and each is placed in charge of a certain district. It is his duty to report all cases of infectious diseases, to trace the source of epidemics, to report any unhygienic conditions, to inspect public schools, etc. Each inspector is to receive a salary of $1200 per annum. (3.)

INSPECTION OF SCHOOL CHILDREN IN CHICAGO. —It is proposed in Chicago to thoroughly inspect the school children in each of the city schools. Teachers and principals must report for medical examination any pupils they believe physically defective, deformed, or afflicted with a functional disorder, The rules provide that the examinations shall be made by a school medical inspector in the office of the principal and under the latter's supervision. (3.)

VACCINATION OF PUBLIC SCHOOL CHILDREN in New York State, according to the decision of Attorney-General Cunneen, need not take in order to satisfy the legal requirements. It is evidently sufficient, in New York, to have "the form of godliness without the power thereof."

A PERMANENT EXHIBIT OF A HYGIENIC HOME, containing everything tending to promote the welfare of its inhabitants, particularly designed to meet the requirements of the working man, is maintained in Berlin. This idea might well be adopted in the larger cities in this country.

DR. JOHN N. HURTY, the well known Secretary of the State Board of Health of Indiana, has recently been unanimously reelected for a period for four years. Dr. Hurty is in charge of the Hygienic Exhibit at the St. Louis Exposition.

EPIDEMIC CEREBRO-SPINAL MENINGITIS, known familiarly as "spotted fever," is reported from Hartford, Conn., to the extent of fifty-eight cases and thirty-two deaths in April. Strict measures of isolation have been carried out by the Board of Health.

COMPULSORY REGISTRATION OF TUBERCULOSIS as a contagious disease was voted down by a tie vote in a recent meeting of the Philadelphia County Medical Society.

LECTURES FOR MEDICAL INSPECTORS are being conducted under the auspices of Director Martin of the Philadelphia Board of Health.

TYPHOID BACILLI ISOLATED FROM DRINKING WATER.—In a previous issue we recorded various findings of this organism in water. To make the list more complete, we have below starred a few additional names quoted in the article of Konradi (see below), and have added the references for all.

Fischer and Flatau	Cent. f. Bakt., Ref. Abt. 1,	29
Genersich	" " "	27
Hankin	" "	26
*Hanriot	" " Ref.	29
*Konradi	" " Orig.	35
Kubler and Neufeld	Zeit. f. Hyg., Bd. 31	
Loesener	Arb. a. d. kais. Gesundheit. Bd. 11	
*Tavel	Cent. f. Bakt., Orig.	33
Wesbrook	Rep. Minn. St. Bd. Health for '95-'98	
*Bonhoff (doubtful)	Cent. f. Bakt., Orig. Abt. 1,	33

B. R. RICHARDS.

TYPHOID FEVER DIAGNOSTICUM.—Under this name Ficker has placed in the hands of a manufacturing chemist for sale a slightly turbid fluid for use after the fashion of the Widal test, for the diagnosis of typhoid fever. To a little of this fluid the physician adds a drop of the patient's blood. In a short time the liquid shows a flocculation, and in time becomes clear by sedimentation, if the reaction be present. The test does not require a microscope, and can be applied at the bedside, while the fluid remains good for nine months. (11.)

Ruediger of Chicago has recently recommended for use in the same manner cultures of typhoid bacilli, killed by the addition of formalin. He claims for this method saving in time, as well as in trouble, over the usual method with living cultures. (12.)

TYPHOID BACILLI IN WELL PERSONS.—Juergens, examining the members of households where typhoid fever was present, found the bacilli, not only in the sick members, but also in those but slightly affected, and even in well persons associated with the clinically developed cases. (13.)

TYPHOID FEVER FROM CREAM IN WILLIAMS-TOWN, MASS.—The investigation of thirteen cases of typhoid fever which occurred at Williamstown during November, 1903, among the students of Williams College, shows that the probable source of infection was from a can of heavy cream, this being the only article of diet common to all the patients.

The cream supply was primarily obtained from Hoosick, N. Y., being shipped daily to the North Adams Milk Co., and subsequently delivered by eight different routes, seven of which were in North Adams and the other in Williamstown. No cases of the disease occurred among people using the regular supply at North Adams, and the investigation did not show the exact source of infection in the cream which went to Williamstown. A portion of this cream, returned daily to the milk depot, was used as a special supply for afternoon orders, and seven cases of typhoid fever occurred at North Adams among those who might have received the cream in this way. As additional evidence of the cream being the source of infection it was found that one member of the Tufts College football team, which played at Williamstown during the period when the infection of these patients probably occurred, and who had access to the cream, was subsequently taken ill with the disease.

On account of the length of time which elapsed from the date of the patient's going to bed to the reporting of the cases to the State Board of Health, the investigation could not be called complete, and it was not possible to obtain information which would point to the exact source of infection, on account of this lapse of time and the consequent loss of important connecting facts.—

F. L. MORSE, M. D.

TYPHOID FEVER FROM MILK IN PLYMOUTH, MASS.—On Feb. 1 the attention of the State Board of Health was called by the Board of Health of the town of Plymouth to the presence of an unusual number of cases of typhoid fever in the town, and it was asked that an investigation be made as to the cause of the disease.

From Jan. 2nd to Feb. 3rd 28 patients were found to have gone to bed ill with typhoid fever, 18 of them previous to the 15th of the month, and the remainder up to and including the 26th. All these patients had resided in the town for some time, and none had been away on any vacation, while with but one exception all had taken milk of one producer by the name of Finney. This exception was a young woman to whom the milkman was paying attention.

In the milkman's family five members were sick with the disease on Feb. 1st, the father, mother and three children. The milk barn is located about a mile from the home, and there are accommodations for twenty head of cattle, the milking being done by two of the boys. The milk was brought directly to the house, placed in a 100-qt. mixing can, cooled, and subsequently turned into 8-qt. cans for delivery. A small amount was placed in quart cans for the use of special customers, but ordinarily the milk was dispensed by measure at the house of each customer.

One of the boys doing the milking was taken ill on Jan. 9th, but continued to work until Jan. 15th, when he gave up work entirely, and three days later, on account of the appearance of the disease among the customers the milk supply was voluntarily suspended.

There have been four deaths in the course of the epidemic. One of the early cases to become ill was a patient living in a house located on the shores of Town Brook Pond. The attending physician did not give instructions relating to the disinfection of the discharges, and they had been thrown sometimes into a privy located on the water's edge, and at other times upon the ice which had formed upon the pond.

During the month of January about 1000 tons of ice had been

cut on this pond, 700 tons to be used for refrigerating purposes only, and 300 tons to be used in the fish business. The harvesting of the latter supply was completed on Jan. 28th, and ice was taken from the pond within 20 feet of the privy already mentioned. A sample of ice was obtained at a point near this locality and sent to Lawrence for examination. It showed numerous bacteria present, and upon the advice of the State Board of Health all of the ice was prevented from being used.—

F. L. MORSE, M. D.

TYPHOID EPIDEMIC IN WATERTOWN.—Information from Watertown, N. Y., March 10, says: George A. Soper of New York, the sanitary expert who is in charge of the typhoid fever situation here, says that there is a marked improvement in conditions. The number of cases reported daily shows a decided decrease, and the total number of cases is considerably less. The number of cases now in the city is less than 500. Arrangements have been practically completed for supplying the city with pure spring water. A number of tank wagons will be put into commission, and kept until the filtration plant is in operation next fall.

LEPROSY ON CAPE COD.—A case of leprosy has been discovered at North Harwich, the patient being a Portuguese 38 years of age, who has resided in this country for twelve years. His father, mother and sister are said to have died with the disease before his arrival in this country. His symptoms developed about five years ago with the formation upon the forearms of tubercles, which afterwards ulcerated. He has been treated at New Bedford by two different physicians, but the disease was not recognized by them. At the present time the face is covered with small tubercles the size of the tip of the little finger, with numerous ulcerations on the upper and lower extremities. Numerous cicatrices are present upon the forearms, indicating old ulcers which have subsequently healed. The roof of the mouth and nasal passages are also ulcerated, and there is considerable swelling of the face and hands.

The slight infectious character of this disease must be apparent when it is known that this man has been free to go and come in the past five years, during which time he has been in an infectious state, without giving rise to any other case. He is at present quarantined by the Board of Health of the town.

F. L. MORSE, M. D.

SMALLPOX IN LEOMINSTER.—A case of smallpox was reported from the town of Leominster on May 2nd, this being the first case of the disease existing in the eastern part of the State for a period of about two months. The patient is a French Canadian 34 years of age, who has never been vaccinated.

F. L. MORSE, M. D.

MERCURIC BICHLORIDE, AS A DISINFECTANT, NOT HARMFUL THROUGH VAPOR.—Bertarelli has investigated during two years the effect of disinfection by mercuric bichloride, on the disinfectors, and on the persons living in rooms after such disinfection, in Turin, where solutions of one to one hundred strength are used regularly.

The urine and feces were examined, and animals, enclosed in experimental chambers treated with the solutions, were observed.

He concludes that no risk of mercurial poisoning need be feared from the emanations of premises thus disinfected.

The solutions of "bichloride" used in this country rarely approach in strength the figures quoted for Turin, so that it appears proper to dismiss any haunting qualms which may have existed in their use. Of course, precautions against accidental swallowing of the solutions require the same attention as heretofore. (4.)

COAL SMOKE CONSISTS of solid matter and gases. The solid matter is made up of about equal parts of carbon and coal-ash, rather less than two pounds of each being thrown off in the burning of each ton of coal.

The gaseous matter consists of carbon dioxid, from 2 to 11 per cent by volume; carbon monoxid, .3 to 0 per cent.; oxygen, 7 to 18 per cent.; nitrogen about 80 per cent., and traces of hydrogen and of a large variety of hydrocarbons.

Smoke-consuming devices remove the solid matters largely, but not the gases. The economy of these devices lies, not, as is often supposed, in the saving of the carbon otherwise wasted, which is too small an item to be of much value, but in the added efficiency gained from the use of the methods of firing necessary to secure smokelessness, and in the smaller amount of hired help required. Under ordinary conditions, one pound of coal evaporates from 5 to 6 pounds of water, but under smokeless conditions, from 6 to 7 pounds. The total saving is put at 15 to 30 per cent.—(*From notes furnished by Prof. A. H. Gill.*)

ANTHRAX IN LYNN.—*The Boston Medical and Surgical Journal* of April 21st, 1904, states that fifteen cases of anthrax have occurred in Lynn, Mass., during the last three or four years, and urges investigation, with a view to prevention.

OYSTERS AND CLAMS.—"Seventy-seven samples of oysters have been examined by the New Hampshire State Board of Health Laboratory for boric acid and in thirty-four cases it was present. When the inspection was first commenced every sample of tub oysters contained boric acid, and the results obtained from samples from Dover, Portsmouth, Manchester and Concord showed conclusively that it was the practice of Boston wholesalers to add boric acid, or a preparation known as 'Preservaline' and containing boric acid, to every tub of oysters they sent out. A vigorous correspondence with dealers in Norfolk and Providence River tub oysters produced such beneficial results that on the last inspection of oysters from the above-named cities but little boric acid was found. The practice of preserving oysters by the liberal use of boric acid permitted the small grocer or marketman to keep oysters on his counter, without ice, in warm weather, as long as any remained unsold. We must conclude that a preservative active enough to arrest decay in such perishable articles as oysters, under such conditions, would not fail to arrest, in a like manner, the action of the digestive ferments.

"Clams are equally liable to adulteration by preservatives, and because of their less common use may contain even larger quantities of boric acid.

"The action of the wholesale houses in quickly abandoning the use of boric acid when notified by their customers that they were not allowed to sell goods so treated, proves the practice to be unnecessary." (1.)

NEW MILK REGULATION.—The Boston Board of Health has amended its milk regulations of 1898 by the addition (April 29, 1904,) of a paragraph relating to bacteriological examinations and control as follows:

> Art. IV., sect. 1.—No person, by himself or by his servant or agent, or as the servant or agent of any other person, firm, or corporation, shall bring into the city of Boston for purposes of sale, exchange or delivery, or sell, exchange, or deliver any milk, or cream which contains more than 500,000 bacteria per cubic centimeter, or which has a temperature higher than fifty degrees Fahrenheit.

Routine bacteriological examinations of the Boston milk supply are now being arranged for at the Boston Board of Health Laboratory.

References.

New Hampshire San. Bull.
    1. January, 1904.
Johns Hopkins Hospital Bull.
    2. February, 1904.
American Medicine.
    3. Feb. 27, 1904.
   14. March 18, 1904.
   16. March 5, 1904.

Zeit. f. Hyg.
    4.   1903, xlii.
    10.   1903, p. 397 (Abs., Pratt, *Boston Medical and Surgical Journal*, April 23, 1904).
British Medical Journal.
    5.   March 21, 1903.
    6.   Feb. 6, 1904.
    7.   Feb. 20, 1904.
Journal American Medical Association.
    8.   March 12, 1904.
    13.   April 23, 1904.
Boston Medical and Surgical Journal.
    9.   March 3, 1904.
Berl. klin. Wochen.
    11.   1903, No. 45.
Journal Infectious Diseases.
    12.   Vol. 1, No. 2, 1904.

BOOKS.

ELEMENTS OF WATER BACTERIOLOGY.—Prescott (S. C.), and Winslow (C. E. A.) John Wiley & Sons. 1904. Price, $1.00.

For a long time there has been an urgent need of a treatise on Water Bacteriology, which would not only give the methods in use in Europe, but also the especially facile procedures which have been worked out in American laboratories. The authors have met this need with a well-arranged and practical volume of 125 pages.

Some criticisms may be made of the mediocre press work, of the ambiguous wording in one or two places and of the rather poor proof reading. For example, in the diagram on Page 7, one of the two "Nitrates" should be "Nitrates." On Page 9, it is stated that "A good river water under favorable conditions should thus contain only a few hundred bacteria." Would not the reader get the impression that all waters with less than a few hundred bacteria are good, and all with a few thousand bacteria (unpolluted muddy streams) are bad?

In the first paragraph on Page 38 there are two indistinct letters and a split infinitive. On Page 45 it would be better to say "more common"; and "the latter" refers to a word four lines back. It would perhaps be better to give the date of Johnson's paper, Page 75.

The subject matter itself in the book is excellent. One can only be impressed with the careful presentation of the subject. Especially praiseworthy is the bibliographical work and the convenience of the references. Especially well balanced are the chapters on the Significance of the Presence of *B. coli* and Other Intestinal Bacteria in Water. The authors take the sound position that a sample of water free from *B. coli* is undoubtedly safe, and that its continued presence in 1-c. c. samples is an index of serious pollution.

Chapter IX, which treats of intestinal bacteria other than *B. coli,* is an excellent summary of the present knowledge of the sanitary significance of this class of bacteria. Much of this chapter is new. The authors say that the presence of *Streptococci* is valuable confirmatory evidence of dangerous pollution.

The methods given for the examination of water are excellent. Many of them are the same as those recommended by the American Public Health Association. The other methods are largely supplementary or are new methods not discussed by the Association. The outline of the methods is very well given and is in general very clear. One might ask if double dilution (Page 28) were not the best method for handling samples rich in bacteria. On Page 44 it is stated that bacteria develop very little at the body temperature after 24 hours of incubation. Can this be strictly true?

While reading Page 54 one will ask if natural immunity does not protect the human race to some extent.

In the last chapter the value of bacterial methods is set forth very well. However, the authors are inclined to overestimate the accuracy of the various methods. The reading is easier than the doing. Again, there is perhaps a tendency to forget that while the bacterial examination in many cases is a sanitary *sine qua non,* it is seldom the *ne plus ultra.*

Everyone interested in the analysis of water should own a copy of this little book. It is the best of its kind in any language, and with the minor errors eliminated in the future editions, should have a wide circulation.—*R. S. W.*

GENERAL PATHOLOGY.—By Sidney Martin, M. D., F. R. S., F. R. C. P., Professor of Pathology at University College; Physician to University College Hospital, London. With numerous woodcuts from micro-photographs, and other illustrations, including many in colors. Philadelphia, 1904. P. Blakiston's Son & Co. Pages, 495, with index, preface and introduction.

Based on lectures delivered at University College, and intended primarily for students, this book seems to us better fitted for those already somewhat familiar with the subject than it is for the beginner, to whom detailed explanations are necessary if he is to secure any consecutive and logical view of the whole. Nevertheless the author has succeeded in covering the chief fields of modern pathology in clear language. We are particularly pleased with his advocacy of physiological pathology, believing that the term pathology is too often restricted to the mere anatomy of disease. Disease is a process in a machine, the autopsy revealing merely a vertical section through the process, with the machine stopped. The divorcement of clinical research and teaching from pathological research and teaching not infrequently results in the student receiving the impression, not formularized, but latent, that every disease possesses a dual personality; he carries two distinct pictures of pneumonia, say, with him; one, the pneumonia of his clinical teacher, existing only in the hospital ward; the other, the pneumonia of his pathological teacher, existing only in the autopsy room. To substitute a proper composite picture these two are the real basis of successful medical teaching.

SANITARY ENGINEERING NOTES.

ROBERT SPURR WESTON, M. A.,
Assoc. M. Boston Soc. C. E.

REPORT OF THE SPECIAL COMMISSION ON THE WATER SUPPLY OF SPRINGFIELD, MASS., 1904.—The present Ludlow and Jabish Brook supplies are subject to very numerous growths of organisms, principally anabæna, which give rise to disagreeable tastes and odors in the water. Consequently the improvement of the present supply, or the taking of a new supply from another source, is becoming a pressing question.

The recent report by Samuel M. Gray, M. Am. Soc. C. E., and George W. Fuller, Assoc. M. Am. Soc. C. E., with the appended report of E. E. Lochridge, Resident Engineer, discusses the whole problem in a thorough manner.

Experiments by Mr. Lochridge demonstrated that the present supply could be purified by double filtration, together with repeated aeration. This purified supply would be good for 15,000,-000 gals. per diem, and could be supplemented by filtered Connecticut River water from above Holyoke. This combination would be the cheapest method of supplying the city with 25,000,-000 gals. per diem.

The engineers considered supplementing the Ludlow water with that of the Scantic River (filtered), and investigated the practicability of supplying the city solely with filtered Connecticut River water. They also studied the Westfield River at Huntington.

The estimated cost of the various supplies per million gallons, on a basis of 25,000,000 gals. per day, is as follows:

Ludlow Reservoir and Connecticut River . . . $25.44
Westfield at Huntington 27.76
Ludlow and Scantic 26.89
Connecticut River 27.08

In view of the extreme difficulty of purifying the Ludlow water, the necessity of pumping the Connecticut River supply, the small amount of pollution of the Westfield—a gravity supply

—and the slight differences in cost, the engineers have recommended the most desirable supply, namely, the Westfield River at Huntington. The estimated cost of this construction is $4,303,990, which, although about $1,000,000 above the cost of the Ludlow and Connecticut River scheme, is well within the means of the Water Department, particularly if the excessive consumption of water be lessened.

It is gratifying to note that the engineers have recommended that all water, even the upland water, be filtered. However, the names of the engineers were a guarantee that this modern position would be taken. The so-called "unpolluted" watersheds which are available for water supply are not numerous.

THE EFFECT OF POLLUTED RIVERS UPON THE NEIGHBORING GROUND WATER.—Wolf, K. (Arb. aus den Kgl. hygien. Instituten zu Dresden. Vol I, 1903, p. 291.)— The Dresden water supply is taken from the gravel layers, which extend underneath the Elbe River. At times of flood the numbers of bacteria in the ground water rises to several thousand per cubic centimeter. Several of these bacteria were isolated from the ground water. Two of them were determined to be *B. coli* and *B. vulgaris,* respectively. The author suggests that the water of filter galleries and wells adjacent to rivers should be analyzed at all stages of the river before deciding upon the ground water as a source of supply.

NEW METHOD FOR THE DETERMINATION OF THE VELOCITY OF GROUND WATER FLOW.—Slichter. (Jour. f. Gas. und Wasserversorgung, 1903, No. 12, p. 230.) —In place of studying the rate of passage of salt or dye stuff through the ground, the author introduces ammonium chloride at the higher of the two points in the ground water table, and brings them into an electric circuit, thus measuring the electro-conductivity of the soil, which, on the appearance of the ammonium chloride at the second and lower observation point, shows a sudden change.

A NEW COAGULANT FOR USE WITH RAPID FIL-TERS.—In several rapid filter plants, for example, Lorain, O., and Danville, Ill., the use of sulphate of alumina has been stopped and lime and ferrous sulphate have been used in its place, thereby effecting a considerable cost saving, with continuance of good bacterial results. A. C. Brown (Engineering Record, Vol. 48, p. 701, 1903) describes his experience with this coagulant as used at Lorain.

BACTERIA IN SOIL IN RELATION TO INFILTRA-TION GALLERIES FOR WATER SUPPLY. G. C. Whipple. (Engineering Record, Vol. 48, p. 501-2.)—Experiments were made to determine the efficiency of the soil for removing bacteria from water collected by filter galleries, which galleries were constructed of vitrified pipe, laid with open joints, in trenches from 10 to 20 ft. deep, and surrounded with gravel or broken stone. One typical experiment is selected for an example.

Depth Below Surface (Ft.)	Bacteria per Gram of Soil.
0.	136,000
0.5	115,800
1	6,800
2	2,850
3	885
4	380
5	60
6	00
7	00
8	00

Mr. Whipple concludes that "The sand below 5 ft. in depth never contains more than a very small number of bacteria. Tests for *B. coli* were negative."

These experiments confirm the belief that wells are most frequently contaminated from the surface, and seldom through sandy soils. Fissured soils, however, may allow the direct passage of water from a source of pollution to a well.

SEWAGE DISPOSAL IN IOWA. A. Marston. (Jour. Western Soc. E.)—Reviewed in American Chemical Research, Vol. X, No. 4, by L. P. Kinnicutt.) This paper gives a detailed account of the eleven sewage disposal plants in the State of Iowa. They are all modern plants, using the septic tank. The reader is referred to Prof. Kinnicutt's review or the original paper for a fuller account.

FILTERS, VERSUS CONTACT BEDS AND SEWAGE PURIFICATION. *Municipal Engineer.* Vol. XXVI, p. 111-117; also Journ. Am. Chem. Research, Vol. X, No. 4.)—In this paper the author concludes that the septic tank is a necessary preliminary to sewage purification. It is to be noted that the English practice is to provide from one to one and one-half days' storage in the septic tank, while the American practice is to store the sewage from one-half to one day only. Regarding the treatment of the septic tank effluent, whether by means of sand beds, contact beds, or trickling beds, the author states that the tendency of the English practice is away from the contact beds and toward the trickling bed. These latter are built of coarse material, and the sewage is applied continuously in the form of a spray. In cold climates there would be danger of freezing were trickling beds used.

THE TARRING OF MACADAMIZED ROADS TO PREVENT DUST. Schottelius and Guglielminetti (Muench, med. Wochenschrift, 1903, No. 25, p. 1068.)—The authors note that pneumonia, influenza, diphtheria, etc., are increased by breathing dust. They show this by adequate statistics. They describe the process for preventing the same by covering the road with a layer of tar in the following manner.

On a dry and warm day the cleaned and rolled macadam is given one or two coats of coal tar previously heated to 60 degrees C. After two to three hours the tar is strewn with dry sand. The tar absorbs rapidly, and it is claimed that dust is diminished. It is said that one pound of tar will cover 5 sq. ft., and that it would cost about $150 to tar a mile of road 18 ft. wide. Petroleum is not a satisfactory substitute for tar.

CIDER VINEGAR AND SUGGESTED STANDARDS OF PURITY. (Albert E. Leach and Herman C. Lythgoe. *Journal American Chemical Society,* Vol. XXVI. p. 375.)—The authors give analyses of many true and also many sophisticated vinegars, and describe the methods used for analyzing the same. As a result of their experience they suggest the following standard:

"The acetic acid shall be more than 4.50 per cent.; the cider vinegar solids more than 2 per cent.; the ash should constitute at least 6 per cent. of the solids; the alkalinity of 1 gram of ash should be equivalent to at least 65 c. c. of tenth-normal acid; at least 50 per cent. of the phosphates in the ash should be soluble in water. The reducing sugars should be the same in amount after as before inversion, and should not exceed 25 per cent. of the solids. The polarization, expressed in terms of 200 mm. of undiluted vinegar, should lie between -0.1 degree and -4.0 degree Ventzke. Malic acid should be indicated by both calcium chloride and the lead acetate test."

"Aside from the test for acid and total solids, by far the most important tests are the polarization and the tests for malic acid."

POPULAR ESSAYS ON HYGIENE AND SANITATION.

(A Series of Leaflets designed to teach in simple language some of the more important Lessons of the Time concerning Health and Disease.)*

SERIES A. ON DIRT AND DISEASE.

No. 1. WHY DIRT IS DANGEROUS.

Dirt and disease are apt to go together, but until lately no one knew why. Today we know that dirt and disease are often closely connected, because dirt is generally not merely dead earth but rather a kind of *living earth,* crowded with unseen and almost countless *germs* or *microbes,* many of which may be dangerous and even deadly.

WHAT IS DIRT? We use the term dirt for various things: for "earth," for "soil," and for "stains" and "spots" of many kinds, but dirty dishes, dirty faces, dirty clothing, dirty shoes and dirty streets often mean something foul or filthy. The word dirt itself comes from an older word drit (meaning dung or excrement), and, strictly speaking, the word "dirt" should not be used for good clean earth, or virgin soil, or sands and gravels, such as are found in sea beaches or sandbanks or deserts. It really ought to be kept for dung or excrement or filth, or for earth, soil or sands polluted or stained with dung, excrement or filth.

---

*Prepared and published by the Sanitary Research Laboratory of the Massachusetts Institute of Technology in Boston, at the request and by the Gift of a Friend of Science and Education.

The present is the first (No. 1) in SERIES A.   ON DIRT AND DISEASE.

Some of those to follow are : —

No. 2.   WHY DIRTY MILK IS DANGEROUS.
No. 3.   WHY DIRTY WATER IS DANGEROUS.
No. 4.   WHY DIRTY STREETS ARE DANGEROUS.
No. 5.   WHY DIRTY PERSONS ARE DANGEROUS.

Other Leaflets may eventually be prepared upon " Microbes, — Good and Bad ; " " Some Common Diseases : How they Come and how to Avoid them ; " " Farm Sanitation ; " " Why Flies are Filthy and Dangerous ; " and other practical sanitary and hygienic topics.

It is hoped that Boards of Health, School Boards, Hospital Authorities, Charity Workers, Health-Education Leagues, Anti-Tuberculosis Societies and other Educators or Philanthropic Persons and Organizations may make use of this Leaflet and those which are to follow in that campaign of Sanitary education in which all civilized peoples must sooner or later participate.

Reprints of the Essay here published (SERIES A, No. 1—WHY DIRT IS DANGEROUS) may be had (postpaid) by addressing the Biological Department, Mass. Institute of Technology, Boston, Mass., and enclosing postage stamps according to the following schedule : —

> One to fifty copies . . . . .2 cents each.
> Fifty or more copies . . . . .1 cent   "

WHY DIRT IS DANGEROUS. Dirt is dangerous chiefly because it is very often dung, excrement or filth, and as such may be the carrier of disease germs or microbes from diseased human beings or other animals to persons who, though well, are able to catch a disease.

In typhoid fever, for example, germs peculiar to that disease are thrown off (excreted) in the bowel discharges, urine and spit of the patient. These excreta, as they are called, may thus become carriers of typhoid fever, because they carry its germs, and linen, bed-pans, spittoons, handkerchiefs and the like, soiled or dirtied by any of these excreta, may be bearers of the living poisonous germs of this terrible disease from a patient to a laundress, a maidservant, a nurse, or to anyone whose hands become dirty by handling such articles or excreta. From hands so soiled contagion may be carried to plates, cups, saucers, spoons, and above all, food.

HOW DIRT IS DANGEROUS. Dirt being often really dung, excrement or filth, is dangerous because it passes so readily and in so many ways from the patient to the public. We have just spoken of laundresses and others whose hands may become dirty by handling dirty linen, dirty bedpans and the like. Such persons are themselves in great danger from this dirt and often actually "catch" the disease. But if the urine or bowel discharges of typhoid fever patients are thrown into a brook leading to a reservoir of drinking water, the lives of all the people of the town or city using that water are endangered. Again, if such dirt finds its way into milk there is grave danger for anyone who drinks that milk, or if into a sewer emptying upon an oyster bed for anyone eating oysters thus sewage-polluted; or if such sewage is used to water a celery or lettuce or strawberry patch then anyone eating such dirtied celery, lettuce or strawberries may run the risk of losing his life.

WHY DIRTY STREETS ARE DANGEROUS. Dirty streets are dangerous because the dirt in this case may cling to shoes or other articles of footwear and be carried from the streets into houses where, either as fresh dirt or more often as dry dirt (dust), it may find its way to foods or other articles which either enter or touch the mouths of members of the household. Street dirt is also dangerous when dried up and pulverized or turned into dust, which may be readily lifted and blown about by winds, thus finding its way perhaps directly into the mouths of human beings, or through cracks and crevices or open doors and windows into human habitations and finally into human bodies upon articles of food or drink.

Insects, such as flies and mosquitoes, may also carry dirty particles from dirty streets into houses and deposit them upon food materials in the pantry or upon the table.

We need only stop to think for a moment how really dirty the dirt of a street may be, to understand how dangerous it may become. If we remember that the streets are constantly used by dirty horses, dogs, cats, birds (such as sparrows and pigeons) and occasionally by other animals, when we remember how many people of all sorts thoughtlessly spit in the streets or on the sidewalks,—using the gutter as a kind of spittoon,— when we consider how many loads of manure and other dirty materials are hauled through the streets and how many careless people throw into the streets rubbish of all sorts, such as papers, orange-peel, banana-skins, cigar-stubs and the like, when we realize that a certain number of the animals or human beings whose droppings, spit or rubbish are cast into the streets are suffering from diseases (and sometimes loathsome diseases) and especially from consumption, diphtheria, colds or other complaints, then we can easily see how and why it is that street dirt is dangerous.

WHY DIRTY WATER IS DANGEROUS. It is still easier to understand that water which contains dirt or excreta may be very dangerous, because in no way are the germs of disease more readily taken into the human body than with food and drink. We shall shortly publish in this series a special circular upon drinking water and disease and all who are interested may procure and read that leaflet.

WHY DIRTY MILK IS DANGEROUS. Dirty milk is dangerous because the dirt most often found in milk is cow dung or else dirt derived from dirty milkmen who have handled the milk with dirty hands. Then, too, milk is good food for some germs or microbes, very much as it is for human beings, and germs will therefore grow and multiply in milk more readily than in water. There will be later a special leaflet in this series upon this subject and all who are interested may procure a copy of it.

DIRTY HANDS AND FACES AND WHY THESE ARE DANGEROUS. Human hands go only too readily almost everywhere and thus very easily become dirty. Children, for example, having soiled their hands may perhaps the next minute put their fingers upon their faces or into their mouths and thus carry dirt, and with that the germs of disease, directly into the body itself, Frequent washing of the hands is a great sanitary safeguard, and for this reason no one should sit down to a meal at which food will be "handled" without having first carefully washed his hands. Workingmen away from home, taking their dinners from a dinner-pail, should be particularly careful to wash their hands, especially if they have been handling paints or other poisonous substances, or dirt in any of its thousand forms.

CLEANLINESS IS NEXT TO GODLINESS. This is an old saying which has come down to us as a result of long and painful experience. Why, of all things, should cleanliness be placed next to godliness? Why should not honesty, or industry, or any one of a thousand things rather than cleanliness, be placed there? The reason probably is that very much as godliness is believed to give to the godly eternal life in the world to come, so cleanliness, as shown by experience, tends to give to the cleanly long life in this world. Dirt and disease, danger and death have been found by hard experience to go together, while cleanliness tends toward safety, health, comfort and long life.

HOW DIRTY PEOPLE KEEP HEALTHY. Everybody who stops to think knows that some dirty people do appear to keep healthy and live long, and some may wonder that this is so. The reason appears to be this: Some people are so strong, robust, hearty and healthy that they can resist almost all ordinary causes of disease. They can get "soaked through" in a rain without catching cold; they can go with wet shoes and stockings, or thinly clad, and yet seem to be none the worse: they may even sometimes be exposed to contagious or infectious diseases without catching them. All this is at first sight hard to explain, but if we remember that the human body is after all a good deal like a machine, such, for example, as a watch or a wagon, we can perhaps realize that, like most machines, some specimens are stronger than others and when exposed to rough usage stand the strain wonderfully well, while some, though looking just as strong, break down easily. It is true that some few human beings are so strong and robust that they can thrive for a time, even in dirt, but these are the exception and not the rule, and even for them dirt is always a danger; for if these same strong people get overworked, or run down, or become dissipated in any way, they, too, generally suffer, just like their weaker neighbors, from dirt and filth.

Contributors of Regular Papers.

SAMUEL W. ABBOTT, M. D.,
Sec. Mass. State Bd. of Health.

DAVID D. BROUGH, M.D.
Med. Inspec. Boston Bd. Health.

ALEXANDER BURR, D. V. S.,
Veterinarian, Boston Bd. of Health.

PAUL CARSON, M. D.,
Boston Port Physician.

CHARLES V. CHAPIN, M. D.,
Supt. Health, Providence, R. I.

W. H. CHAPIN, M. D.,
Springfield.

H. LINCOLN CHASE, M. D.,
Agent, Brookline Bd. of Health.

H. W. CLARK,
Chemist, Mass. State Bd. of Health.

JAMES C. COFFEY,
Ex. Officer Worcester Bd. of Health.

FRANCIS G. CURTIS, M. D.,
Newton.

ELBRIDGE G. CUTLER, M. D.,
Boston.

FRANCIS P. DENNY, M. D.,
Brookline Bd. Health Bact. Lab.

SAMUEL H. DURGIN, M. D.,
Chairman, Boston Board of Health.

HARRISON P. EDDY,
Worcester Sewage Disposal Plant.

GEORGE H. ELLIS,
Wauwinet Farm.

PROF. HAROLD C. ERNST,
Harvard Medical School.

W. S. EVERETT, M. D.,
Hyde Park.

JAMES B. FIELD, M. D.,
Lowell.

G. W. FITZ, M. D.,
Cambridge.

X. H. GOODNOUGH, C. E.,
Engineer, Mass. State Bd. of Health.

CHARLES HARRINGTON, M. D.
Milk Inspector, Boston Bd. of Health.

ROBERT W. HASTINGS, M. D.,
Brookline.

H W. HILL, M. D.,
Boston Bd. of Health Bact. Lab.

MAY S. HOLMES, M. D.,
Worcester Isolation Hospital.

S. C. KEITH, S. B.,
Boston.

PROF. L. P. KINNICUTT,
Worcester Polytechnic Institute.

ATHERTON P. MASON, M. D.,
Fitchburg Bd. of Health Bact. Lab.

JOHN H. McCOLLOM, M. D.,
Boston City Hospital.

WILLIAM H. MITCHELL,
Boston.

FRANK L. MORSE, M. D.,
Med. Inspec., Mass. State Bd. of Health.

COL. WILLIAM F. MORSE,
New York.

J. ALBERT C. NYHEN,
Brookline Bd. of Health Bact. Lab.

W. H. PARK, M. D.,
New York Board of Health Lab.

AUSTIN PETERS. M. R. C. V. S.,
Mass. State Cattle Dept.

MRS. ELLEN H. RICHARDS,
Mass. Institute Technology.

MARK W. RICHARDSON, M. D.,
Boston.

B. R. RICKARDS, S. B.,
Boston Bd. of Health Bact. Lab.

PROF. WILLIAM T. SEDGWICK,
Mass. Institute Technology.

T. B. SHEA, M. D.,
Member, Boston Bd. Health.

PROF. THEOBALD SMITH,
Pathologist, Mass. State Bd. Health.

F. HERBERT SNOW, C. E.,
Brockton.

W. LYMAN UNDERWOOD,
Mass. Institute Technology.

JOHANNA VON WAGNER,
Yonkers, N Y.

HENRY P. WALCOTT, M. D.,
Chairman, Mass. State Bd. Health.

EDWARD R. WARREN,
Boston.

ROBERT SPURR WESTON,
Boston.

FRANKLIN W. WHITE, M. D.
Boston.

C. E. A. WINSLOW, M. SC.,
Mass. Inst. Technology.

PUBLIC HEALTH
IN
AMERICA

An Arno Press Collection

Ackerknecht, Erwin H[einz]. **Malaria In the Upper Mississippi Valley: 1760-1900.** 1945

Bowditch, Henry I[ngersoll]. **Consumption In New England Or, Locality One of Its Chief Causes** and **Is Consumption Contagious, Or Communicated By One Person to Another In Any Manner?** 1862/1864. Two Vols. in One.

Buck, Albert H[enry] (Editor). **A Treatise On Hygiene and Public Health.** 1879. Two Vols.

Boston Medical Commission. **The Sanitary Condition of Boston:** The Report of a Medical Commission. 1875

Budd, William. **Typhoid Fever:** Its Nature, Mode of Spreading, and Prevention. 1931

Chapin, Charles V[alue]. **A Report On State Public Health Work,** Based On a Survey of State Boards of Health: Made Under the Direction of the Council on Health and Public Instruction of the American Medical Association. [1915]

Davis, Michael M[arks], Jr. and Andrew R[obert] Warner. **Dispensaries:** Their Management and Development. 1918

Dublin, Louis I[srael] and Alfred J. Lotka. **The Money Value of a Man.** 1930

Dunglison, Robley. **Human Health.** 1844

Emerson, Haven. **Local Health Units for the Nation.** 1945

Emerson, Haven. **A Monograph On the Epidemic of Poliomyelitis (Infantile Paralysis) In New York City In 1916.** 1917

Fish, Hamilton. **Report of the Select Committee of the Senate of the United States On the Sickness and Mortality On Board Emigrant Ships.** 1854

Frost, Wade Hampton. **The Papers of Wade Hampton Frost, M.D.:** A Contribution to Epidemiological Method. 1941

Gardner, Mary Sewall. **Public Health Nursing.** 1916

Greenwood, Major. **Epidemics and Crowd Diseases:**
An Introduction to the Study of Epidemiology. 1935

Greenwood, Major. **Medical Statistics From Graunt to Farr.**
1948

Hartley, Robert M. **An Historical, Scientific and Practical Essay On Milk, As an Article of Human Sustenance:**
With a Consideration of the Effects Consequent Upon the Unnatural Methods of Producing It for the Supply of Large Cities. 1842

Hill, Hibbert Winslow. **The New Public Health.** 1916

Knopf, S. Adolphus. **Tuberculosis As a Disease of the Masses & How To Combat It.** 1908

MacNutt, J[oseph] Scott. **A Manual for Health Officers.** 1915

Richards, Ellen H. [Swallow]. **Euthenics:** The Science of Controllable Environment. 1910

Richardson, Joseph G[ibbons]. **Long Life and How To Reach It.** 1886

Rumsey, Henry Wyldbore. **Essays On State Medicine.** 1856

Shryock, Richard Harrison. **National Tuberculosis Association 1904-1954:** A Study of the Voluntary Health Movement In the United States. 1957

Simon, John. **Filth-Diseases and Their Prevention.** 1876

Sternberg, George M[iller]. **Sanitary Lessons of the War and Other Papers.** 1912

Straus, Lina Gutherz. **Disease In Milk:** The Remedy Pasteurization. The Life Work of Nathan Straus. 1917

Wanklyn, J[ames] Alfred and Ernest Theophron Chapman. **Water Analysis:** A Practical Treatise on the Examination of Potable Water. 1884

Whipple, George C. **State Sanitation:** A Review of the Work of the Massachusetts State Board of Health. 1917. Two Vols. in One.

Selections From Public Health Reports and Papers Presented at the Meetings of the American Public Health Association (1873-1883). 1977

Selections From Public Health Reports and Papers Presented at the Meetings of the American Public Health Association (1884-1907). 1977